Nanotechnology in Diabetes

Nanotechnology in Diabetes: Advancements in Diagnosis, Therapy, and Personalized Care explores the applications of nanotechnology in the diagnosis, treatment, and long-term management of diabetes. The introductory chapters present an outline of diabetes, its prevalence, complexities, and the limitations of current management techniques. The book also explores the role of nanotechnology in regenerative medicine, particularly its potential in pancreatic islet cell regeneration. It further reviews the development of nano-biosensors for continuous glucose monitoring, highlighting their potential for accurate, real-time blood sugar monitoring, thus improving patient outcomes. Further, the chapters discuss the role of nanotechnology in personalized medicine by tailoring treatment plans based on individual patient profiles, providing a customized approach to diabetes care. In turn, the text examines the ethical, regulatory, and practical considerations associated with integrating nanotechnology into clinical practice. The book concludes with discussions on emerging trends and future innovations in the field, highlighting ongoing research that holds promise for the future of diabetes management.

Key Features

- Examines the potential of nanotechnology in transforming diabetes management, from glucose monitoring to advanced drug delivery systems.
- Explores the potential of nanotechnology to personalize diabetes treatment based on individual patient profiles for more effective care.
- Delivers cutting-edge insights into the use of nanotechnology for pancreatic islet cell regeneration, offering promising long-term solutions for diabetes.
- Discusses the ethical, regulatory, and practical challenges of integrating nanotechnology into clinical settings for diabetes care.
- Highlights emerging research, future innovations, and trends set to revolutionize the future of diabetes treatment through nanotechnology.

As such, this book is useful for researchers and professionals of nanotechnology, pharmaceutical sciences, biomedical engineering, and regenerative medicine.

Nanotechnology in Diabetes

Advancements in Diagnosis, Therapy, and Personalized Care

Edited by
Pankaj Sharma, Shashi Ravi Suman Rudrangi, and Vinay Jain

CRC Press
Taylor & Francis Group
Boca Raton London New York

CRC Press is an imprint of the
Taylor & Francis Group, an **informa** business

Designed cover image: **Shutterstock**

First edition published 2027
by CRC Press
2385 NW Executive Center Drive, Suite 320, Boca Raton FL 33431

and by CRC Press
4 Park Square, Milton Park, Abingdon, Oxon, OX14 4RN

CRC Press is an imprint of Taylor & Francis Group, LLC

ISBN: 978-1-032-98434-6 (hbk)
ISBN: 978-1-032-98435-3 (pbk)
ISBN: 978-1-003-59865-7 (ebk)

DOI: 10.1201/9781003598657

Typeset in Times
by KnowledgeWorks Global Ltd.

Contents

Preface

Diabetes mellitus has emerged as one of the most important global health challenges of the 21st century, affecting millions of people worldwide and placing an immense burden on healthcare systems. Despite considerable advances in pharmacological therapies, diagnostic technologies, and lifestyle interventions, effective long-term management of diabetes and its associated complications remain a complex and evolving challenge. In recent years, nanotechnology has gained increasing attention as a transformative scientific approach capable of addressing these challenges through innovative diagnostic and therapeutic solutions.

Nanotechnology in Diabetes: Advancements in Diagnosis, Therapy, and Personalized Care aims to present a comprehensive overview of the emerging role of nanotechnology in improving diabetes management. The integration of nanoscale materials, smart drug delivery systems, biosensors, and regenerative nanomedicine has opened new opportunities for enhancing treatment precision, improving therapeutic outcomes, and enabling personalized healthcare strategies. By combining advances in nanoscience with biomedical and pharmaceutical research, nanotechnology has the potential to significantly transform the future of diabetes diagnosis and therapy.

This edited volume brings together contributions from researchers, clinicians, and scientists working at the intersection of nanotechnology and metabolic disease research. The chapters included in this book explore a wide range of topics, including the fundamentals of nanotechnology, nano-enabled biosensors for glucose monitoring, nanocarriers for targeted drug delivery, encapsulation of antidiabetics agents, regenerative nanomedicine, and emerging trends in nano-based therapeutics. In addition, the book also addresses important aspects such as regulatory frameworks, ethical points, and practical challenges associated with the clinical translation of nanotechnology-based solutions.

One of the strengths of this volume is its interdisciplinary perspective. Integrating knowledge from material science, pharmaceutical technology, biomedical engineering, and clinical research, the book aims to provide readers with a holistic understanding of the potential applications of nanotechnology in diabetes care. The content is intended to serve as a valuable resource for researchers, healthcare professionals, graduate students, and policymakers interested in emerging technologies in diabetes management.

We sincerely thank all contributing authors for their scholarly efforts and valuable insights, which made this book possible. We hope this volume will stimulate further research and innovation in nanotechnology-driven approaches for improving diabetes diagnosis, therapy, and personalized care.

Acknowledgments

The completion of this book, *Nanotechnology in Diabetes: Advancements in Diagnosis, Therapy, and Personalized Care*, has been a rewarding academic journey that would not have been possible without the encouragement, support, and collaboration of many individuals and institutions. As the lead editor, I, **Dr. Pankaj Sharma**, would like to express my sincere gratitude to everyone who contributed to the successful development of this volume.

First and foremost, I am deeply thankful to all the contributing authors who shared their expertise and research insights to make this comprehensive and impactful. Their scholarly contributions have enriched this work and helped present a multidimensional understanding of the role of nanotechnology in diabetes diagnosis, therapy, and personalized healthcare.

I would also like to acknowledge the valuable guidance and support provided by my co-editors, **Dr. Shashi Ravi Suman Rudrangi** and **Dr. Vinay Jain**, whose supervision, critical insights, and academic experiences greatly contributed to shaping the direction and quality of this book. Their encouragement and thoughtful suggestions throughout the editorial process helped maintain the scientific rigor and interdisciplinary perspective of the volume.

On a personal note, I would like to express my heartfelt gratitude to my beloved **Maa** and **Papa**, whose blessings, sacrifices, and constant encouragement have been the strongest foundation of my academic and professional journeys. Their unwavering faith in me has always motivated me to strive for excellence.

I am especially grateful to my wife, **Kirti**, for her patience, understanding, and continuous support during the long hours dedicated to this project. Her encouragement and positivity have been a constant source of strength throughout this journey.

My deepest affection goes to my sons, **Chiku** and **Piku**, whose innocent smiles and joyful presence bring balance and happiness to my life. They are my greatest inspiration and remind me of the importance of perseverance and purpose.

Finally, I extend my appreciation to the publisher and all reviewers for their valuable support in bringing this book to fruition. I hope this text will inspire further research, innovation, and collaboration in the field of nanotechnology-driven solutions for diabetes management.

Pankaj Sharma

About the Editors

Pankaj Sharma is a professor of pharmaceutics and head of the Department at ShriRam College of Pharmacy, Banmore, Morena (MP), India, with over 14 years of teaching and research experience in pharmaceutical sciences. He earned his PhD in pharmaceutical sciences from Jiwaji University, Gwalior, where his doctoral research focused on the development of nanoemulsion-based transdermal drug delivery systems for malaria therapy. He also holds an MPharm in pharmaceutics, supported by an AICTE–GPAT fellowship.

Dr. Sharma's research interests span nanomedicine, smart polymers, transdermal and targeted drug delivery systems, pharmaceutical nanotoxicology, artificial intelligence in healthcare, and advanced formulation development. He has made significant contributions to academia through 60+ peer-reviewed publications, including articles in Scopus- and Web of Science-indexed journals, along with numerous book chapters published by leading international publishers.

He is the editor/author of multiple international books published and accepted by CRC Press (Taylor & Francis), Elsevier, Apple Academic Press, and Bentham Science, and actively contributes to interdisciplinary research at the intersection of nanotechnology, AI, and personalized medicine. Dr. Sharma is also an approved MPharm mentor, having successfully supervised several postgraduate research projects.

In recognition of his academic excellence, he has received the Best Doctorate Award from the Indian Pharma Educational Society and holds a UK design patent for a smart pharmaceutical monitoring system. His commitment to teaching, research mentorship, and innovation continues to support the advancement of pharmaceutical education and translational research.

Shashi Ravi Suman Rudrangi, PhD, FRSC, CChem, CSci, is a chartered scientist and senior pharmaceutical leader with over 14 years of international experience spanning formulation research and development, manufacturing science and technology (MSAT), end-to-end chemistry, manufacturing, and controls (CMC) strategy, and the commercialization of oral solid dosage products. He currently serves as associate director, CMC Drug Product Manufacturing at Olema Oncology, Dublin, Ireland, where he leads strategic CMC manufacturing activities supporting the development and commercialization of innovative oncology therapies.

Prior to joining Olema Oncology, Dr. Rudrangi served as the Senior Drug Product Development and Commercialization Manager (Technical Head) at Kent-Athlone Pharma Group, UK and Ireland, where he led multidisciplinary teams responsible for the development and scale-up of oral solid dosage formulations. Throughout his career, he has directed complex technology transfer programs and contributed to the successful commercial launch of pharmaceutical products in multiple European markets. His expertise includes formulation and process development, quality by design (QbD), process validation, GMP manufacturing, and product lifecycle management.

Dr. Rudrangi earned his PhD in pharmaceutics and MSc in formulation science from the University of Greenwich, UK, and a Bachelor of Pharmacy from Kakatiya University, India. His research interests include advanced drug delivery systems, solubility enhancement technologies, amorphous solid dispersions, particle engineering, pharmaceutical process optimization, and the translation of innovative formulations from laboratory development to commercial manufacturing. Earlier in his career, he served as a lecturer in pharmaceutics at universities in the UK.

An internationally recognized scientist, Dr. Rudrangi is a fellow of the Royal Society of Chemistry (FRSC), a chartered chemist (CChem), and a chartered scientist (CSci). He is an active member of several leading international scientific and professional organizations. His professional recognition includes the Royal Society of Chemistry Inspirational Committee Award and the Best Young Researcher Forum Award at the World Drug Delivery Summit (USA). He has also served as conference chair for multiple Royal Society of Chemistry Formulation Science & Technology Group conferences, contributing to scientific collaboration and innovation within the global pharmaceutical community.

Vinay Jain has always been astounded by the medicinal properties plants possess. To use them to better mankind has always been a goal of his through his graduation in 2002 from the School of Studies (SOS) in Pharmaceutical Sciences at Jiwaji University, Gwalior. This motivated him to select pharmacognosy as one of his major subjects. He completed an MPharm in 2007 in pharmacognosy from Barkatullah University, Bhopal. Having completed his postgraduation, Dr. Jain started exploring phytochemicals in his professional journey as an assistant professor at ShriRam College of Pharmacy, Banmore. Concurrently, he got a chance to join the training and placement team. This developed his soft skills to a large extent. He successfully defended his thesis, "Phytochemical and Pharmacological Investigation of *Arisaema leschenaultia*" for his PhD and was awarded a PhD in pharmaceutical science and technology from Berhampur University, Odisha. Dr. Jain was a co-convener of an Indo-Caribbean conference hosted by ShriRam College of Pharmacy in 2018 and was also the organizing secretary of the national conference on "The Future Prospect in Pharma Marketing," hosted in association with IPGA. To date, Dr. Jain has guided more than 20 undergraduate and post-graduate students in major projects. He has had about 30 papers published in distinguished journals/books of international and national repute, which are indexed in SCI and Scopus. He has presented more than 20 papers in national and international seminars and conferences. He was also privileged to get grants from technical professional bodies like AICTE and MPCST for organizing conferences. He is a lifetime member of the Indian Society of Pharmacognosy. He always tries to keep his staff highly motivated with his open-door policy for grievance redressal and efficient leadership skills because he believes that only a highly motivated team creates a highly efficient institution.

1 Diabetes Essentials
A Gateway to Deeper Understanding

Mahesh Kumar Posa
School of Health and Medical Sciences, Adamas University Barasat, Kolkata, India

Kiran B. Dhamak
PRES's College of Pharmacy (for Women), Chincholi, Nashik, Pune, India

Chanda Ranjan
The Oxford College of Pharmacy, Bengaluru, India

Renu Arya
Government of Haryana, Panchkula, India

Mubeen G.
Al-Ameen College of Pharmacy, Bangalore, India

Ruchi Tiwari
PSIT-Pranveer Singh Institute of Technology (Pharmacy), Kanpur, India

Megha Mishra
Faculty of Pharmacy VNS Group of Institutions, Bhopal, India

1.1 INTRODUCTION

Diabetes mellitus (DM) is one of the major health problems worldwide in the 21st century. Diabetes, beyond its clinical definition as a glucose metabolic disorder, is a multifactorial disease that depends on genetics, lifestyle, and the environment. Its increasing incidence in all age groups and socioeconomic strata serves as evidence for the urgency to have a systematic understanding of the cause, burden, and prevention of this disease [1]. This chapter provides an introduction to the essentials of diabetes and lays the groundwork for more detailed discussion of diabetes mechanisms, diagnosis, management, and directions for the future.

1.1.1 The Global Burden of Diabetes

Diabetes has become an epidemic in each country of the world, with more than 537 million people in the age group 20–79 years diagnosed worldwide in 2021, and the number is expected to increase to 783 million by 2045 (International Diabetes Federation, IDF) [2, 3]. However, close to half remain undiagnosed, which means that treatment is delayed and individuals are at increased

DOI: 10.1201/9781003598657-1

risk of complications. Nearly three-quarters of all cases are in low- and middle-income countries, highlighting inequities in health care and preventive measures [3].

For example, India and China alone account for over one-third of the world's diabetic population, which emphasizes the need for specific public health measures in Asia. In addition, its financial toll is enormous – worldwide health care expenditure related to diabetes surpassed $966 billion in 2021, putting pressure on families and health systems. Thus, diabetes is not only a disease but also a socioeconomic issue, and its prevention and management is a worldwide priority [4].

1.1.2 Historical Perspectives and Evolution

The history of diabetes goes back to 1500 BCE when excessive urine was first documented in ancient Egyptian texts as the primary symptom. The word diabetes (Greek: "to siphon") was given by Aretaeus of Cappadocia in the 2nd century CE and the sweet taste of urine in patients suffering from the disease led to the word "mellitus" (Latin: honeyed) – coined by Thomas Willis in the 17th century [5].

A tipping point was reached in 1921, when Frederick Banting and Charles Best isolated insulin, turning diabetes from a death sentence to a chronic disease. Since then, knowledge has evolved from an exclusive emphasis on insulin deficiency to the identification of the contributions of insulin resistance (IR), genetics, inflammation, and gut microbiota. For instance, the discovery of GLP-1 receptor agonists and SGLT2 inhibitors over the past decades has changed treatment paradigms, showing that historic discoveries keep on reshaping therapeutic environments [6, 7].

1.1.3 Need for Early Awareness and Education

Early education and awareness is key to easing the burden of diabetes. It has already been shown that progression from prediabetes to type 2 diabetes mellitus (T2DM) in high-risk individuals can be reduced by up to 58% by lifestyle intervention (Diabetes Prevention Program, USA). As an example, early interventions like healthy nutrition, regular exercise, and weight control have been shown to be more effective and cost-effective than pharmacological treatments at a later stage [8, 9].

For instance, the Finish Diabetes Prevention Study showed that those who made moderate lifestyle changes – including reducing the fat content of their diets and getting a minimum of 150 minutes of physical activity per week – dramatically reduced their risk of developing T2DM. National awareness days such as World Diabetes Day (14 November) and school-based health programs also help to show the importance of community engagement in prevention [10].

Education is also important for busting myths, increasing treatment adherence, and promoting use of technologies such as continuous glucose monitoring. By stimulating early recognition, healthcare systems will move from reactive management of complications to proactive approaches to prevent the onset and progression of disease [11].

1.2 FUNDAMENTALS OF GLUCOSE HOMEOSTASIS

Glucose homeostasis is a stable level of blood glucose achieved by the delicate balance between glucose production, glucose utilization, and storage in the body. In healthy people, fasting blood glucose levels are kept fairly steady within the range of 70–100 mg/dL in spite of variations in dietary intake, activity, and energy requirements [12]. This homeostasis is maintained mainly by the hormones insulin and glucagon, secreted by flat, islet cells located in the pancreas, and is addressed by a system of the liver, muscle, adipose tissue, and central nervous system. Imbalance of this leads to metabolic disorders such as DM [12, 13]. Figure 1.1 shows regulation of glucose homeostasis

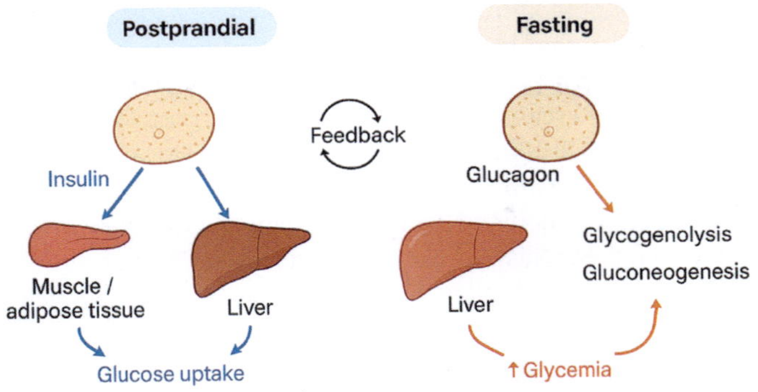

FIGURE 1.1 Mechanisms of glucose homeostasis.

by pancreatic β-cells and α-cells. Insulin is responsible for the uptake and storage of glucose, and glucagon mobilizes glucose during fasting.

1.2.1 Physiology of Insulin and Glucagon

Insulin, which is released by β-cells of the pancreas in response to an increase in blood glucose, is the major anabolic hormone. It increases the uptake of glucose by muscle and adipose tissue (through GLUT4 transporters), increases glycogen synthesis in the liver and muscles, increases lipogenesis, and blunts hepatic glucose production. For example, following a carbohydrate-rich meal, insulin maintains efficient clearance of glucose from circulation and thus prevents postprandial hyperglycemia [14].

However, glucagon, which is released from pancreatic α-cells during hypoglycemia or fasting, is a counter-regulatory hormone. It promotes hepatic glycogenolysis (breakdown of glycogen) and gluconeogenesis (production of glucose from non-carbohydrate precursors), and thus restores blood glucose levels. Together, insulin and glucagon act like a biological "yin and yang" to make sure there is glucose when we are fasting and glucose storage when we are fed [15].

1.2.2 Function of Pancreatic β-Cells and α-Cells

Pancreatic β-cells, in the islets of Langerhans, are specialized blood glucose sensors. Insulin secretion occurs via a glucose-stimulated pathway that involves adenosine triphosphate (ATP)-sensitive potassium channels (KATP) and voltage-gated calcium channels, resulting in insulin vesicle exocytosis. β-cell dysfunction, whether by autoimmune destruction (in type 1 diabetes mellitus [T1DM]) or progressive exhaustion (in T2DM), is at the core of diabetes pathogenesis [16].

In contrast, glucagon secretion from the α-cells is triggered by low levels of glucose and serves to prevent hypoglycemia in fasting, exercise, and illness. For instance, during extended fasting, the liver promotes gluconeogenesis from amino acids and glycerol, driven by glucagon. This process supplies almost all of the glucose needed to fuel the high-energy demands of the brain. Dysregulation of α-cell function, including inappropriate glucagon secretion, is further responsible for hyperglycemia and progression of disease in T2DM [17].

1.2.3 Metabolic Balance in Health

Glucose homeostasis is regulated by a complicated interplay between insulin and glucagon and other modulators (cortisol, catecholamines, growth hormone, incretins). After meals insulin is dominant, and stores nutrients and maintains an anabolic state. During fasting, the glucose-releasing hormone, glucagon, becomes predominant and mobilizes energy-sustaining substrates in order to maintain the vital organs' functions [14].

A good example is the "dawn phenomenon" with a physiological increase in early-morning glucose as a consequence of increased growth hormone and cortisol secretion. Glucose is normal because in healthy persons, insulin secretion compensates. However, in diabetes, this effect is enhanced as a result of impaired insulin action and results in hyperglycemia in the morning. Thus, metabolic balance represents the body's adaptive mechanisms to achieve energy homeostasis in various possible situations: feeding, fasting, exercise, and stress. This harmony is therefore critically important to understand the pathophysiological derangements underlying diabetes [18].

1.3 CLASSIFICATION OF DIABETES MELLITUS

DM is a heterogeneous metabolic disorder of chronic hyperglycemia, due to defects in insulin secretion, insulin action, or both. Diabetes is clinically classified because the classification has implications for diagnosis, management, and complication prediction [19]. According to the American Diabetes Association (ADA) and the World Health Organization (WHO), there are four broad categories of diabetes – T1DM, T2DM, gestational diabetes mellitus (GDM), and other specific types [20].

1.3.1 Type 1 Diabetes: Autoimmune Cellular Destruction of β-Cells

T1DM is a predominantly autoimmune disease that leads to selective destruction of pancreatic β-cells and leads to absolute insulin deficiency. It usually appears in childhood or adolescence, but can appear at any age. Autoantibodies directed against β-cell antigens, such as glutamic acid decarboxylase (GAD), insulin, and islet antigen-2 (IA-2), are assumed to be of crucial importance for its pathogenesis [21]. Genetic susceptibility (especially HLA class II alleles, HLA-DR3 and DR4) and environmental triggers (viral infections) are thought to be involved in disease pathogenesis. Clinically, T1DM patients commonly present with polyuria, polydipsia, unexplained weight loss, and in severe cases, diabetic ketoacidosis (DKA). Exogenous insulin therapy is a lifelong necessity for maintaining euglycemia and preventing both acute and chronic complications [22, 23].

1.3.2 Type 2 Diabetes: Insulin Resistance and β-Cell Dysfunction

T2DM is the most common type of diabetes, which represents >90% of the total cases in the world. It is defined by a mixture of peripheral tissue IR and progressive β-cell dysfunction leading to relative insulin insufficiency. Risk factors include obesity, physical inactivity, increasing age, family history, and ethnicity [24]. Unlike T1DM, T2DM is often long and latent, and the diagnosis is made in the course of a regular health check or after the late emergence of complications. Clinical management focuses on lifestyle interventions, oral hypoglycemic agents, and at an advanced stage, insulin treatment. Chronic hyperglycemia is associated with microvascular (retinopathy, nephropathy, neuropathy) and macrovascular (cardiovascular, cerebrovascular) complications in T2DM [25].

1.3.3 Gestational Diabetes Mellitus (GDM)

GDM is defined as glucose intolerance with onset or first recognition during pregnancy in the second or third trimester. GDM develops because of pregnancy-associated changes in hormones that create IR, together with inadequate β-cell compensation. Risk factors include advanced maternal age, obesity, familial history of diabetes, and previous history of GDM. Untreated GDM predisposes to maternal complications like preeclampsia, cesarean delivery, and subsequent T2DM and fetal complications like macrosomia, neonatal hypoglycemia, and long-term metabolic disorders.

Routinely, screening is done with oral glucose tolerance tests (OGTT) and treatment is done mainly with dietary changes, exercise, and insulin treatment, if needed [26, 27].

1.3.4 Other Specific Types (Monogenic, Secondary, Drug-Induced)

Other special types of diabetes include rare or secondary diabetes that occur due to some different underlying genetic or external reasons. Monogenic diabetes, which includes maturity-onset diabetes of the young (MODY) and neonatal diabetes, is due to mutations in single genes that affect β-cell function. Secondary diabetes is a result of pancreatitis, cystic fibrosis, or hormonal disorders such as Cushing's syndrome and acromegaly. Also, drug-induced diabetes may result from long-term use of medications that integrate glucocorticoids, thiazide diuretics, or antipsychotics, which inhibit insulin action or secretion. These distinct forms need to be identified since the treatment strategies may be different from more standard T1DM or T2DM treatment [28].

1.4 PATHOPHYSIOLOGY AND MECHANISTIC INSIGHTS

DM is not due to a single defect, but a complex interaction of molecular, genetic, and environmental factors. At the heart are abnormalities in insulin action, β-cell function, inflammatory pathways, and metabolic regulation. The research of these mechanisms is the scientific foundation of therapy development. Figure 1.2 illustrates the pathophysiological mechanisms of the relationship between chronic hyperglycemia and microvascular and macrovascular complications in diabetes [29].

1.4.1 Insulin Resistance and Cellular Mechanisms

IR is the hallmark of T2DM and occurs when peripheral tissues (skeletal muscle, liver, and adipose tissue, mainly) do not respond to circulating insulin at a sufficient rate [30]. At the level of the cell, IR is characterized by:

Defective insulin receptor signaling: Down-modulation of insulin receptor substrate (IRS) proteins impairs downstream PI3K-Akt signaling [31].
Impaired GLUT4 translocation: In skeletal muscle and adipose tissue, defective recruitment of glucose transporters causes impaired glucose transport [32].
Hepatic insulin resistance: In this case, the liver's ability to utilize glucose is compromised. This leads to increased gluconeogenesis and decreased glycogenesis, causing hyperglycemia during fasting [33].

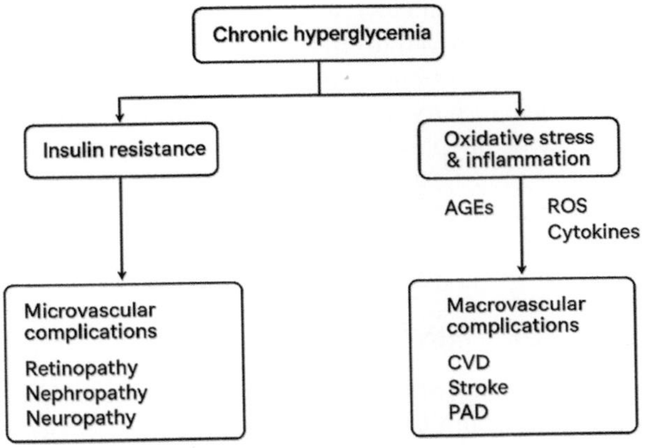

FIGURE 1.2 Pathophysiology of diabetes and complications.

Likewise, obesity is associated with lipotoxicity, an increased concentration of free fatty acids that activates protein kinase C (PKC) and serine kinases that interfere with insulin receptor signaling. This mechanistic connection accounts for the fact that obesity is one of the major causes of T2DM [34, 35].

1.4.2 Chronic Inflammation and Oxidative Stress

Low-grade chronic inflammation is now accepted as one of the pivotal mechanisms of diabetes pathogenesis. The adipose tissue in obesity recruits pro-inflammatory macrophages and secretes cytokines (TNF-a, IL-6, MCP-1) that interfere with insulin signaling. Concomitantly, the oxidative stress, which is characterized by an imbalance between reactive oxygen species (ROS) and antioxidant protection, leads to the destruction of β-cells, which are especially susceptible because of their low antioxidant potential [36].

For example, hyperglycemia promotes the generation of advanced glycation end-products (AGEs) that bind to RAGE (receptors for AGEs), activating NF-kB and contributing to a regenerative cycle of oxidative stress and inflammation. This "metabolic inflammation" further increases insulin resistance and β-cell failure, and ties poor glycemic control to microvascular and macrovascular complications [37].

1.4.3 Genetic and Epigenetic Factors

A large amount of diabetes susceptibility is attributed to genetic predisposition. Genome-wide association studies (GWAS) have identified more than 400 loci associated with glucose regulation, β-cell function, and insulin sensitivity. For instance, polymorphisms in the TCF7L2 gene modestly increase the risk of T2DM, and HLA class II genes are major determinants of T1DM [38].

Beyond genetics, epigenetic alterations (e.g., DNA methylation, histone modifications, and non-coding RNAs) link environmental exposures to heritable metabolic risk. For example, maternal obesity or under nutrition can program offspring through epigenetic changes that predispose for insulin resistance in offspring later in life. These observations imply that inherited and acquired risk mechanisms are important in diabetes [39].

1.4.4 Gut Microbiota and Metabolic Regulation

Gut microbiota has become a key regulator of glucose homeostasis. Healthy humans tend to have a diverse microbiome, dominated by Firmicutes and Bacteroidetes, that produce short-chain fatty acids (SCFAs) like butyrate, which enhance insulin sensitivity and decrease inflammation. In contrast, dysbiosis (lowering of microbial diversity and enrichment of pro-inflammatory species, such as *Ruminococcus gnavus*, *Bacteroides vulgatus*) is linked to insulin resistance and T2DM [40]. For instance, the decrease in butyrate-producing bacteria leads to a defect in gut barrier function, resulting in leakage of lipopolysaccharide (LPS), which then causes systemic inflammation. Prebiotics, probiotics, and fecal microbiota transplantation are currently under active investigation as adjunct therapies for diabetes, with such trials spurring translational research into the microbiome [41, 42].

1.5 DIAGNOSIS AND SCREENING

Correct diagnosis and early screening of diabetes are important for early treatment, prevention of complications, and reduction of health care burden. Diagnostic strategies have changed over the years from the sole utilization of glucose measurements to the inclusion of long-term glycemic indicators, novel biomarkers, and risk stratification models [43].

1.5.1 Diagnostic Criteria (FPG, HbA1c, OGTT)

The three most commonly accepted diagnostic tests are fasting plasma glucose (FPG), oral glucose tolerance test (OGTT), and glycated hemoglobin (HbA1c) [44].

Fasting plasma glucose (FPG): A fasting blood glucose of ≥ 126 mg/dL (7.0 mmol/L) confirms diabetes; 100–125 mg/dL indicates impaired fasting glucose (prediabetes) [45].
Oral glucose tolerance test (OGTT): After consumption of 75 g glucose, a 2 h plasma glucose >= 200 mg/dL (11.1 mmol/L) is diabetes, and 140–199 mg/dL is impaired glucose tolerance [46].
HbA1c: A result of HbA1c >= 6.5% (48 mmol/mol) = diabetes. HbA1c is most useful for the long-term glycemic evaluation, although it can be influenced by hemoglobinopathies or anemia [47].

For instance, a patient with FPG 128 mg/dL and HbA1c 7.1% would be considered to have diabetes even without an OGTT. Conversely, if results are discordant, then repeat testing may be necessary. These criteria are recommended by the WHO and the ADA, and are the accepted international gold standard. Table 1.1 shows standardized diagnostic criteria for diabetes and prediabetes following the ADA and WHO recommendations [48].

1.5.2 Biomarkers of Early Detection

Conventional diagnostic tools recognize the presence of diabetes when dysglycemia is well established and usually fail to identify early pathologic changes [43]. Promising new biomarkers for early detection:

C-peptide: C-peptide is an index of endogenous insulin secretion and β-cell function [52, 53].
Adiponectin and leptin: Change in levels are associated with insulin resistance [54].
Inflammatory markers (CRP, IL-6, TNF-a): Metabolic inflammation is associated with preceding diabetes [55].
MicroRNAs (miR-375, miR-29 family): Epigenetic markers that have been involved in the dysfunction of β-cells [56].
1,5-Anhydroglucitol (1,5-AG): A short-term glycemic indicator that is sensitive to postprandial excursions [56].

For instance, low levels of adiponectin have been found in years prior to the development of overt diabetes and thus demonstrate their predictive role. Such biomarkers have the potential to supplement conventional diagnostics to allow earlier detection of high-risk individuals [57].

TABLE 1.1
Diagnostic Criteria for Diabetes and Prediabetes

Test	Normal Range	Prediabetes	Diabetes	Notes	Reference
FPG	<100 mg/dL (5.6 mmol/L)	100–125 mg/dL (5.6–6.9 mmol/L)	≥126 mg/dL (7.0 mmol/L)	Fasting ≥ 8 h	[49]
OGTT, 2-h)	<140 mg/dL (7.8 mmol/L)	140–199 mg/dL (7.8–11.0 mmol/L)	≥200 mg/dL (11.1 mmol/L)	75 g glucose load	[50]
HbA1c	<5.7% (39 mmol/mol)	5.7–6.4% (39–46 mmol/mol)	≥6.5% (48 mmol/mol)	Reflects 2–3 months average glucose	[51]
Random plasma glucose	N/A	N/A	≥200 mg/dL (11.1 mmol/L) with symptoms	Used in symptomatic patients	[45]

1.5.3 Determining Risk Factors and Prediabetes

Prediabetes is an intermediate stage of dysglycemia (FPG 100–125 mg/dL, HbA1c 5.7–6.4%, or OGTT 140–199 mg/dL), which is an important time for intervention [58]. Key risk factors include:

Non-modifiable: Age > 45 years, family history of diabetes, ethnicity (South Asians, Hispanic, African-Americans at increased risk) [59].
Modifiable: Obesity, sedentary lifestyle, diets high in calories, smoking, and hypertension [60].
Special conditions: Gestational diabetes, PCOS (polycystic ovarian syndrome), metabolic syndrome [61].

For example, an overweight woman, 38 years old with a history of gestational diabetes and HbA1c 6.2% would be classified as prediabetic with the need for lifestyle intervention and close monitoring. In such cases, early detection prevents conversion of diabetes into T2DM [62].

1.5.4 Screening Guidelines: Global Perspectives

Screening methods are different in a variety of organizations but have the same purpose:

ADA: It recommends screening for all adult subjects >=45 years or earlier in overweight/obese subjects with risk factors [63].
WHO: It recommends population-based screening in high prevalence areas, and targets those >40 years or with cardiovascular risk factors [64].
International Diabetes Federation (IDF): Opportunistic screening using simple tools such as random glucose and risk scores should be recommended in resource-limited settings [65].

For instance, in India, there's a simple, low-cost community-based method, the Indian Diabetes Risk Score (IDRS), which uses age, waist circumference, family history, and physical activity to identify high-risk individuals for further examination [66]. It is clear that globally there is a move toward risk-based, individualized, and community-oriented screening models. Combination of AI-based prediction models, continuous glucose monitoring (CGM), and mobile health (mHealth) will likely hone screening strategies in the foreseeable future.

1.6 CLINICAL MANIFESTATIONS AND COMPLICATIONS

DM has many acute and chronic manifestations. While acute complications are caused by rapid glucose spikes, chronic complications result gradually from a continued state of hyperglycemia and metabolic imbalance. These effects not only have physical health consequences but also cause a significant detriment to quality of life and mental wellness [67].

1.6.1 Acute Manifestations: Hyperglycemia, Hypoglycemia, Ketoacidosis

Hyperglycemia: It is the acute presentation of the DM syndrome, and includes polyuria, polydipsia, polyphagia, blurred vision, and fatigue. If left untreated, chronic hyperglycemia results in dehydration, electrolyte imbalance, and increased risk of infection. For instance, uncontrolled T2DM is frequently complicated by recurrent urinary tract or skin infections because the glucose-rich microenvironments are suitable for microbial growth [68].
Hypoglycemia: It is seen most often in insulin-treated patients/patients on sulfonylureas. Symptoms include shaking, confusion, coma, and in serious cases, seizures. A real-life example of this is hypoglycemia unawareness, whereby patients on long-term insulin therapy don't recognize the warning signs, resulting in a sudden loss of consciousness [69].

Diabetic ketoacidosis (DKA): This is a life-threatening complication that's usually seen in type 1 diabetics, and is caused by the lack of insulin that leads to the overproduction of ketone bodies. Clinically, it presents with nausea, abdominal pain, Kussmaul breathing, and fruity odor breath. Laboratory results include metabolic acidosis with increased anion gap [70].

Hyperosmolar hyperglycemic state (HHS): Hyperglycemia is not always accompanied by ketosis, as evident in HHS seen in type 2 diabetics who present with extreme hyperglycemia (>600 mg/dL) with dehydration in the absence of any significant ketosis [71].

1.6.2 Chronic Microvascular Complications (Retinopathy, Nephropathy, Neuropathy)

Chronic hyperglycemia harms the small blood vessels through various mechanisms, including, AGEs, oxidative stress, and the activation of the polyol pathway [72].

Diabetic retinopathy: It is the world's leading cause of blindness in adults microaneurysms, hemorrhages, cotton wool spots, and neovascularization. Proliferative diabetic retinopathy (PDR) causes vitreous hemorrhage and retinal detachment if left untreated [73].

Diabetic nephropathy: It is the leading cause of end-stage renal disease (ESRD). At the earliest stages, microalbuminuria is evident and with time, it leads to overt proteinuria and decrease in glomerular filtration rate (GFR). Early detection is possible through annual screening using urinary albumin-to-creatinine ratio (UACR) [74].

Diabetic neuropathy: Up to 50% of people with long-term diabetes develop diabetic neuropathy. It is composed of peripheral neuropathy (paresthesias, numbness, burning pain in extremities), autonomic neuropathy (orthostatic hypotension, gastroparesis, erectile dysfunction), and focal neuropathies (cranial nerve palsies). A good example is the "diabetic foot" caused by combined neuropathy, ischemia, and infection, which frequently ends up in amputation [75].

1.6.3 Macrovascular Complications (Cardiovascular Disease, Stroke, Peripheral Arterial Disease)

Macrovascular complications are the main cause of morbidity and mortality in diabetes and are caused by atherosclerosis, endothelial dysfunction, and chronic inflammation.

Cardiovascular disease (CVD): Diabetics are at a two- to four-fold higher risk for coronary artery disease (CAD). For example, myocardial infarction (MI) often affects atypically (silent MI) and this can make early diagnosis difficult [76].

Stroke: Ischemic stroke is increased two-fold for people with diabetes. Hyperglycemia during acute stroke exacerbates neuronal injury and decreases the potential recovery [75].

Peripheral arterial disease (PAD): PAD, defined by claudication, non-healing ulcers, and gangrene, puts patients at risk of lower limb amputation. The most common example is critical limb ischemia in long-term diabetics with a history of concurrent smoking [77].

Together, these complications emphasize diabetes as a cardiometabolic syndrome, which is more than just a dysregulation of glucose.

1.6.4 Psychological and Quality-of-Life Impacts

Besides physical issues, diabetes has major psychological and lifestyle impacts:

Psychological burden: High levels of depression, anxiety, and diabetes-related distress have been reported, usually from lifetime disease management and fear of complications. For instance, adolescents requiring frequent monitoring and insulin injections suffer from "diabetes burnout," which is common [78].

Social and economic impact: Self-monitoring things every day, dietary restrictions, and health care costs place a real burden. In low- and middle-income countries, inequities are compounded by a lack of access to medicines such as insulin [79].

Quality of life (QoL): The patient is left severely disabled by chronic complications like loss of vision, dialysis dependency, or amputation. Multidisciplinary management with mental health counseling and patient education is an important part of improving outcomes [80].

1.7 THERAPEUTIC AND MANAGEMENT STRATEGIES

Diabetes management is a complex and patient-centric process. It involves a multimodal approach that combines lifestyle changes, pharmacologic therapies, technology-based monitoring, and preventative care. The main objectives are optimal glycemic control, complication reduction, and improvement of the QoL. The modern management focuses on precision medicine, according to individual needs based on age, comorbidities, genetics, and patient preferences [81]. Table 1.2 summarizes the comparison of diabetes management options, mechanisms, and clinical advantages.

1.7.1 Lifestyle Modification (Nutrition, Exercise, and Stress Management)

Lifestyle interventions are the mainstay of diabetes care and are usually the initial treatment after diagnosis, for individuals at high risk for diabetes.

Nutrition: A healthy diet based on the concept of low-glycemic index foods, whole grains, fruits, vegetables, lean proteins, and healthy fats is recommended. Caloric restriction, and Mediterranean or dietary approaches to stop hypertension (DASH) diets are associated with improved glycemic control and reduced cardiovascular risk [82]. For example, the Look AHEAD (action for health in diabetes) trial showed that aggressive lifestyle intervention with caloric restriction and physical activity resulted in meaningful weight loss and improvement in glycemic parameters. Medical nutrition therapy (MNT) by registered dietitians is now a standard recommendation of the ADA [83].

TABLE 1.2
Summary of Major Diabetes Management Strategies

Approach	Mechanism/Description	Clinical Benefits	Examples
Lifestyle modification	Nutrition, physical activity, stress management	Weight reduction, improved insulin sensitivity, lower HbA1c	Mediterranean diet, 150 min/week aerobic exercise
Oral antidiabetic agents	Target hepatic glucose output, insulin secretion, or insulin sensitivity	Moderate HbA1c reduction, low-cost	Metformin, sulfonylureas, DPP-4 inhibitors
Insulin therapy	Exogenous insulin supplementation	Achieves glycemic targets in T1DM and advanced T2DM	Basal, bolus, or basal-bolus regimens; analogs reduce hypoglycemia
Newer agents	GLP-1 receptor agonists, SGLT2 inhibitors	Weight loss, cardiovascular and renal protection, improved glycemic control	Liraglutide, semaglutide, empagliflozin
Technology-assisted care	CGM, insulin pumps, smart wearables	Improved glucose monitoring, reduced hypoglycemia, personalized therapy	Dexcom G6, Freestyle Libre, hybrid closed-loop systems
Integrative/Preventive approaches	Mind-body therapies, community programs, early lifestyle intervention	Delay or prevent diabetes onset, enhance QoL	Yoga, mHealth programs, diabetes prevention program (DPP)

Exercise: Combination exercise consisting of at least 150 minutes per week of moderate intensity aerobic exercise (e.g., brisk walking, cycling) and resistance training twice a week leads to insulin sensitivity improvement and HbA1c reduction of ~0.7%. For example, very simple postprandial interventions such as taking a 15-minute walk markedly reduce postprandial glucose spikes. Also, make efforts to break sedentary activity by taking breaks from sitting for a long time [84].

Stress management: Persisting stress increases cortisol and catecholamines that aggravate insulin resistance and glycemic control. Modifications in lifestyle have been beneficial for glucose variability and patient well-being, such as yoga, mindfulness-based stress reduction, and cognitive-behavioral therapy (CBT) [85].

1.7.2 Pharmacological Intervention: Oral Antidiabetics, Insulin, Newer Drugs

Lifestyle measures are the first step, and when these are inadequate, pharmacological therapy is started. The selection of therapy is determined by glycemic goals, comorbidities (cardio-renal-hepatic), and patient preferences [86, 87].

Oral antidiabetic agents

Metformin: It is used as first-line treatment of T2DM. It decreases hepatic gluconeogenesis and increases insulin sensitivity.

Sulfonylureas (e.g., glimepiride): They stimulate insulin secretion but have the potential risks of hypoglycemia and weight gain.

DPP-4 inhibitors (sitagliptin): It enhances incretin action, lowers glucose mildly, and has mild adverse effects [88].

Insulin therapy: Insulin is a must for all type 1 diabetics and type 2 diabetics with severe hyperglycemia or β-cell failure. Basal, bolus, and basal-bolus insulin regimens are based on patients' lifestyle and carbohydrate consumption. Insulin analogs (glargine, degludec, lispro) offer improved glycemic stability and less risk for hypoglycemia [89].

Newer agents

GLP-1 receptor agonists (GLP-1RAs): Liraglutide and semaglutide are used to achieve glycemic control, weight loss, and reduction of cardiovascular risk.

SGLT2 inhibitors (e.g., empagliflozin, dapagliflozin): They increase renal excretion of glucose, reduce HbA1c, and show advantages in heart failure and chronic kidney disease; these are dual-purpose drugs.

Combination therapies (GLP-1RA + insulin or SGLT2 + metformin) are emerging treatment options for patients with complex metabolic requirements [90].

1.7.3 Role of Technology: Continuous Glucose Monitoring, Insulin Pumps, Smart Wearables

Technology is transforming diabetes management with the rise of real-time monitoring and personalized care.

CGM: It offers dynamic glucose profiles that include postprandial excursions and hypoglycemia during the night, which is missed by finger-stick testing. In T1DM and T2DM alike, devices such as Dexcom G6 and Freestyle Libre are shown to improve adherence and reduce HbA1c [91].

Insulin pumps and hybrid closed-loop systems: Insulin pumps provide continuous subcutaneous infusion of insulin in a pattern similar to physiological patterns. Advanced artificial pancreas (AP) systems combine CGM with pumps and algorithms to automate insulin delivery. For example, the Medtronic MiniMed 780G is a hybrid closed-loop control to minimize hypoglycemia [92].

Smart wearables and digital health: Smartwatches monitor physical activity, sleep, and heart rate and combine this data to deliver a personalized diabetes coaching experience. Mobile apps act as central hubs where users can log daily blood glucose levels, track dietary intake, monitor physical activity, and calculate insulin doses. Many of these applications sync directly with medical devices like CGM. AI-powered prediction algorithms are now coming to the market for predicting the occurrence of the hypoglycemia event and for optimizing insulin dosage [93].

1.7.4 Integrative and Preventative Approaches

Integrative and preventative approaches include holistic medicine:

Preventive models: Diabetes prevention trials (DPP, Finnish DPS) demonstrate that interventions in prediabetes reduce the incidence by 40–60%. Community-based programs particularly in low-income settings emphasize dietary education, physical activity promotion, and obesity control [94].

Integrative therapies: Some herbal medicines (e.g., fenugreek, bitter melon, cinnamon) have demonstrated modest blood glucose lowering effects but standardization and regulation have proven problematic. Tai chi and yoga, or other mind-body practices, enhance glycemic control and adaptive response to stress [95].

Precision medicine and future perspectives: Pharmacogenomics is already beginning to inform treatment – CYP2C9 variants may affect metabolism of sulfonyl urease and SLC5A2 variants may affect SGLT2 response. Other regenerative strategies, such as β-cell replacement therapy, islet-based stem cells, and immune modulation, are currently being studied [96, 97].

1.8 PREVENTION STRATEGIES AND SOCIAL AND PUBLIC HEALTH POINTS

The best way to treat diabetes is to prevent it as the complications are more difficult and costly to treat. With the increasing global burden, the public health response has focused on reducing avoidable risk factors, promoting awareness at the community level, and incorporating prevention into health systems. Prevention models are classified into primary, secondary, and tertiary with the backing of global health [10, 98].

1.8.1 Primary and Secondary Prevention Models

Primary prevention: The objective is to prevent the development of diabetes in people at high risk of the disease. Lifestyle changes are still the best solution. For instance, the Diabetes Prevention Program (DPP; USA) showed that the incidence of T2DM could be reduced by 58% by lifestyle intervention compared with 31% by metformin monotherapy. Nutrient education, physical activity promotion, weight control, and anti-obesity campaigns are key elements of primary prevention [99].

Secondary prevention: It aims to achieve early detection and prevent progression to the disease in prediabetes or undiagnosed diabetes:

- Screening (HbA1c, fasting glucose, or risk score (e.g., IDRS)) identifies cases earlier in their course.
- Early treatment and lifestyle interventions can slow or even reverse prediabetes.
- For example, in the Finnish Diabetes Prevention Study, modest weight loss (~5–7%) led to a substantially decreased progression rate from prediabetes to diabetes [100].

1.8.2 Community-Based Interventions

Community engagement is critical to sustainable diabetes prevention:

Education programs: School-based nutrition classes and workplace wellness initiatives encourage healthy eating and exercise [101].

Peer support groups: It can offer encouragement and compliance, especially for low-resource settings [102].

Culturally tailored interventions: For example, yoga-based diabetes prevention programs in India, or walking clubs in African and Latin American communities, adapt strategies to local traditions [103].

mHealth: Text messaging, telemedicine, and mobile apps enable large-scale education and self-monitoring. India's mDiabetes campaign sent health-conscious SMSes to more than one million people, helping to raise awareness and change lifestyle habits [104].

1.8.3 Policies and WHO Guidelines for Global Health

International organizations are important players for the standardization and dissemination of prevention measures:

WHO: It supports "best buys" framework: policies to address unhealthy diet, physical inactivity, tobacco and alcohol use. It also supports universal access to medicines and technologies, including insulin as an essential medicine, as well as STEPwise surveillance (STEPS) for non-communicable disease (NCD) risk factor surveillance [105].

IDF: World Diabetes Day is an annual awareness day. It suggests low-cost interventions, such as primary care opportunistic screening and dietary interventions (reducing sugar-sweetened beverages) [106].

National policies: In the US, a National Diabetes Prevention Program (CDC-led) has incorporated lifestyle coaching into primary care. The National Programme for Prevention and Control of Cancer, Diabetes, Cardiovascular Diseases and Stroke (NPCDCS) in India involves screening, education, and mobilization of the community [107].

1.8.4 Future of Diabetes Prevention

The future of diabetes prevention is precision public health – purposeful interventions that bring together genetic, behavioral, and environmental data.

Digital health and artificial intelligence (AI): High-impact algorithms for personalized interventions can be used to identify high-risk individuals [108].

Nutrigenomics: Genetic-based personalized nutrition can be used to maximize prevention [109].

Modulating the microbiome: Probiotics, prebiotics, and fecal microbiota transplantation can help in preventing metabolic disease [110].

Policy innovations: Taxation on sugar-sweetened beverages (Mexico and the UK) has already proven to reduce consumption; as such it can be a blueprint for policy action elsewhere in the world [111].

Youth-centered prevention: Because childhood obesity is a strong predictor of diabetes in adults, programs in schools that combine healthy eating, exercise, and digital activity will be at the heart [112].

1.9 EMERGING TRENDS AND FUTURE DIRECTIONS

Science and technology are revolutionizing the way diabetes is managed. Precision medicine, AI, nanotechnology, and regenerative approaches are emerging from the shadows of traditional therapy as the field seeks to prevent, treat, and possibly cure diabetes. These innovations offer tailored, effective, and less invasive care for patients around the world [113]. Figure 1.3 shows the comprehensive diabetes management model that combines lifestyle, pharmacological, technological, and emerging therapeutic interventions.

1.9.1 Precision Medicine and Pharmacogenomics

The concept of precision medicine uses personalized approach to treatment depending on genetic, epigenetic, and metabolic profile of each individual instead of the common one-size-fits-all approach [114].

Pharmacogenomics: Genetic differences in CYP2C9, KCNJ11, TCF7L2, and SLC5A2 affect the response to sulfonylureas, metformin, and SGLT2 inhibitors [115].

Example: TCF7L2 polymorphic patients can potentially have decreased insulin secretion, thus less responsive to sulfonylureas but better respondent to incretin-based therapy [116].

Metabolomics and multi-omics integration enables disease onset prediction and treatment response and as such, can be used to prevent and treat diseases on an individual basis [117].

In precision medicine, the subtypes of diabetes in addition to type 1 and type 2 that include maturity-onset diabetes of the young (MODY) or latent autoimmune diabetes of adults (LADA) are determined, and the correct choice of therapy is guaranteed [118].

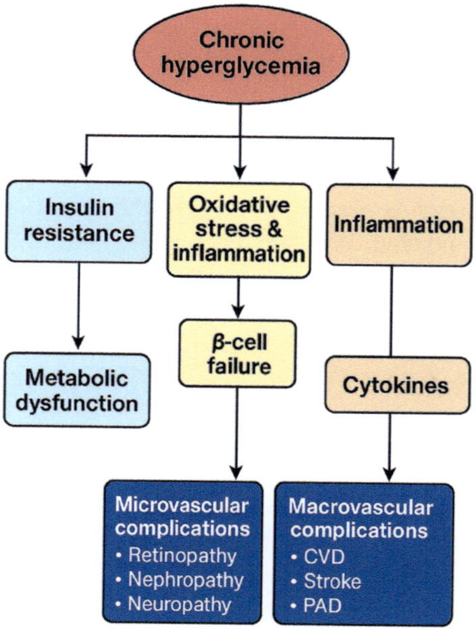

FIGURE 1.3 Integrated diabetes management and emerging therapeutic strategies.

1.9.2 Artificial Intelligence and Digital Health in Diabetes Care

Disease monitoring, prediction, and self-management are being transformed by AI and digital platforms:

Predictive analytics: AI is used to forecast hyperglycemia, hypoglycemia, and risk of complication based on CGM, electronic health record (EHR), and lifestyle data [119].

Decision support system: Machine learning models can help clinicians customize therapy, optimize insulin doses, and choose the right combinations of pharmacological therapy [120].

Remote monitoring and telemedicine: Digital devices, mobile apps, and cloud-connected glucose monitors allow real-time feedback that enhances adherence and glycemic control. Diabetes digital coaches combine AI-based recommendations, behavioral nudges, and teleconsultation as the means of sustaining lifestyle interventions within the high-risk populations [121].

1.9.3 Regenerative Medicine and β-Cell Replacement Therapy

Regenerative therapies are meant to reinstate the natural production of insulin and possibly to cure diabetes:

Stem cell-derived -cells: Human pluripotent stem cells are developed into insulin producing -cells and implanted to rejuvenate the pancreas.

Islet transplantation: T1DM patients are able to survive longer on immune rejection due to encapsulation technologies.

Gene therapy and immunomodulation: Techniques are intended to address autoimmune destruction of -cells and increase -cell proliferation in clinical trials.

Example: Vertex phase I/II trial showed that encapsulated stem-cell derived 0-cells could normalize glucose in a small number of patients with T1DM, but only without immunosuppression [122].

1.9.4 Nanotechnology and Advanced Drug Delivery Systems

Nanotechnology provides accurate delivery of drug, enhances penicillin efficacy, and reduces side effects:

Insulin nanoparticle delivery: Insulin formulations are delivered to the body orally or through transdermal routes bypassing the drawbacks of subcutaneous injection.

Glucose-responsive systems: Smart nanoparticles are fed with insulin, which is released when the glucose level changes, simulating the physiological regulation [123, 124].

Indeed, insulin- or GLP-1 analog-loaded polymeric nanocarriers and liposomes have shown prolonged glucose regulation in preclinical models, which opens the way to non-invasive, patient-friendly therapy [125].

1.10 CONCLUSION

DM is a multifactorial and complex disease which presents a major clinical, societal, and economic problem on an international basis. Between the molecular complexity of insulin resistance and eight-cell dysfunction, on the one hand, and the systemic effects of chronic complications, on the other hand, the disease can only be understood in an integrated view that cuts across biology, lifestyle, and technology.

Developments in diagnostics, treatment, and policies in public health have largely enhanced the control of the disease, but the increasing incidence highlights the importance of early diagnosis, patient-centered care, and prophylaxis. The future of diabetes management is characterized by innovations in precision medicine, digital health, regenerative therapies, and nanotechnology that can transform diabetes care and enable more effective, patient-centered, and potentially curative treatment.

Finally, diabetes needs to be fought by a multidisciplinary approach, including clinicians, researchers, policymakers, and communities, to bring together scientific and practical strategies. This chapter offers an overall roadmap to the interpretation and management of one of the most urgent health issues of the present day by combining the insights into the pathophysiology, clinical presentation, prevention, and the latest forms of treatment.

ACKNOWLEDGMENTS

The authors express special thanks to editors for providing necessary facilities and motivation.

REFERENCES

1. Hossain MJ, Al-Mamun M, Islam MR. Diabetes mellitus, the fastest growing global public health concern: Early detection should be focused. Health Science Reports. 2024;7(3):e2004.
2. Sun H, Saeedi P, Karuranga S, Pinkepank M, Ogurtsova K, Duncan BB, Stein C, Basit A, Chan JC, Atlas JM. Global, regional and country-level diabetes prevalence estimates for 2021 and projections for 2045. 2022, 183. https://doi.org/10.1016/j.diabres.2021.109119.
3. Kumar A, Gangwar R, Ahmad Zargar A, Kumar R, Sharma A. Prevalence of diabetes in India: A review of IDF diabetes atlas 10th edition. Current Diabetes Reviews. 2024;20(1):105–14.
4. Sun H, Saeedi P, Karuranga S, Pinkepank M, Ogurtsova K, Duncan BB, Stein C, Basit A, Chan JC, Mbanya JC, Pavkov ME. IDF Diabetes Atlas: Global, regional and country-level diabetes prevalence estimates for 2021 and projections for 2045. Diabetes Research and Clinical Practice. 2022;183:109119.
5. Pollak M. Diabetes in Native Chicago: An Ethnography of Identity, Community, and Care. University of Nebraska Press; 2021.
6. Simoni RD, Hill RL, Vaughan M. The discovery of insulin: The work of Frederick Banting and Charles Best. Journal of Biological Chemistry. 2002 Jun 28;277(26):e1–2.
7. Lambert C, Delgado E. 100 years since the discovery of insulin, from its discovery to the insulins of the future. Biomedicines. 2024 Feb 27;12(3):533.
8. An X, Zhang Y, Sun W, Kang X, Ji H, Sun Y, Jiang L, Zhao X, Gao Q, Lian F, Tong X. Early effective intervention can significantly reduce all-cause mortality in prediabetic patients: A systematic review and meta-analysis based on high-quality clinical studies. Frontiers in Endocrinology. 2024;15:1294819.
9. Diabetes Prevention Program (DPP) Research Group. The diabetes prevention program (DPP) description of lifestyle intervention. Diabetes Care. 2002;25(12):2165–71.
10. Galaviz KI, Narayan KV, Lobelo F, Weber MB. Lifestyle and the prevention of type 2 diabetes: A status report. American Journal of Lifestyle Medicine. 2018;12(1):4–20.
11. Klupa T, Czupryniak L, Dzida G, Fichna P, Jarosz-Chobot P, Gumprecht J, Mysliwiec M, Szadkowska A, Bomba-Opon D, Czajkowski K, Malecki MT. Expanding the role of continuous glucose monitoring in modern diabetes care beyond type 1 disease. Diabetes Therapy. 2023;14(8):1241–66.
12. Hantzidiamantis PJ, Awosika AO, Lappin SL. Physiology, Glucose. In StatPearls. StatPearls Publishing; 2024.
13. Nakrani MN, Wineland RH. F. Anjum Physiology, Glucose Metabolism. 2023.
14. Dimitriadis GD, Maratou E, Kountouri A, Board M, Lambadiari V. Regulation of postabsorptive and postprandial glucose metabolism by insulin-dependent and insulin-independent mechanisms: An integrative approach. Nutrients. 2021;13(1):159.
15. Haedersdal S, Andersen A, Knop FK, Vilsbøll T. Revisiting the role of glucagon in health, diabetes mellitus and other metabolic diseases. Nature Reviews Endocrinology. 2023;19(6):321–35.
16. Sarmiento BE, Santos Menezes LF, Schwartz EF. Insulin release mechanism modulated by toxins isolated from animal venoms: From basic research to drug development prospects. Molecules. 2019 May 14;24(10):1846.
17. Rix I, Nexøe-Larsen C, Bergmann NC, Lund A, Knop FK. Glucagon physiology. 2015.

18. Poggiogalle E, Jamshed H, Peterson CM. Circadian regulation of glucose, lipid, and energy metabolism in humans. Metabolism. 2018;84:11–27.
19. Marchetti P, Baronti W, Boggi U, Marselli L. Diabetes Mellitus: Classification and Diagnosis. In Transplantation of the Pancreas (pp. 3–12). Springer International Publishing; 2023.
20. Solis-Herrera C, Triplitt C, Reasner C, DeFronzo RA, Cersosimo E Classification of diabetes mellitus. Endotext [Internet]. 2018. https://www.ncbi.nlm.nih.gov/books/NBK279119/.
21. Roep BO, Thomaidou S, Van Tienhoven R, Zaldumbide A. Type 1 diabetes mellitus as a disease of the β-cell (do not blame the immune system?). Nature Reviews Endocrinology. 2021;17(3):150–61.
22. Alves Abrantes JJ, Veríssimo de Azevedo JC, Fernandes FL, Duarte Almeida V, Custódio De Oliveira LA, Ferreira de Oliveira MT, Galvão De Araújo JM, Lanza DC, Bezerra FL, Andrade VS, Araújo de Medeiros Fernandes TA. Viruses as a potential environmental trigger of type 1 diabetes mellitus. Biomedical Reports. 2024;20(5):81.
23. Addissouky TA, Ali MM, El Sayed IE, Wang Y. Type 1 diabetes mellitus: Retrospect and prospect. Bulletin of the National Research Centre. 2024;48(1):42.
24. Goyal R, Singhal M, Jialal I. Type 2 diabetes. StatPearls [Internet]. 2023. https://www.ncbi.nlm.nih.gov/books/NBK513253/.
25. Serbis A, Giapros V, Kotanidou EP, Galli-Tsinopoulou A, Siomou E. Diagnosis, treatment and prevention of type 2 diabetes mellitus in children and adolescents. World Journal of Diabetes. 2021;12(4):344.
26. Jiang L, Tang K, Magee LA, von Dadelszen P, Ekeroma A, Li X, Zhang E, Bhutta ZA. A global view of hypertensive disorders and diabetes mellitus during pregnancy. Nature Reviews Endocrinology. 2022;18(12):760–75.
27. Choudhury AA, Rajeswari VD. Gestational diabetes mellitus: A metabolic and reproductive disorder. Biomedicine & Pharmacotherapy. 2021;143:112183.
28. Bhattacharya S, Fernandez CJ, Kamrul-Hasan AB, Pappachan JM. Monogenic diabetes: An evidence-based clinical approach. World Journal of Diabetes. 2025;16(5):104787.
29. Tamarai K, Bhatti JS, Reddy PH. Molecular and cellular bases of diabetes: Focus on type 2 diabetes mouse model-TallyHo. Biochimica et Biophysica Acta (BBA)-Molecular Basis of Disease. 2019; 1865(9):2276–84.
30. Dilworth L, Facey A, Omoruyi F. Diabetes mellitus and its metabolic complications: The role of adipose tissues. International Journal of Molecular Sciences. 2021;22(14):7644.
31. Zheng M, Wang P. Role of insulin receptor substance-1 modulating PI3K/AKT insulin signaling pathway in Alzheimer's disease. 3 Biotech. 2021;11(4):179.
32. Klip A, McGraw TE, James DE. Thirty sweet years of GLUT4. Journal of Biological Chemistry. 2019;294(30):11369–81.
33. Zhang X, Yang S, Chen J, Su Z. Unraveling the regulation of hepatic gluconeogenesis. Frontiers in Endocrinology. 2019;9:802.
34. Chandrasekaran P, Weiskirchen R. Cellular and molecular mechanisms of insulin resistance. Current Tissue Microenvironment Reports. 2024;5(3):79–90.
35. Seböková E, Klimes I, Stolba P. Cellular and molecular mechanisms of insulin resistance. Vnitrni Lekarstvi. 1995;41(2):76–83.
36. Rohm TV, Meier DT, Olefsky JM, Donath MY. Inflammation in obesity, diabetes, and related disorders. Immunity. 2022;55(1):31–55.
37. Hayden MR. Overview and new insights into the metabolic syndrome: Risk factors and emerging variables in the development of type 2 diabetes and cerebrocardiovascular disease. Medicina. 2023;59(3):561.
38. Imamura M, Maeda S. Perspectives on genetic studies of type 2 diabetes from the genome-wide association studies era to precision medicine. Journal of Diabetes Investigation. 2024;15(4):410–22.
39. Mahmoud AM. An overview of epigenetics in obesity: The role of lifestyle and therapeutic interventions. International Journal of Molecular Sciences. 2022;23(3):1341.
40. Rinninella E, Tohumcu E, Raoul P, Fiorani M, Cintoni M, Mele MC, Cammarota G, Gasbarrini A, Ianiro G. The role of diet in shaping human gut microbiota. Best Practice & Research Clinical Gastroenterology. 2023;62:101828.
41. Virk MS, Virk MA, He Y, Tufail T, Gul M, Qayum A, Rehman A, Rashid A, Ekumah JN, Han X, Wang J. The anti-inflammatory and curative exponent of probiotics: A comprehensive and authentic ingredient for the sustained functioning of major human organs. Nutrients. 2024;16(4):546.
42. Guo H, Pan L, Wu Q, Wang L, Huang Z, Wang J, Wang L, Fang X, Dong S, Zhu Y, Liao Z. Type 2 diabetes and the multifaceted gut-X axes. Nutrients. 2025;17(16):2708.
43. Zhang J, Zhang Z, Zhang K, Ge X, Sun R, Zhai X. Early detection of type 2 diabetes risk: Limitations of current diagnostic criteria. Frontiers in Endocrinology. 2023;14:1260623.

44. Hjellestad ID, Astor MC, Nilsen RM, Søfteland E, Jonung T. HbA1c versus oral glucose tolerance test as a method to diagnose diabetes mellitus in vascular surgery patients. Cardiovascular Diabetology. 2013; 12(1):79.
45. ElSayed NA, McCoy RG, Aleppo G, Balapattabi K, Beverly EA, Briggs Early K, Bruemmer D, Ebekozien O, Echouffo-Tcheugui JB, Ekhlaspour L, Gaglia JL. Diagnosis and classification of diabetes: Standards of care in diabetes—2025. Diabetes Care. 2025; 48.
46. Athanasiadou KI, Paschou SA, Markozannes G, Vasileiou V, Kanouta F, Mitropoulou M, Antsaklis P, Theodora M, Psaltopoulou T, Daskalakis G, Goulis DG. Gestational diabetes mellitus subtypes according to oral glucose tolerance test and pregnancy outcomes. Endocrine. 2025:1–9.
47. World Health Organization. In Use of Glycated Haemoglobin (HbA1c) in the Diagnosis of Diabetes Mellitus Abbreviated Report of a WHO Consultation (pp. 25–25). 2011.
48. Kim DL, Kim SD, Kim SK, Park S, Song KH. Is an oral glucose tolerance test still valid for diagnosing diabetes mellitus? Diabetes & Metabolism Journal. 2016;40(2):118–28.
49. Janghorbani M, Amini M. Normal fasting plasma glucose and risk of prediabetes and type 2 diabetes: The Isfahan diabetes prevention study. The Review of Diabetic Studies: RDS. 2012;8(4):490.
50. Eyth E, Basit H, Swift C. Glucose Tolerance Test. StatPearls; 2023.
51. Incani M, Sentinelli F, Perra L, Pani MG, Porcu M, Lenzi A, Cavallo MG, Cossu E, Leonetti F, Baroni MG. Glycated hemoglobin for the diagnosis of diabetes and prediabetes: Diagnostic impact on obese and lean subjects, and phenotypic characterization. Journal of Diabetes Investigation. 2015;6(1):44–50.
52. Leighton E, Sainsbury CA, Jones GC. A practical review of C-peptide testing in diabetes. Diabetes Therapy. 2017;8(3):475–87.
53. Gregory EL, Jones C A Practical Review of C-Peptide Testing in Diabetes. 2017.
54. Szumilas K, Wilk A, Szumilas P, Dziedziejko V, Pawlik A. Role of leptin and adiponectin in the pathogenesis of post-transplant diabetes mellitus. Prostaglandins & Other Lipid Mediators. 2024; 174:106876.
55. Wang X, Bao W, Liu J, OuYang YY, Wang D, Rong S, Xiao X, Shan ZL, Zhang Y, Yao P, Liu LG. Inflammatory markers and risk of type 2 diabetes: A systematic review and meta-analysis. Diabetes Care. 2013;36(1):166–75.
56. Turko R, Hajja A, Magableh AM, Omer MH, Shafqat A, Khan MI, Yaqinuddin A. The emerging role of miRNAs in biological aging and age-related diseases. Non-Coding RNA Research. 2025. https://doi.org/10.1016/j.ncrna.2025.05.002.
57. Fajkić A, Jahić R, Ejubović M, Đešević M, Ejubović AJ, Lepara O. The trend of changes in adiponectin, resistin, and adiponectin–Resistin index values in type 2 diabetic patients with the development of metabolic syndrome. Medicina. 2024;60(11):1795.
58. Bergman M, Chetrit A, Roth J, Dankner R. One-hour post-load plasma glucose level during the OGTT predicts mortality: Observations from the Israel study of glucose intolerance, obesity and hypertension. Diabetic Medicine. 2016;33(8):1060–66.
59. Kanaya AM. Diabetes in South Asians: Uncovering novel risk factors with longitudinal epidemiologic data: Kelly West award lecture 2023. Diabetes Care. 2024;47(1):7–16.
60. Leggio M, Lombardi M, Caldarone E, Severi P, D'emidio S, Armeni M, Bravi V, Bendini MG, Mazza A. The relationship between obesity and hypertension: An updated comprehensive overview on vicious twins. Hypertension Research. 2017;40(12):947–63.
61. Yao K, Bian C, Zhao X. Association of polycystic ovary syndrome with metabolic syndrome and gestational diabetes: Aggravated complication of pregnancy. Experimental and Therapeutic Medicine. 2017;14(2):1271–76.
62. Davies MJ, Aroda VR, Collins BS, Gabbay RA, Green J, Maruthur NM, Rosas SE, Del Prato S, Mathieu C, Mingrone G, Rossing P. Management of hyperglycaemia in type 2 diabetes, 2022. A consensus report by the American Diabetes Association (ADA) and the European Association for the Study of Diabetes (EASD). Diabetologia. 2022;65(12):1925–66.
63. Fang M, Wang D, Coresh J, Selvin E. Undiagnosed diabetes in US adults: Prevalence and trends. Diabetes Care. 2022;45(9):1994–2002.
64. Balakumar P, Maung-U K, Jagadeesh G. Prevalence and prevention of cardiovascular disease and diabetes mellitus. Pharmacological Research. 2016;113:600–9.
65. Fichadiya NC, Kadri AM, Dave BB. Evaluation of Indian diabetes risk score and random blood sugar testing for opportunistic screening of type 2 diabetes patients at a district Hospital of Gujarat. Indian Journal of Community Medicine. 2022;47(4):517–21.
66. Rajput M, Garg D, Rajput R. Validation of simplified Indian diabetes risk score for screening undiagnosed diabetes in an urban setting of Haryana. Diabetes & Metabolic Syndrome: Clinical Research & Reviews. 2017;11:S539–42.

67. Dwivedi M, Pandey AR. Diabetes mellitus and its treatment: An overview. J Adv Pharmacol. 2020; 1(1):48–58.
68. Kishore P. Diabetes mellitus (DM)-endocrine and metabolic disorders-MSD manual professional edition. Merck Manual, Professional Version. 2015.
69. Nakhleh A, Shehadeh N. Hypoglycemia in diabetes: An update on pathophysiology, treatment, and prevention. World Journal of Diabetes. 2021;12(12):2036.
70. Lowie BJ, Bond MC. Diabetic ketoacidosis. Emergency Medicine Clinics of North America. 2023;41(4): 677–86.
71. Pasquel FJ, Umpierrez GE. Hyperosmolar hyperglycemic state: A historic review of the clinical presentation, diagnosis, and treatment. Diabetes Care. 2014;37(11):3124–31.
72. Li Y, Liu Y, Liu S, Gao M, Wang W, Chen K, Huang L, Liu Y. Diabetic vascular diseases: Molecular mechanisms and therapeutic strategies. Signal Transduction and Targeted Therapy. 2023;8(1):152.
73. Yang Z, Tan TE, Shao Y, Wong TY, Li X. Classification of diabetic retinopathy: Past, present and future. Frontiers in Endocrinology. 2022;13:1079217.
74. Natesan V, Kim SJ. Diabetic nephropathy–a review of risk factors, progression, mechanism, and dietary management. Biomolecules & Therapeutics. 2021;29(4):365.
75. Glow D, Moore P. Assessing diabetic peripheral neuropathy in primary care. BPJ Issue. 2014;61:37–47.
76. Aronson D, Edelman ER. Coronary artery disease and diabetes mellitus. Cardiology Clinics. 2014; 32(3):439.
77. Uccioli L, Gandini R, Giurato L, Fabiano S, Pampana E, Spallone V, Vainieri E, Simonetti G. Long-term outcomes of diabetic patients with critical limb ischemia followed in a tertiary referral diabetic foot clinic. Diabetes Care. 2010;33(5):977–82.
78. Kiriella DA, Islam S, Oridota O, Sohler N, Dessenne C, de Beaufort C, Fagherazzi G, Aguayo GA. Unraveling the concepts of distress, burnout, and depression in type 1 diabetes: A scoping review. EClinicalMedicine. 2021;40:1–9.
79. Patel MR. Financial toxicity in diabetes: The state of what we know. Current Diabetes Reports. 2025;25(1):32.
80. Adepu R, Rasheed A, Nagavi B. Effect of patient counseling on quality of life in type-2 diabetes mellitus patients in two selected South Indian community pharmacies: A study. Indian Journal of Pharmaceutical Sciences. 2007;69(4):519–24.
81. Bain SC, Cummings MH, McKay GA. Multidisciplinary approach to management and care of patients with type 2 diabetes mellitus. Diabetes. 2019;7:73–81.
82. Widmer RJ, Flammer AJ, Lerman LO, Lerman A. The Mediterranean diet, its components, and cardiovascular disease. The American Journal of Medicine. 2015;128(3):229–38.
83. Vitolins MZ, Anderson AM, Delahanty L, Raynor H, Miller GD, Mobley C, Reeves R, Yamamoto M, Champagne C, Wing RR, Mayer-Davis E. Action for health in diabetes (Look AHEAD) trial: Baseline evaluation of selected nutrients and food group intake. Journal of the American Dietetic Association. 2009;109(8):1367–75.
84. Bassin SR, Srinath R. The impact of physical activity in patients with type 2 diabetes. American Journal of Lifestyle Medicine. 2025;19(1):147–61.
85. Hamasaki H. The effects of mindfulness on glycemic control in people with diabetes: An overview of systematic reviews and meta-analyses. Medicines. 2023;10(9):53.
86. Kolhe RC, Chaudhari PS, Ghadage PK. Yoga as a holistic approach to diabetes management: Addressing stress, metabolic balance and glycemic control. Journal of Ayurveda and Integrated Medical Sciences. 2025;10(2):263–72.
87. Schroeder EB. Management of type 2 diabetes: Selecting amongst available pharmacological agents. [Updated 2026, Apr 12]. In: Feingold KR, Adler RA, Ahmed SF, et al., editors. Endotext [Internet]. South Dartmouth (MA): MDText.com, Inc.; 2000. Available from: https://www.ncbi.nlm.nih.gov/books/NBK425702/.
88. Feingold KR. Oral and injectable (non-insulin) pharmacological agents for the treatment of type 2 diabetes. [Updated 2025, Dec 29]. In: Feingold KR, Adler RA, Ahmed SF, et al., editors. Endotext [Internet]. South Dartmouth (MA): MDText.com, Inc.; 2000. Available from: https://www.ncbi.nlm.nih.gov/sites/books/NBK279141/.
89. Donnor T, Sarkar S. Insulin-pharmacology, therapeutic regimens and principles of intensive insulin therapy. [Updated 2023, Feb 15]. In: Feingold KR, Adler RA, Ahmed SF, et al., editors. Endotext [Internet]. South Dartmouth (MA): MDText.com, Inc.; 2000. Available from: https://www.ncbi.nlm.nih.gov/sites/books/NBK278938/.
90. Rolek B, Haber M, Gajewska M, Rogula S, Pietrasik A, Gąsecka A. SGLT2 inhibitors vs. GLP-1 agonists to treat the heart, the kidneys and the brain. Journal of Cardiovascular Development and Disease. 2023;10(8):322.

91. Freckmann G, Pleus S, Grady M, Setford S, Levy B. Measures of accuracy for continuous glucose monitoring and blood glucose monitoring devices. Journal of Diabetes Science and Technology. 2019;13(3):575–83.
92. Avari P, Lumb A, Flanagan D, Rayman G, Misra S, Choudhary P, Dhatariya K. Insulin pumps and hybrid close loop systems within hospital: A scoping review and practical guidance from the Joint British Diabetes Societies for Inpatient Care. Journal of Diabetes Science and Technology. 2023;17(3):625–34.
93. Gershkowitz BD, Hillert CJ, Crotty BH. Digital coaching strategies to facilitate behavioral change in type 2 diabetes: A systematic review. The Journal of Clinical Endocrinology & Metabolism. 2021;106(4):e1513–20.
94. Demissie GD, Birungi J, Shrestha A, Haregu T, Thirunavukkarasu S, Oldenburg B. The effectiveness of lifestyle interventions in reducing cardiovascular risk and risk factors in people with prediabetes: A systematic review and meta-analysis. Nutrition, Metabolism and Cardiovascular Diseases. 2025:104130.
95. Alshali KZ. Review of herb supplement use in type 2 diabetes. Archives of Pharmacy Practice. 2020;11(2-2020):42–9.
96. Gieroba B, Kryska A, Sroka-Bartnicka A. Type 2 diabetes mellitus–conventional therapies and future perspectives in innovative treatment. Biochemistry and Biophysics Reports. 2025;42:102037.
97. Venkatachalapathy P, Padhilahouse S, Sellappan M, Subramanian T, Kurian SJ, Miraj SS, Rao M, Raut AA, Kanwar RK, Singh J, Khadanga S. Pharmacogenomics and personalized medicine in type 2 diabetes mellitus: Potential implications for clinical practice. Pharmacogenomics and Personalized Medicine. 2021;13:1441–55.
98. Narayan KV, Gregg EW, Fagot-Campagna A, Engelgau MM, Vinicor F. Diabetes—a common, growing, serious, costly, and potentially preventable public health problem. Diabetes Research and Clinical Practice. 2000;50:S77–84.
99. Tuomilehto J, Uusitupa M, Gregg EW, Lindström J. Type 2 diabetes prevention programs—From proof-of-concept trials to national intervention and beyond. Journal of Clinical Medicine. 2023;12(5):1876.
100. Cosic V, Jakab J, Pravecek MK, Miskic B. The importance of prediabetes screening in the prevention of cardiovascular disease. Medical Archives. 2023;77(2):97.
101. Berry L, Mirabito AM, Baun WB What's the hard return on employee wellness programs?. SSRN; 2020.
102. Kaur J, Singh P. Exploring the potential of Peer support group for family planning needs of women in resource-constrained settings in India. Proceedings of the ACM on Human-Computer Interaction. 2025;9(2):1–25.
103. Abu S, Llahana S. Factors influencing the uptake of culturally tailored diabetes self-management education and support programmes among ethnic minority patients with type 2 diabetes: A systematic review. Primary Care Diabetes. 2025;19(2):103–10.. https://doi.org/10.1016/j.pcd.2025.01.010.
104. Ramachandran A, Kumar R, Nanditha A, Raghavan A, Snehalatha C, Krishnamoorthy S, Joshi P, Tesfaye F. mDiabetes initiative using text messages to improve lifestyle and health-seeking behaviour in India. BMJ Innovations. 2018;0:1–8.. https://doi.org/10.1136/ bmjinnov-2017-000265.
105. Khaltaev N, Axelrod S. Countrywide" best buy" interventions for noncommunicable diseases prevention and control in countries with different level of socioeconomic development. Chronic Diseases and Translational Medicine. 2023;9(01):44–53.
106. Shahbazian H. World diabetes day; 2013. Journal of Renal Injury Prevention. 2013;2(4):123.
107. Insamran W, Sangrajrang S. National cancer control program of Thailand. Asian Pacific Journal of Cancer Prevention: APJCP. 2020;21(3):577.
108. Bucher A, Blazek ES, Symons CT. How are machine learning and artificial intelligence used in digital behavior change interventions? A scoping review. Mayo Clinic Proceedings: Digital Health. 2024;2(3):375–404.
109. Marcum JA. Nutrigenetics/nutrigenomics, personalized nutrition, and precision healthcare. Current Nutrition Reports. 2020;9(4):338–45.
110. Ciernikova S, Sevcikova A, Drgona L, Mego M. Modulating the gut microbiota by probiotics, prebiotics, postbiotics, and fecal microbiota transplantation: An emerging trend in cancer patient care. Biochimica et Biophysica Acta (BBA)-Reviews on Cancer. 2023;1878(6):188990.
111. Colchero MA, Molina M, Guerrero-López CM. After Mexico implemented a tax, purchases of sugar-sweetened beverages decreased and water increased: Difference by place of residence, household composition, and income level. The Journal of Nutrition. 2017;147(8):1552–57.
112. Scott J, Agarwala A, Baker-Smith CM, Feinstein MJ, Jakubowski K, Kaar J, Parekh N, Patel KV, Stephens J. Cardiovascular health in the transition from adolescence to emerging adulthood: A scientific statement from the American Heart Association. Journal of the American Heart Association. 2025;14(9):e039239.

113. Guan Z, Li H, Liu R, Cai C, Liu Y, Li J, Wang X, Huang S, Wu L, Liu D, Yu S. Artificial intelligence in diabetes management: Advancements, opportunities, and challenges. Cell Reports Medicine. 2023;4(10):1–20.
114. Strianese O, Rizzo F, Ciccarelli M, Galasso G, D'Agostino Y, Salvati A, Del Giudice C, Tesorio P, Rusciano MR. Precision and personalized medicine: How genomic approach improves the management of cardiovascular and neurodegenerative disease. Genes. 2020;11(7):747.
115. Nasykhova YA, Tonyan ZN, Mikhailova AA, Danilova MM, Glotov AS. Pharmacogenetics of type 2 diabetes—Progress and prospects. International Journal of Molecular Sciences. 2020;21(18):6842.
116. Zimdahl H, Ittrich C, Graefe-Mody U, Boehm BO, Mark M, Woerle HJ, Dugi KA. Influence of TCF7L2 gene variants on the therapeutic response to the dipeptidylpeptidase-4 inhibitor linagliptin. Diabetologia. 2014;57(9):1869–75.
117. Chen C, Wang J, Pan D, Wang X, Xu Y, Yan J, Wang L, Yang X, Yang M, Liu GP. Applications of multi-omics analysis in human diseases. MedComm. 2023;4(4):e315.
118. Parveen S, Khan M, Odigwe CC, Qureshi F, Iroegbu N. Latent autoimmune diabetes of adult masquerading as type 2 diabetes mellitus. Journal of Medical Cases. 2015;6(7):327–29.
119. Abdelaal A, Ibrahim AF, Elkatatny S. Data-driven approach for resistivity prediction using artificial intelligence. Journal of Energy Resources Technology. 2022;144(10):103003.
120. Fujihara K, Sone H. Machine learning approach to drug treatment strategy for diabetes care. Diabetes & Metabolism Journal. 2023;47(3):325–32.
121. Amante DJ, Harlan DM, Lemon SC, McManus DD, Olaitan OO, Pagoto SL, Gerber BS, Thompson MJ. Evaluation of a diabetes remote monitoring program facilitated by connected glucose meters for patients with poorly controlled type 2 diabetes: Randomized crossover trial. JMIR Diabetes. 2021;6(1):e25574.
122. Kumar BR. Case 23 Vertex Pharmaceuticals. In Rising Stars: Integrative Case Studies on the 100 Fastest-Growing Companies (pp. 177–183). Springer International Publishing; 2024.
123. Karmakar S, Bhowmik M, Laha B, Manna S. Recent advancements on novel approaches of insulin delivery. Medicine in Novel Technology and Devices. 2023;19:100253.
124. Caturano A, Nilo R, Nilo D, Russo V, Santonastaso E, Galiero R, Rinaldi L, Monda M, Sardu C, Marfella R, Sasso FC. Advances in nanomedicine for precision insulin delivery. Pharmaceuticals. 2024;17(7):945.
125. Andreadi A, Lodeserto P, Todaro F, Meloni M, Romano M, Minasi A, Bellia A, Lauro D. Nanomedicine in the treatment of diabetes. International Journal of Molecular Sciences. 2024;25(13):7028.

2 Recent Advancements in Glucose-Responsive Insulin Delivery Systems

M. Kishore Babu
QIS College of Pharmacy, Ongole, India

Vaishali Shirsat and Safala Malvankar
Bombay College of Pharmacy (Autonomous), Mumbai, India

Umadevi A.
School of Pharmaceutical Sciences, Vels Institute of Science Technology and Advanced Studies, Chennai, India

Vema Kiran
MB School of Pharmaceutical Sciences, Mohan Babu University, Tirupati, India

Ranjit Gadhave
Dr. Vishwanath Karad MIT World Peace University, School of Health Sciences and Technology, Pune, India

Neeraj Verma
Hygia College of Pharmacy, Lucknow, India

2.1 INTRODUCTION

Diabetes mellitus – both type 1 (T1DM) and insulin-treated type 2 (T2DM) – remains a major global health burden because safe, physiologic insulin replacement is difficult to achieve with current therapies. Patients must balance frequent glucose monitoring, carbohydrate counting, and manually timed insulin dosing; even with modern insulin formulations and delivery devices, many people spend large portions of each day outside the target glucose range and remain at risk for both chronic complications from hyperglycemia and immediate danger from hypoglycemia. These care gaps leave unanswered needs: simpler regimens that reduce user burden, faster/dynamic responses to changing glucose, and safety mechanisms that reduce hypoglycemia. Recent reviews and meta-analyses emphasize that while technology has improved outcomes, a substantive clinical gap remains between current therapy and the biologic performance of endogenous pancreatic β-cells [1].

Traditional insulin injection (basal/bolus injections or pump therapy) is intrinsically open-loop, meaning dosing is planned or triggered manually, and cannot readily adapt to rapid increases or decreases in ambient glucose. Continuous glucose monitors (CGMs) and smart insulin pumps have closed that gap by making hybrid closed-loop (HCL) "artificial pancreas" systems that algorithmically adjust insulin delivery in real time [2]. These systems greatly reduce patient workload and

DOI: 10.1201/9781003598657-2

improve the metrics such as time-in-range (TIR) for many users, yet they still rely on sensor accuracy, algorithm tuning, and exogenous insulin pharmacokinetics, which introduce lag and residual risk, especially for unpredictable events like meals or exercise. Thus, engineering insulin delivery systems that are intrinsically glucose-responsive – i.e., drug formulations or materials that change release or activity in direct response to ambient glucose – is a complementary strategy for device-based automation [3].

"Glucose-responsive" approaches aim to replicate fundamental aspects of the native endocrine pancreas: rapid sensitivity to rising glucose, graded release proportional to the stimulus, and automatic cessation of action during glucose normalization. Mechanistic strategies encompass enzyme-based triggers (glucose oxidase), reversible covalent chemistries (phenylboronic acid or PBA), affinity-related-binders (Concanavalin A or Con A and aptamers), and chemically modified "smart" insulin molecules whose activity depends on glucose concentration or on local biochemical signals. These materials and molecular tactics are usually embedded in hydrogels, nanoparticles, microneedle (MN) arrays, or in depot implants so that the formulation itself becomes a self-regulating controller – effectively providing a molecular closed-loop that does not require electronic sensors or external pumps. Recent authoritative reviews summarize these modalities and map to practical challenges of kinetics, biocompatibility, and manufacturability [4].

Concrete recent examples illustrate the promise and current stage of translation. Glucose-responsive MN patches have produced robust, glucose-triggered insulin release and extended normoglycemia in rodent models, demonstrating minimally invasive transdermal delivery with rapid responsiveness. Several different MN designs combining enzyme-sensing vesicles or boronate-containing gels have been reported in the 2023–2025 literature with reproducible in vivo glycemic control. Separately, new "smart" insulin constructs have been engineered to switch activity on and off with glucose, reducing hyperglycemia and lowering the incidence of dangerous hypoglycemia in animal studies – a crucial proof-of-principle for clinical benefit. These advances make clear that glucose-responsive strategies are approaching translational frontiers, where safety, sensor reliability, and regulatory pathways will determine which concepts reach patients [5, 6].

Together, the clinical imperative (simpler, safer glycemic control) and the maturing science of glucose-sensing materials create a compelling rationale for continued development of glucose-responsive insulin (GRI) delivery systems as either standalone therapeutics or as synergistic complements to electronic closed-loop platforms [7].

2.2 HISTORICAL EVOLUTION AND DESIGN GOALS

From simple injectables to self-regulating materials, insulin delivery has moved steadily from passive dosing toward active, glucose-responsive systems that aim to mimic key behavior of pancreatic β-cells. Early practical advances – long acting basal analogs and programmable insulin pumps – allowed finer pharmacokinetic (PK) control but remained fundamentally open-loop systems: dose timing and amount still require patient action or external algorithmic input. Over the last decade, the field has bifurcated along two complementary paths: device-centric closed-loop systems (CGM + algorithms + pump) that automate dosing, and chemistry/material-centric glucose-responsive formulations that change insulin release or activity in direct response to ambient glucose. Both approaches seek the same endpoint – safe, more physiologic glycemic control with less user burden – but they attack different parts of the problem (sensor/algorithm limits versus molecular response kinetics) [8].

Material and molecular strategies trace a clear historical progression. Protein-based sensors such as glucose oxidase (GOx) and affinity binders like Con A were among the first mechanisms that were used to transduce glucose changes into altered release; later work introduced reversible covalent chemistries (PBA) and engineered "smart" insulin analogs that change their activity or availability when glucose concentration changes. These sensing motifs have been integrated into hydrogels, nanoparticles, MNs, and depot implants, shifting the control logic from electronics back into the formulation itself. Contemporary reviews summarize how that evolution trades complexity in electronics for complexity in chemistry and material science [9].

Concrete recent examples highlight where the technology stands. Glucose-responsive MN patches, usually GOx-containing vesicles or PBA-crosslinked hydrogels embedded in dissolvable MNs arrays, have repeatedly produced rapid, glucose-triggered insulin release and prolonged normoglycemia in rodent model; several 2023–2024 studies reported that MN patches reduced the risk of hypoglycemia compared with conventional subcutaneous injections. These minimally-invasive transdermal systems exemplify the shift from passive depot injection to an active, stimulus-responsive system [8, 10, 11].

Key design goals have naturally emerged from both mechanistic constraints and clinical requirements.

Sensitivity: The system must discriminate clinically relevant glucose changes (i.e., 70–180 mg/dL) while avoiding cross-reactivity with other sugars.

Response time: Kinetics must be fast enough to blunt postprandial excursions yet not so fast as to overshoot.

Reversibility: Insulin release or activation should stop as glucose normalizes to prevent hypoglycemia.

Biocompatibility: Enzyme, polymer, or binding protein must provoke inflammation after immunogenicity over repeated dosing.

Storage stability and manufacturability: Formulations must survive cold chain or possess acceptable shelf life and be scalable for clinical translation. Recent perspectives emphasize that balancing these metrics – rather than optimizing a single parameter – determines translational readiness [12].

In short, the historical arc runs from passive carriers toward increasingly autonomous, glucose-sensing materials. The remaining challenge is engineering systems that simultaneously meet sensitivity, speed, safety, and stability requirements so they can move beyond compelling animal studies into trials, and ultimately, into routine care.

2.3 MOLECULAR SENSING MECHANISMS

GRI systems convert a change in local glucose concentration into a predictable change in insulin availability or activity. The principal motifs sensing explored to date, are enzyme-based triggers (notably GOx), reversible covalent boronate chemistries (PBA), affinity-based lectins (Con A), chemically engineered "smart" insulins, and emerging molecular recognition elements such as aptamers and synthetic receptors. Each approach trades off sensitivity, speed, reversibility, biocompatibility, and manufacturability in different ways; successful platforms typically combining a sensing motif with a delivery scaffold (hydrogel, nanoparticle, microneedle, depot) to shape release kinetics and protect payloads [7, 13]. The major glucose-sensing mechanisms employed in GRI systems, along with their performance characteristics, are summarized in Table 2.1. As shown schematically in Figure 2.1, glucose-responsive systems employ enzymatic, affinity-based, or molecular modification strategies to modulate insulin release or activity.

2.3.1 Enzyme-Based Systems – Glucose Oxidase (GOx)

Glucose oxidase is the oldest and most widely used enzymatic trigger for GRIs. GOx catalyzes oxidation of glucose to gluconic acid and hydrogen peroxide; the local production of acid (pH drop) and/or H_2O_2 can be transduced into insulin release by pH-sensitive polymers, H_2O_2-cleavable linkers, or volume changes in enzyme-containing vesicles. GOx-based MN patches and nanogels have

TABLE 2.1
Comparative Summary of Glucose-Sensing Mechanisms Used in GRI Delivery Systems

Sensing Mechanism	Glucose Sensitivity Range	Response Time	Key Advantages	Key Drawbacks	Representative Recent Examples (Preclinical)	Reference
GOx	Physiological to hyperglycemic range (5–25 mM)	Fast (minutes)	High sensitivity due to enzymatic amplification; well-studied chemistry; strong postprandial response	Oxygen dependence; H_2O_2 generation causing oxidative stress; enzyme instability over time	GOx-based nanogels and MN patches showing rapid glucose-triggered insulin and normoglycemia in rodents	[14, 15]
PBA/boronate chemistry	Moderate-high glucose (typically > 8–10 mM; tunable)	Moderate (minutes to tens of minutes)	Reversible non-enzymatic; good long-term stability; compatible with polymers and MNs	pH-dependent binding; interference from competing diols (e.g., fructose); requires pKa tuning	PBA-functionalized hydrogels and MNs with improved physiological pH responsiveness (2023–2025)	[16]
Con A	Physiological glucose range	Fast (minutes)	Strong affinity-based competitive binding; sharp glucose responsiveness	Immunogenicity; protein leakage; poor long-term biocompatibility	Affinity-based hydrogels and depot systems (largely proof-of-concept, declining use post-2020)	[9, 17]
Smart insulin (chemically modified insulin)	Tunable activation threshold (physiological to hyperglycemic)	Fast once activated	Molecular-level glucose responsiveness; reduced hypoglycemia risk; no external carrier needed	Synthetic complexity; stability and immunogenicity concerns; early translational stage	NNC2215 and related GRI conjugates demonstrating reversible activation in animal models (2023-2-24)	[18]
Aptamer/synthetic receptor systems	Tunable (design-dependent)	Moderate	High selectivity; programmable affinity; enzyme-free	Early-stage development; limited in vivo validation; stability issues	Aptamer-regulated hydrogels and nanocarriers (mostly exploratory).	[4, 19]

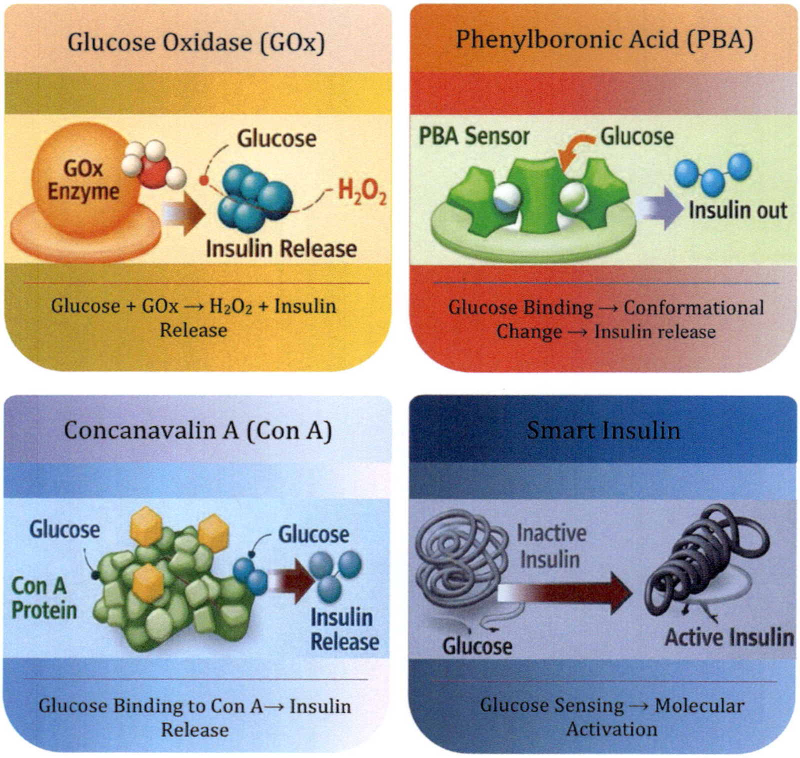

FIGURE 2.1 Schematic overview of glucose-responsive mechanisms (GOx, PBA, Con A, modified insulin).

shown rapid, glucose-triggered release and restored normoglycemia in multiple rodent studies; as the enzyme amplifies the glucose signal, GOx systems can achieve high sensitivity to postprandial excursion. However, enzyme instability, oxygen-dependence, and H_2O_2-mediated oxidative damage remain practical hurdles that many groups now address by co-encapsulating catalase or by engineering H_2O_2-scavenging linkers [20].

2.3.2 Phenylboronics Acids (PBA) and Boronate Chemistries

PBA forms reversible covalent complexes with diols (including glucose), enabling polymer swelling/deswelling or competitive displacement mechanisms that modulate insulin release. PBA-containing hydrogels and MNs are attractive because the chemistry is non-enzymatic (no oxygen requirement) and reversible; recent designs have tuned PBA's apparent pKa and introduced dual pH/glucose responsiveness to improve performance under physiological conditions. Nonetheless, PBA's relatively high intrinsic pKa and potential interference from competing diols (fructose, glycoproteins) require chemical modification (electron-withdrawing substituents, boronate esters) or microenvironment engineering to achieve clinically relevant sensitivity at ~7.4. Contemporary work includes 3D-printed PBA-bearing implants and pH/glucose dual-responsive networks that show controlled on-demand release in animal models [21].

2.3.3 Plant Lectin (Concanavalin A or Con A)

Con A is a multivalent lectin that binds glucose/mannose residues, and was among the first affinity-based elements used to sequester insulin (via glycosylated carriers) and release it when free glucose competes for binding. Con A platforms can produce sharp, competitive displacement responses, but clinical translation has been constrained by Con A's known immunogenicity, risk of leakage, and limited long-term stability. Recent reviews highlight Con A's utility for mechanistic studies and short-term implants, but they also document efforts to replace or shield Con A to mitigate activation [9, 17, 22].

2.3.4 Smart Insulin (Chemically Modified Insulin That Changes Activity with Glucose)

An alternative paradigm engineers insulin itself to be glucose-sensitive, for example, by attaching glucose-binding moieties, steric "cages" cleavable by glucose-triggered chemistry, or reversible boronate linkers that modulate receptor affinity. The advantage is a truly minimal system: active agent + sensing function in a single molecule. Recent funded programs (T1DM grand challenge projects and several academic consortia) have produced prototype "smart" insulins that activate under hyperglycemic conditions and deactivate as glucose normalizes; in animal models, these constructs reduce the risk of hypoglycemia and – in theoretical formulations – could allow much less frequent dosing. Remaining challenges include preserving insulin's pharmacokinetics, avoiding immunogenic neo-epitopes, and scaling synthesis under good manufacturing practice (GMP) conditions [23].

2.3.5 Other Approaches: Aptamer-Based, Synthetic Receptor, Competitive Binding Motifs

Aptamers – short nucleic acid sequences selected to bind glucose-correlated biomarkers – offer highly tunable affinity and the potential for binding with fast off-rates. Synthetic small-molecule receptors and engineered proteins (including computationally designed glucose binders) are also emerging as alternatives that avoid enzymatic instability and lectin immunogenicity. While many such systems currently serve as sensors rather than release actuators, hybrid designs linking conformational change to hydrogel porosity, or to blocker displacement, show promise in preliminary reports [24].

2.3.6 Kinetics, pH Effects, Interference, and Durability

Kinetics: Clinically relevant GRIs must match physiological timescales – ideally initiating significant release within minutes of a glucose rise and halting release as glucose returns to baseline. Enzymatic systems amplify the signal and can be fast if the polymer network is thin (MNs/nanogels) but slow in bulk depots.

pH and interference: GOx produces local acidification, which can be exploited but it also causes protonation-dependent behavior and may damage surrounding tissue; PBA sensitivity is pH-dependent (apparent pKa tuning is essential). Cross-reactivity with other diols (fructose, glycoproteins) and with oxidative by-products (H_2O_2) can generate false triggers or biocompatibility issues.

Durability: Long-term function demands enzyme stabilization (PEGylation, co-encapsulation), ligand/receptors stability (avoidance of proteolysis or denaturation), and resistance biofouling in vivo. Consequently, most translational efforts favor composite approaches – combining a sensing motif with a protective scaffold and increasingly, with electronic/algorithmic hybrids to balance speed, specificity, and safety [25].

2.4 MATERIALS AND PLATFORMS FOR A GLUCOSE-RESPONSIVE INSULIN DELIVERY

The translation of the molecular glucose sensing into clinically useful control of insulin depends critically on the material platform that hosts the sensor and the drug. Over the past five years, research has been shifted from large, slow bulk matrices to engineered micro- and nanoscale carriers and minimally invasive interfaces that prioritize fast kinetics, biocompatibility, and manufacturability. The major platform – hydrogels/microgels, nanoparticles/nanogels, MN patches, implantable depots, and emerging oral/pulmonary systems – trade-offs responsiveness, longevity, and regulatory complexity in different ways [5, 26]. Figure 2.2 gives an overview of the major material and devices platforms used to translate glucose-sensing mechanisms into functioning insulin delivery systems.

2.4.1 Hydrogels and Microgels

Hydrogels remain a foundational platform because their hydrated, porous networks can be chemically tuned to swell or collapse in response glucose-triggered stimuli (pH, boronate binding, redox). Two dominant design strategies are (i) enzyme-triggered pH changes, where glucose oxidase (GOx) converts glucose into gluconic acid and lowers local pH to drive protonation-dependent swelling, and (ii) reversible boronate (PBA) binding, where glucose binding alters polymer crosslink density and mesh size. Bulk hydrogels offer high loading capacity but often suffer slow mass transfer and limited reversibility; injectable microgels (micron-scale hydrogel particles) address this by shortening diffusion distances and improving on/off kinetics, making them attractive for subcutaneous depot injections. Recent reviews and studies highlight progress in pKa-tuned PBA derivatives and GOx-stabilization strategies (co-encapsulated catalase, enzyme immobilization) to extend in vivo durability [27].

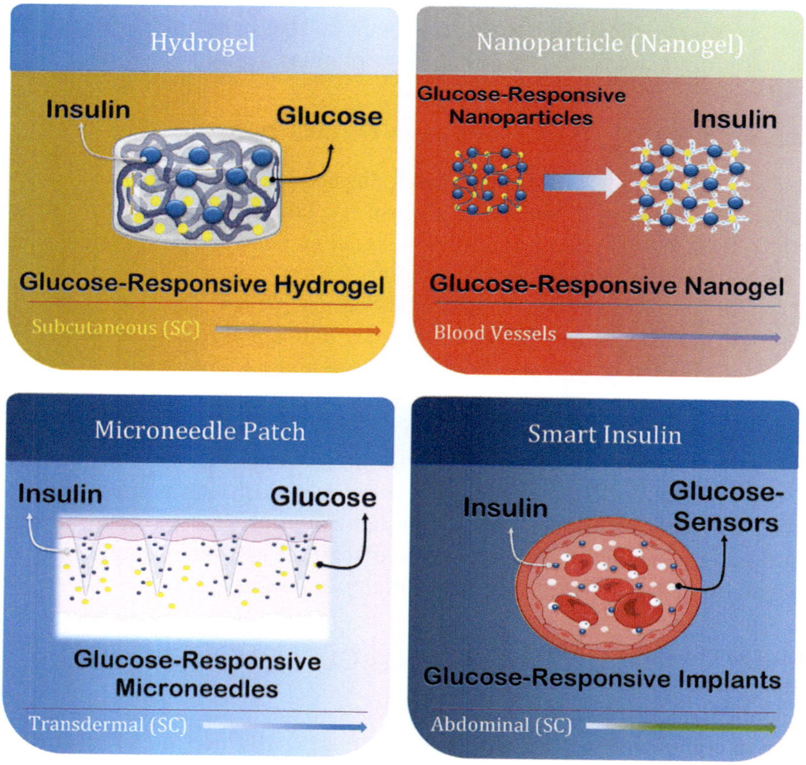

FIGURE 2.2 Representative platforms: hydrogel, nanoparticle, MN, implant.

2.4.2 Nanoparticles and Nanogels

Nanogels and polymeric nanoparticles give finer control over insulin protection and triggered release. By embedding sensing motifs – GOx, PBA moieties, or cleavable linkers – inside a nanoscale matrix, designers exploit short diffusion lengths to achieve faster, graded release and improved reversibility compared with bulk gels. Examples include GOx-loaded polymeric nanogels that generate local acid or H_2O_2 to cleave redox-sensitive linkers and release insulin and PBA-functionalized nanogels that swell or disassemble at hyperglycemic concentrations. Lipid-polymer hybrid nanoparticles have also been pursued to combine biocompatibility with responsive chemistry. Preclinical studies report that nanogel carriers can maintain normoglycemia at lower doses and with fewer hypoglycemia episodes than free insulin in rodent models, although concerns about long-term clearance and bioaccumulation persist [28].

2.4.3 Microneedle Patch (Solid, Dissolving, and Swellable)

MN patches have emerged as one of the most promising clinical interfaces for glucose-responsive systems because they can combine minimally invasive transdermal access with thin responsive matrices that greatly expedites kinetics. Two broad MN approaches dominate: (a) dissolvable MNs carrying insulin in a glucose-sensitive matrix dissolve faster at high glucose levels (iGOx or PBA-based), and (b) swellable or core-shell MNs where a small responsive reservoir at the needle tip controls release. Multiple 2022–2024 reports demonstrate MN patches that restore normoglycemia in diabetic rodents for hours to a day and reduce hypoglycemia risk versus injections. Reviews summarizing clinical translation potential emphasize MN patches' manufacturability and patient acceptability while noting regulatory and sterility challenges that remain prior to human trials [29].

2.4.4 Implantable Depots and Cannula/Catheter Concepts

Implantable depots and catheterized reservoirs aim to provide longer-term, stable GRI delivery (weeks to months). These systems typically combine a protective reservoir with a responsive membrane or actuator that gates insulin flux in response to interstitial glucose. Some implant designs use GOx-based sensing in an enclosed chamber; others leverage boronate membranes or mechanically actuated valves. While implants can offer durable control and enable higher payloads, they carry greater safety and regulatory burdens – foreign-body response, infection risk, and explantation logistics – and therefore have been slower to move toward clinical testing than MN or injectable formats. Recent translational reviews discuss prototype's robust long-term biocompatibility data [30].

2.4.5 Oral and Pulmonary Formulations

Oral and inhaled insulin remain highly desirable for patient convenience, and researchers are exploring glucose-responsive formulation for these routes. Oral strategies rely on protecting insulin from enzymatic degradation and crossing the intestinal barrier; smart hydrogels that swell and release insulin in a high-glucose microenvironment have been trialed in rodents, often combined with permeation enhancers or mucoadhesive carriers. Pulmonary delivery benefit from fast absorption must control dose variability and lung tolerability; glucose-triggered dry-powder particles or nanocarriers are under early investigation. Both routes face steep translational barriers to stability in complex biological milieus, off-target triggers by other sugars, and tight safety requirements that currently keep them at a preclinical stage compared with MNs and subcutaneous depots [31].

2.5 "SMART" INSULIN MOLECULES AND PRODRUGS

2.5.1 Concept and Rationale of Smart Insulin

"Smart" insulin systems aim to integrate glucose sensing and insulin action into a single molecular entity or prodrug, eliminating the need for external sensors or delivery devices. Unlike material-based glucose-responsive platforms, smart insulin approaches chemically modify insulin so that its bioavailability, receptor binding, or activity changes dynamically with ambient glucose concentration. The overarching goal is to mimic endogenous β-cell function – enhancing insulin action during hyperglycemia while minimizing activity during normoglycemia – thereby reducing hypoglycemia risk and patients' intervention [32].

2.5.2 Chemical Modifications Conferring Glucose Sensitivity

2.5.2.1 Boronate-Modified Insulin

PBA chemistry has been extensively explored because boronate groups reversibly bind cis-diols, including glucose. By conjugating PBA moieties directly to insulin or via linker arms, researchers have created insulin derivatives whose solubility, aggregation state, or receptor accessibility varies with glucose concentration. At higher glucose levels, boronate-glucose complexation alters conformation or carrier association, increasing insulin bioavailability. Recent refinements focus on pKa tuning and steric engineering to enable glucose responsiveness at physiological pH (~7.4), addressing earlier limitations of PBA systems. Despite promising in vitro and in vivo results, challenges remain related to competing diols (e.g., fructose) and pH-dependent binding equilibria [33].

2.5.2.2 Protecting-Groups and Caged Insulin Strategies

An alternative approach involves temporarily masking insulin's activity using cleavable or reversible protecting groups. These "caged" insulin prodrugs remain pharmacologically inert under normoglycemic conditions and become activated only when glucose levels rise. Activation may occur acute through glucose-dependent chemical reactions or enzymatic cascades triggered by hyperglycemia [34].

Such strategies inhibit basal insulin activity and hence hypoglycemia risk. Several academic consortia and global efforts are actively developing protecting-groups-based smart insulin candidates with extended circulations time, aiming to reduce dosing frequency while preserving tight glycemic control [34].

2.5.3 Pharmacodynamics and in Vivo Proof-of-Concept

Recently, animal studies have provided compelling proof-of-concept that smart-insulin constructs exhibit glucose-dependent pharmacodynamics. For example, engineered insulin conjugates such as NNC2215 have proven graded activation on hyperglycemia and deactivation as glucose normalizes, resulting in improved postprandial glucose control and fewer hypoglycemic episodes as compared with standard insulin in rodent models. These findings confirm that chemical modification can preserve insulin's therapeutic effect while adding autonomous glucose sensitivity. However, pharmacodynamic success is only achieved with balance between activation threshold, duration of action, and receptor affinity, which are affected by the nature and position of chemical modifications [35].

2.5.4 Stability, Safety, and Translation Challenges

Despite encouraging clinical data, significant challenges remain before smart insulin molecules can reach clinical use. Chemical modifications may destabilize insulin's tertiary structure, reduce shelf life, or introduce neo-epitopes that raise immunogenicity concerns. Boronate linkage and cleavable chemistries can be hydrolysis, oxidation, and off-target reactions in complex biological environments [36].

Manufacturing at GMP scale is another critical hurdle, as reproducibility and long-term storage stability must meet regulatory standards. Consequently, many smart insulin programs combine molecular designs with formulation strategies such as PEGylation, depot systems, and MN delivery to improve stability, control pharmacokinetics, and enhance translational feasibility [37].

2.6 INTEGRATION WITH ELECTRONICS AND CLOSED-LOOP HYBRID SYSTEMS

2.6.1 Evolution from Mechanical Delivery to Electronic Closed-Loop Control

Electronic closed-loop insulin delivery systems – often called artificial pancreas systems – represent the most clinically advanced form of automated glucose control. These systems combine three essential elements: a CGM, an insulin pump, and a control algorithm that automatically adjusts insulin delivery. Commercial HCL platforms including Medtronic MiniMed 780G, Tandem Diabetes Care Control-IQ, and Insulet Omnipod 5 have been shown to provide our patients with notable improvements in glycemic outcomes most notably higher TIR and nocturnal hypoglycemia in both T1DM and insulin-dependent T2DM populations [38].

Large multicenter trials and real-world registry data from 2022 to2024 report 10–15% absolute increases in TIR and 30–40% reductions in time spent below range (<70 mg/dL) when patients switch from conventional pump therapy to HCL systems. However, these platforms are still hybrid in nature, requiring manual meal announcements, calibration, and interaction. Their performance is limited by the insulin pharmacokinetics and sensor lag [39].

2.6.2 Rationale for Hybridization with Glucose-Responsive Materials

While electronic closed-loop systems excel in algorithmic control, they rely on subcutaneously injected rapid-acting insulin, which still exhibits delayed onset and prolonged tail effects. This mismatch between algorithm speed and insulin actions leads to create residual postprandial hyperglycemia and hypoglycemia risk [40].

Integration of GRI formulation or materials into electronic systems offer a complementary strategy. In hybrid designs, molecular or material-based glucose responsiveness provides local, fast, and autonomous modulation of insulin availability, while electronics manage macroscopic dosing trends and safety constraints. This layered control mimics biological redundancy in pancreatic regulation and reduces reliance on perfect sensor accuracy or user input [40].

2.6.3 Examples of Hybrid Electronic-Material Closed-Loop Systems

Recent experimental platforms combine MN patches or subcutaneous depots containing glucose-responsive nanogels with CGM-driven electronics. For example, glucose-responsive MN patches incorporating GOx-based vesicles have been paired with wearable glucose sensors to provide real-time feedback-informed insulin delivery, achieving faster postprandial correction in animal models compared with electronics alone [11, 41].

Another emerging approach involves electrically gated insulin depots, where glucose-responsive hydrogels or membranes modulate insulin diffusion while an external controller provides overriding capability. These systems allow basal insulin release to be chemically controlled and bolus-level control is algorithmically activated reducing total insulin exposure and frequency of hypoglycemia in preclinical testing [42].

2.6.4 Data-Driven Control, AI, Adaptive Algorithms

Modern closed loop systems increasingly integrate machine learning and adaptive algorithms that learn individual insulin sensitivity pattern over time. When coupled with glucose-responsive materials, these algorithms can adjust delivery thresholds, timing, and safety limits based on both sensor data and intrinsic material response [38].

Recent studies demonstrate that adaptive HCL systems using artificial intelligence (AI)-based controllers reduce glycemic variability more effectively than fixed-rule algorithms, especially during exercise, illness, and circadian transitions. The addition of GRI is expected to further reduce algorithmic burden by offloading rapid correction to chemistry rather than computation [43].

2.6.5 Safety, Regulatory Challenges, and Translational Considerations

Hybrid electronic-materials systems introduce new regulatory complexity, as they combine drug, device, and software components. Key challenges include validating long-term stability of glucose-responsive materials, ensuring predictable interactions between chemical and electronic control layers, and fail-safe mechanisms. Regulatory agencies increasingly favor stepwise hybridization, where glucose-responsive formulations are first tested alongside existing, approved electronic platforms [44].

2.7 PRECLINICAL AND CLINICAL STATUS

Representative preclinical and early translational research of GRI systems is summarized in Table 2.2.

2.7.1 Overall Landscape – Mostly Preclinical, Early Translation

As of 2024–2025 the field of GRI remains predominantly preclinical, with the strongest evidence coming from rodents and large-animal (pig) studies rather than completed human trials. Multiple sensing chemistries (GOx, PBA, Con A, and smart-insulin conjugates) have produced reproducible, glucose-triggered pharmacology in animals, but only a handful of candidates have advanced to large-animal proof-of-concept and none have yet reported on completed pivotal human efficacy studies. Recent comprehensive reviews and roadmaps conclude that while biological proof-of-principle is now well established, clinical translation is limited by safety, durability, and manufacturability requirements [8, 10, 13, 50].

TABLE 2.2
Key Preclinical and Early Translational Studies on Glucose-Responsive Insulin Delivery Systems

Author (Year)	Platform/Strategy	Experimental Model	Key Outcomes
Luo *et al.* 2021 [45]	GOx-based MN patch	Diabetic mice	Rapid glucose-triggered insulin release; improved time-in-range and reduced hypoglycemia versus injection
Morariu 2023 [46]	PBA-functionalized nanogel depot	Diabetic mice	Reversible glucose-dependent insulin release; prolonged normoglycemia with reduced insulin dose
Wang et al. 2020 [47]	GOx-loaded nanovesicles	Diabetic rats	Fast postprandial glucose correction; improved pharmacodynamic control
Liu *et al.* 2024 [48]	Smart insulin (NNC2215)	Rodents and pigs	Glucose-dependent insulin activation; fewer hypoglycemic events versus regular insulin
Martínez-Navarrete *et al.* 2024 [49]	Glucose-responsive MN patch	Rodents (preclinical)	Sustained glycemic control with minimally invasive transdermal delivery

2.7.2 Notable Preclinical Successes – Molecular and Device Examples

One of the highest-profile molecular advances is NNC2215, which is a chemically engineered insulin that switches between less active and more active conformation in response to glucose changes. In published large-animal and rodent studies, the construct demonstrated graded activation with increasing glucose (insulin receptor affinity increased ~3.2-fold when the glucose rose from ~3 mM to 20 mM) and produced improved postprandial control with fewer hypoglycemic excursions versus regular insulin. These data represent a watershed for "smart-insulin" chemistry, but developers report that further work is needed on immunogenicity and GMP-compatible synthesis before human trials [35, 51].

On the device/material side, glucose-responsive MN patches and nanogel depots have shown repeated success in animals. Numerous studies between 2022 and 2024 report that MN patches (GOx- or PBA-based matrices) restore normoglycemia within minutes of hyperglycemia and sustain control for hours, with several reports demonstrating efficacy in both rodents and pig – highlighting MNs as a leading translational platform due to kinetics and acceptability. Still, human trials of glucose-responsive MNs are sparse and largely limited to safety/feasibility rather than efficacy endpoints [5].

2.7.3 Where Clinical Activity Exists

Direct human clinical data for bona fide GRIs or fully autonomous GRIs are minimal. Most clinical activity in the broader insulin-delivery space remains focused on device-based closed-loop systems and improves long-acting insulin analogs (e.g., once-weekly basal insulins in late-phase trials), rather than chemically self-regulating insulins. This gap explains the current strategy among many groups: advancing GRI candidates through preclinical studies using robust large-animal toxicology and GMP formulation, while planning first-in-human trials that emphasize safety, pharmacokinetics, and immunogenicity. [52].

2.7.4 Key Translational Bottlenecks Supported by Data

Leading obstacles to clinical translation are (1) safety and biocompatibility, for example, H_2O_2 generation from GOx and potential immune responses to novel conjugates; (2) durability- maintaining enzyme activity or sensor responsiveness over weeks/months; (3) manufacturability and stability-scaling complex chemistries (boronate linkers, macrocycles) into reproducible GMP products with acceptable shelf life; and (4) regulatory complexity for drug-device hybrids. Reviews and preclinical reports consistently identify these areas as the primary gating items before human trials can be undertaken [53].

2.7.5 Near-Term Outlook (Next 2–5 Years)

Expect a two-track translational progression: (a) molecule-first candidates (smart insulins like NNC2215) will complete goods laboratory practices (GLP) toxicology and early (phase 1) human studies focused on safety and glucose-dependent pharmacology; (B) platform/device candidates (MN patches, nanogel depots) will move into first-in-human feasibility/safety studies often integrated with existing electronic CGM/pump systems for conservative stepwise testing. If early human safety and predictable pharmacokinetics are demonstrated, randomized proof-of-concept trials measuring TIR and hypoglycemia reduction should follow. Continued cross-disciplinary investment (chemistry, materials, regulatory science) is the critical enabler for this transition [10, 54].

2.8 SAFETY, IMMUNOGENICITY, AND REGULATORY CONSIDERATIONS

2.8.1 Safety Profile: Chemical By-Products and Local Effects

Glucose-responsive systems introduce new chemical or enzymatic activities at the delivery site, which pose certain safety risks. Enzyme-based sensors like GOx produce gluconic acid and hydrogen peroxide (H_2O_2) as reaction products; H_2O_2 is cytotoxic at sufficient concentrations and local acidification can damage surrounding tissue or to destabilize carrier materials, so many designs now co-encapsulate catalase or H_2O_2-scavenging to mitigate oxidative injury. These issues are a key to biocompatibility testing strategies for GOx-based MNs and depots [40, 55].

2.8.2 Immunogenicity and Neo-Epitopes Formation

Any chemical modification to insulin (smart insulins) or any modification by incorporation of non-human proteins (Con A, microbial GOx) increases the theoretical risk of immune recognition. Recent preclinical research (e.g., engineered insulin conjugates) explicitly measures anti-drug antibody in large-animal models because neo-epitopes can alter pharmacokinetics, neutralize activity, or provoke hypersensitivity. Immunogenicity readouts (binding and neutralizing antibodies, T-cell assays) and long-term repeat-dose studies are therefore required before first-in-human trials. Evidence from the prototype smart-insulin shows promising efficacy but stresses the rigorous GLP toxicology focused on immune endpoints [8].

2.8.3 Material-Related Risks and Biofouling

Polymers, nanoparticles, and implanted membranes can elicit foreign-body responses that degrade sensor function (biofouling), alter release kinetics, or cause fibrosis around implants. MN platforms minimize deep-tissue foreign body risk but still require sterility assurance, skin-compatibility testing, and studies on the local effects of repeated use. Recent MN safety reviews report generally favorable acute tolerability in animals and early human feasibility studies but they highlight gaps in chronic safety data [56].

2.8.4 Regulatory Classification and Pathway Complexity

Most glucose-responsive therapeutics are combination products (drug + device ± biologic). Regulatory authorities therefore assign a primary mode of action (PMOA) to determine lead review center and expectations. In the United States, the U.S. Food and Drug Administration (FDA) and its Office of Combination Products provide guidance on the premarket pathway, GMP expectations, and device-component validation; developers must coordinate both drug and device regulatory strategies (including CMC for the drug, bench and biocompatibility testing for the device, and software validation if electronics are involved). Early regulatory engagement to define the PMOA, pivotal endpoints, and non-clinical packages needs is essential [57].

2.8.5 Data Requirements and Translational Gating Items

Regulators will expect a staged evidence base: robust in vitro characterization (mechanism, off-target triggers, degrades), GLP toxicology (systemic and local), repeat-dose immunogenicity, biodistribution/clearance for particulate systems, and sterility/end-of-shelf-life data. For drug-device hybrids (e.g., MN patches containing a novel GRI), sponsors commonly pursue modular submissions. They first demonstrate safety and PK in small human trials, followed by randomized efficacy trials that measure TIR and hypoglycemia incidence. Recent reviews emphasize that manufacturability and stability (shelf-life, cold-chain dependence) often become the main gating issues before efficacy can be tested clinically [58].

2.8.6 Risk-Mitigation Strategies and Best Practices

Practical mitigations include: (1) replace or shield reactive enzymes (e.g., GOx) with stabilized or catalytic-scavenging systems; (2) minimize novel epitopes via careful linker chemistry and in silico epitope scanning; (3) design fail-safe behaviors (material that defaults to inert on malfunction); and (4) engage regulators early to agree on non-clinical packages. Combining these scientific and regulatory strategies will be essential to move promising glucose-responsive candidates from animal models into safe, informative human studies [59].

2.9 LIMITATIONS, CHALLENGES, AND TRANSLATIONAL BOTTLENECKS

Despite amazing advances, GRI systems face substantial scientific and translation challenges that have, to date, kept them from going beyond preclinical promise to enter routine clinical use. These challenges include aspects of biological performance, materials durability, manufacturability, and regulatory acceptance and are routinely cited and summarized in recent reviews and translation assessments (2023–2025) [60].

2.9.1 Biological and Physiological Limitations

A central challenge is achieving physiologically relevant response kinetics. Many GRI systems respond on the scale of tens of minutes rather than the near-instantaneous insulin secretion of native β-cells. This lag can result in incomplete suppression of postprandial hyperglycemia. Conversely, overly sensitive systems risk overshooting, increasing hypoglycemia if insulin release continues after glucose levels normalize. Additionally, interstitial glucose – the target for most systems – lags behind blood glucose, compounding timing errors [61].

Another limitation is specificity. Boronate-based systems can be activated by competing diols (e.g., fructose, glycoproteins), while enzyme-based platforms produce by-products such as hydrogen peroxide that may perturb local tissue or alter sensor behavior to take place over time. Such effects make it difficult to achieve reliable long-term performance [62].

2.9.2 Durability and Long-Term Stability

Most reported GRI platforms demonstrate efficacy over hours to days, whereas clinical insulin treatment requires regular performance over weeks to months. Enzyme-based systems suffer from gradual loss of activity, oxygen dependence, and oxidative degradation. Polymer matrices can undergo mechanical fatigue, hydrolysis, or biofouling, leading to a drift in insulin release profiles. For smart-insulin molecules, chemical modifications may reduce shelf life, or destabilize insulin's tertiary structure during storage and circulation [18, 32, 48].

2.9.3 Manufacturing and Scalability Challenges

Translation requires GMP-compatible and reproducibility manufacturing, which remains a major bottleneck. Complex chemistries (i.e., boronate linkers, multi-component nanogels) are hard for scale-up with tight batch-to-batch consistency. Sterilization (gamma irradiation, filtration) can inactivate enzymes or damage responsive polymers, while cold chain dependence adds cost and limits accessibility. Several recent translational analyses identify manufacturability – not efficacy – as the dominant hurdle preventing clinical entry [63].

2.9.4 Regulations and Clinical Trials Barriers

Most GRIs are combination products (drugs-device or drug-material hybrids), which increases regulatory complexity. Safety requirements for the demonstration are more rigorous than those for conventional insulin, mandating repeat-dose toxicology, immunogenicity, biodistribution, and failure-mode analysis. Clinically, proving superiority of existing hybrid closed-loop systems is challenging, as modern electronic platforms already deliver substantial benefits in TIR and hypoglycemia reduction [64].

2.9.5 Translational Outlook

Consequently, the field is shifting toward incremental translation: coupled substrates of glucose responsiveness and approved pumps or instruments, and first-in-human trials designed more for safety and pharmacology than for full autonomy. Overcoming these bottlenecks will require more than just better chemistry and materials; it will call for early regulatory exposure and realistic clinical placement along with existing technologies [65].

2.10 FUTURE DIRECTIONS AND RESEARCH PRIORITIES

The near-term trajectory of GRI research is convergent: refine molecular sensors and material for fast, reproducible biochemical responsiveness while simultaneously de-risking translation through staged integration with existing electronic systems and rigorous regulatory planning. Efforts supported by large consortia (e.g., the T1DM Grand Challenge) are underway to advance smart-insulin molecules and novel microneedle/nanogel formulations through GLP toxicology and first-in-human studies [66].

Key scientific priorities

- Improve kinetics and specificity: Prioritize chemistries and architectures that initiate insulin availability within minutes of hyperglycemia and reliably stop as glucose glycemia normalizes. Examples include thin, MN-hosted GOx or tuned PBA chemistries and molecular smart-insulin constructs like NNC2215 that show reversible glucose-dependent activation in large-animal models.
- Enhance durability and biocompatibility: Stabilize enzymes (PEGylation, co-encapsulation with catalase), minimize oxidative by-products, and design anti-biofouling surfaces for implants to preserve months-long function.
- Mitigate immunogenicity and off-target triggers: Use in silico epitope screening, improved linker chemistry, and selective microenvironments to reduce neo-epitopes and diol cross-reactivity (e.g., fructose/glycoproteins).

Translational and regulatory priorities

- Adopt modular, stepwise clinical paths: Safety-first human studies pharmacokinetic-pharmacodynamic (PK-PD and immunogenicity), and randomized efficacy trials (TIR, hypoglycemia endpoints) often pair new material with approved CGM/pump platforms to reduce regulatory risk.
- Early regulatory engagement: Define PMOA, required GLP packages, and combination-products expectations with agencies to streamline CMC, biocompatibility, and software requirements.
- Completing GLP toxicology for lead smart-insulin candidates, first-in-human safety, and PK studies for microneedle or nanogel GRIs and demonstrating hybrid material responsiveness measurably reduce the need for algorithmic correction, as well as the frequency of hypoglycemia, in controlled trials. Achieving these milestones will transform promising preclinical advances into clinically deployable, patient-centric therapies.

2.11 CONCLUSION

GRI delivery systems represent a transformative approach toward achieving safer, more physiological glycemic control in diabetes management. Over the past decade, substantial progress has been made in molecular sensing mechanisms, smart insulin chemistries, and advanced material platforms such as nanogels and MN patches demonstrating robust glucose-dependent insulin action in preclinical studies. These innovations address clinical limitations of conventional insulin therapy, especially delayed pharmacokinetics and hypoglycemia risk. However, translation to clinical practice remains constrained by challenges related to long-term stability, immunogenicity, manufacturability, and regulatory complexity. Current evidence supports a pragmatic, stepwise pathway in which glucose-responsive systems are first evaluated as adjuncts to established electronic closed-loop technologies. Continued interdisciplinary collaboration across chemistry, materials science, clinical pharmacology, and regulatory science will be essential to advance these technologies from proof-of-concept toward routine clinical use. With sustained investment and rigorous translational strategies, GRI systems have potential to redefine the future of autonomous diabetes care.

ACKNOWLEDGMENTS

I would like to express my sincere gratitude to Hygia College of Pharmacy, Lucknow, India, for providing the necessary facilities and a supportive environment to complete this book chapter. I am also thankful to my colleagues and the editorial team for their constant encouragement and technical guidance throughout this process.

REFERENCES

1. Pang H, Chen Z, Han FY. Nano-based therapy for type 1 diabetes: From immuno-intervention to insulin delivery. Acta Biomaterialia. 2025;201:101–20. https://doi.org/10.1016/j.actbio.2025.06.016.
2. Rimon MT, Hasan MW, Hassan MF, Cesmeci S. Advancements in insulin pumps: A comprehensive exploration of insulin pump systems, technologies, and future directions. Pharmaceutics. 2024; 16(7):944.
3. Tian T, Aaron RE, Yeung AM, Huang J, Drincic A, Seley JJ, Wallia A, Gilbert G, Spanakis EK, Masharani U, Faulds E. Use of continuous glucose monitors in the hospital: The diabetes technology society hospital meeting report 2023. Journal of Diabetes Science and Technology. 2023;17(5): 1392–418.
4. Webber MJ, Anderson DG. Smart approaches to glucose-responsive drug delivery. Journal of Drug Targeting. 2015;23(7–8):651–55.
5. Guo X, Wang W. Challenges and recent advances in the subcutaneous delivery of insulin. Expert Opinion on Drug Delivery. 2017;14(6):727–34.
6. Wang S, Yang C, Zhang W, Zhao S, You J, Cai R, Wang H, Bao Y, Zhang Y, Zhang J, Ji K. Glucose-responsive microneedle patch with high insulin loading capacity for prolonged glycemic control in mice and minipigs. ACS Nano. 2024;18(38):26056–65.
7. Kurtzhals P, Nishimura E, Haahr H, Høeg-Jensen T, Johansson E, Madsen P, Sturis J, Kjeldsen T. Commemorating insulin's centennial: Engineering insulin pharmacology towards physiology. Trends in Pharmacological Sciences. 2021;42(8):620–39.
8. Pal S, Rakshit T, Saha S, Jinagal D. Glucose-responsive materials for smart insulin delivery: From protein-based to protein-free design. ACS Materials Au. 2025;5(2):239–52.
9. Bercea M, Lupu A. Recent insights into glucose-responsive concanavalin A-based smart hydrogels for controlled insulin delivery. Gels. 2024;10(4):260.
10. Yao Y, Ji K, Wang Y, Gu Z, Wang J. Materials and carriers development for glucose-responsive insulin. Accounts of Materials Research. 2022;3(9):960–70.
11. Chen G, Yu J, Gu Z. Glucose-responsive microneedle patches for diabetes treatment. Journal of Diabetes Science and Technology. 2019;13(1):41–8.
12. Ceriello A, Prattichizzo F, Phillip M, Hirsch IB, Mathieu C, Battelino T. Glycaemic management in diabetes: Old and new approaches. The Lancet Diabetes & Endocrinology. 2022;10(1):75–84.
13. VandenBerg MA, Webber MJ. Biologically inspired and chemically derived methods for glucose-responsive insulin therapy. Advanced Healthcare Materials. 2019;8(12):1801466.
14. Danquah MK, Jeevanandam J. Emerging Nanomedicines for Diabetes Mellitus Theranostics. Elsevier; 2022.

15. Yin R, Wang K, Du S, Chen L, Nie J, Zhang W. Design of genipin-crosslinked microgels from concanavalin a and glucosyloxyethyl acrylated chitosan for glucose-responsive insulin delivery. Carbohydrate Polymers. 2014;103:369–76.
16. Das BC, Chokkalingam P, Masilamani P, Shukla S, Das S. Stimuli-responsive boron-based materials in drug delivery. International Journal of Molecular Sciences. 2023;24(3):2757.
17. Lin K, Yi J, Mao X, Wu H, Zhang LM, Yang L. Glucose-sensitive hydrogels from covalently modified carboxylated pullulan and concanavalin A for smart controlled release of insulin. Reactive and Functional Polymers. 2019;139:112–19.
18. Gonzalvo JD. Introduction to basal insulin therapy: Clinical management of diabetes. The American Journal of Managed Care. 2018;24(6 Suppl):S87–92.
19. Bakh NA, Cortinas AB, Weiss MA, Langer RS, Anderson DG, Gu Z, Dutta S, Strano MS. Glucose-responsive insulin by molecular and physical design. Nature Chemistry. 2017;9(10):937–44.
20. Bauer JA, Zámocká M, Majtán J, Bauerová-Hlinková V. Glucose oxidase, an enzyme "Ferrari": Its structure, function, production and properties in the light of various industrial and biotechnological applications. Biomolecules. 2022;12(3):472.
21. Ma Q, Zhao X, Shi A, Wu J. Bioresponsive functional phenylboronic acid-based delivery system as an emerging platform for diabetic therapy. International Journal of Nanomedicine. 2021:297–314.
22. Yin R, Bai M, He J, Nie J, Zhang W. Concanavalin A-sugar affinity based system: Binding interactions, principle of glucose-responsiveness, and modulated insulin release for diabetes care. International Journal of Biological Macromolecules. 2019;124:724–32.
23. Yu J, Zhang Y, Yan J, Kahkoska AR, Gu Z. Advances in bioresponsive closed-loop drug delivery systems. International Journal of Pharmaceutics. 2018;544(2):350–57.
24. Mayol B, Qubbaj IZ, Nava-Granados J, Vasquez K, Keene ST, Sempionatto JR. Aptamer and oligonucleotide-based biosensors for health applications. Biosensors. 2025;15(5):277.
25. Yang Y, Sun H, Sun X, Wang Y, Xu F, Xia W, Chen L, Li M, Yang T, Qiao Y, Geng D. From mechanism to applications: Advanced microneedles for clinical medicine. Bioactive Materials. 2025;51:1–45.
26. Zhao J, Xu G, Yao X, Zhou H, Lyu B, Pei S, Wen P. Microneedle-based insulin transdermal delivery system: Current status and translation challenges. Drug Delivery and Translational Research. 2022; 12(10):2403–27.
27. Ünlü B, Ropero-Vega JL, Alvarez-Caballero JM, Flórez-Castillo JM, Türk S. Smart hydrogels for treatment of microbial diseases. Pharmaceutics 2026, 18, 198. https://doi.org/10.3390/pharmaceutics18020198
28. Li C, Wu G, Ma R, Liu Y, Liu Y, Lv J, An Y, Shi L. Nitrilotriacetic acid (NTA) and phenylboronic acid (PBA) functionalized nanogels for efficient encapsulation and controlled release of insulin. ACS Biomaterials Science & Engineering. 2017;4(6):2007–17.
29. Naik K, Singh K. Microneedle strategies for diabetic wound management: A comprehensive review of materials, mechanisms, and therapeutic outcomes. Materials Today Advances. 2026;29:100684.
30. Chu MK, Gordijo CR, Li J, Abbasi AZ, Giacca A, Plettenburg O, Wu XY. In vivo performance and biocompatibility of a subcutaneous implant for real-time glucose-responsive insulin delivery. Diabetes Technology & Therapeutics. 2015;17(4):255–67.
31. Mansoor S, Kondiah PP, Choonara YE, Pillay V. Polymer-based nanoparticle strategies for insulin delivery. Polymers. 2019;11(9):1380.
32. Wang Z, Wang J, Kahkoska AR, Buse JB, Gu Z. Developing insulin delivery devices with glucose responsiveness. Trends in Pharmacological Sciences. 2021;42(1):31–44.
33. Kang H, Yang R, Wei W, Liu K, Xu Y, Wu X, Dai H. Phenylboronic acid biomaterials: From chemical principles to material design. Coordination Chemistry Reviews. 2026;548:217166.
34. Franc S, Daoudi A, Pochat A, Petit MH, Randazzo C, Petit C, Duclos M, Penfornis A, Pussard E, Not D, Heyman E. Insulin-based strategies to prevent hypoglycaemia during and after exercise in adult patients with type 1 diabetes on pump therapy: The DIABRASPORT randomized study. Diabetes, Obesity and Metabolism. 2015;17(12):1150–57.
35. Hoeg-Jensen T, Kruse T, Brand CL, Sturis J, Fledelius C, Nielsen PK, Nishimura E, Madsen AR, Lykke L, Halskov KS, Koščová S. Glucose-sensitive insulin with attenuation of hypoglycaemia. Nature. 2024;634(8035):944–51.
36. Yang Y, Shahinozzaman M, Shin H, Bupp S, Sourbier C. Impact of structure and formulation changes on the function of insulin products. Frontiers in Endocrinology. 2025;16:1601119.
37. Lombardi L, Genio VD, Albericio F, Williams DR. Advances in peptidomimetics for next-generation therapeutics: Strategies, modifications, and applications. Chemical Reviews. 2025;125(15):7099–166.
38. Templer S. Closed-loop insulin delivery systems: Past, present, and future directions. Frontiers in Endocrinology. 2022;13:919942.

39. Nattero-Chávez L, Lorenzo M, Ruiz de Adana MS, Simó-Servat O, Abad M, Quirós C, Durán Martínez M, Quintero Tobar A, Bayona A, Ruiz Gracia T, de la Calle de la Villa E. Prospective multicenter evaluation of glycemic and patient-reported outcomes following transition to a next-generation continuous glucose monitoring system in users of advanced hybrid closed-loop technology. Therapeutic Advances in Endocrinology and Metabolism. 2026;17:20420188251407515.
40. Liu J, Yi X, Zhang J, Yao Y, Panichayupakaranant P, Chen H. Recent advances in the drugs and glucose-responsive drug delivery systems for the treatment of diabetes: A systematic review. Pharmaceutics. 2024;16(10):1343.
41. McAlister E, Kirkby M, Dominguez-Robles J, Paredes AJ, Anjani QK, Moffatt K, Vora LK, Hutton AR, McKenna PE, Larrañeta E, Donnelly RF. The role of microneedle arrays in drug delivery and patient monitoring to prevent diabetes induced fibrosis. Advanced Drug Delivery Reviews. 2021;175:113825.
42. Mohanty AR, Ravikumar A, Peppas NA. Recent advances in glucose-responsive insulin delivery systems: Novel hydrogels and future applications. Regenerative Biomaterials. 2022;9:rbac056.
43. Chen J, Yi Q, Wang Y, Wang J, Yu H, Zhang J, Hu M, Xu J, Wu Z, Hou L, Zhang Z. Long-term glycemic variability and risk of adverse health outcomes in patients with diabetes: A systematic review and meta-analysis of cohort studies. Diabetes Research and Clinical Practice. 2022;192:110085.
44. Fan X, Gu S, Lei J, Gu S, Yang L. Controlled release of insulin based on temperature and glucose dual responsive biomicrocapsules. Molecules. 2022;27(5):1686.
45. Luo FQ, Chen G, Xu W, Zhou D, Li JX, Huang YC, Lin R, Gu Z, Du JZ. Microneedle-array patch with pH-sensitive formulation for glucose-responsive insulin delivery. Nano Research. 2021;14(8):2689–96.
46. Morariu S. Advances in the design of phenylboronic acid-based glucose-sensitive hydrogels. Polymers. 2023;15(3):582.
47. Wang J, Wang Z, Yu J, Kahkoska AR, Buse JB, Gu Z. Glucose-responsive insulin and delivery systems: Innovation and translation. Advanced Materials. 2020;32(13):1902004.
48. Liu Y, Wang S, Wang Z, Yu J, Wang J, Buse JB, Gu Z. Recent progress in glucose-responsive insulin. Diabetes. 2024;73(9):1377–88.
49. Martínez-Navarrete M, Pérez-López A, Guillot AJ, Cordeiro AS, Melero A, Aparicio-Blanco J. Latest advances in glucose-responsive microneedle-based systems for transdermal insulin delivery. International Journal of Biological Macromolecules. 2024;263:130301.
50. Ravaine V, Ancla C, Catargi B. Chemically controlled closed-loop insulin delivery. Journal of Controlled Release. 2008;132(1):2–11.
51. Sacks DB. Smart insulin switches itself off in response to low blood sugar. Nature. 2024;634:785–87. https://doi.org/10.1038/d41586-024-03286-5.
52. Jarosinski MA, Dhayalan B, Rege N, Chatterjee D, Weiss MA. 'Smart'insulin-delivery technologies and intrinsic glucose-responsive insulin analogues. Diabetologia. 2021;64(5):1016–29.
53. Bai L, Su J. Converging technologies in biomaterial translational research. Biomaterials Translational. 2023;4(4):197.
54. Bratlie KM, York RL, Invernale MA, Langer R, Anderson DG. Materials for diabetes therapeutics. Advanced Healthcare Materials. 2012;1(3):267–84.
55. Liu M, Wang R, Hoi MP, Wang Y, Wang S, Li G, Vong CT, Chong CM. Nano-based drug delivery systems for managing diabetes: Recent advances and future prospects. International Journal of Nanomedicine. 2025:6221–52.
56. Kyriakides TR, Kim HJ, Zheng C, Harkins L, Tao W, Deschenes E. Foreign body response to synthetic polymer biomaterials and the role of adaptive immunity. Biomedical Materials. 2022;17(2):022007.
57. Lee Y, Srivastava I, Feibus KB, Bielski ER, Sterrett L, Harris D, Luke MC. Development of drug-device combination products and generic substitution in the United States: An overview. Innovations in Pharmacy. 2025;16(2):1–10. https://doi.org/10.24926/iip.v16i2.6461.
58. Neadle S, Wallenstein M. Combination Products Current Good Manufacturing Practices (cGMPs). In The Combination Products Handbook (pp. 81–154). CRC Press; 2023.
59. Correa S, Grosskopf AK, Lopez Hernandez H, Chan D, Yu AC, Stapleton LM, Appel EA. Translational applications of hydrogels. Chemical Reviews. 2021;121(18):11385–457.
60. Kapustina O, Burmakina P, Gubina N, Serov N, Vinogradov V. User-friendly and industry-integrated AI for medicinal chemists and pharmaceuticals. Artificial Intelligence Chemistry. 2024;2(2):100072.
61. Skelin Klemen M, Dolenšek J, Slak Rupnik M, Stožer A. The triggering pathway to insulin secretion: Functional similarities and differences between the human and the mouse β cells and their translational relevance. Islets. 2017;9(6):109–39.
62. Yang J, He X, Chen L, Zhang Y. The selective detection of galactose based on boronic acid functionalized fluorescent carbon dots. Analytical Methods. 2016;8(47):8345–51.

63. Kolahi Azar H, Gharibshahian M, Rostami M, Mansouri V, Sabouri L, Beheshtizadeh N, Rezaei N. The progressive trend of modeling and drug screening systems of breast cancer bone metastasis. Journal of Biological Engineering. 2024;18(1):14.
64. Baghban R, Namvar E, Attar A, Mortazavi M. Progressing nanotechnology to improve diagnosis and targeted therapy of diabetic retinopathy. Biomedicine & Pharmacotherapy. 2025;183:117786.
65. Yang JF, Yang S, Gong X, Bakh NA, Zhang G, Wang AB, Cherrington AD, Weiss MA, Strano MS. In silico investigation of the clinical translatability of competitive clearance glucose-responsive insulins. ACS Pharmacology & Translational Science. 2023;6(10):1382–95.
66. Krishnamurthy A, Goswami R. Glucose-responsive smart insulin. Annals of the National Academy of Medical Sciences (India). 2018;54(02):064–73.

3 Foundational Principles and Molecular Mechanisms of Nanotechnology

Vikram T. Choudhary
The Oxford College of Pharmacy, Bangalore, India

Jyothirmayee Devineni
KVSR Siddhartha College of Pharmaceutical Sciences, Vijayawada, India

D. Thangamani
Institute of Forest Genetics and Tree Breeding, Coimbatore, India

Pavan Kumar Sreenivasal
College of Dentistry, King Faisal University, Al-Ahsa, Saudi Arabia

Shipra Omar
School of Pharmaceutical Sciences, Shri Guru Ram Rai University, Dehradun, India

Anita A.
Dayananda Sagar University, Bengaluru, India

3.1 INTRODUCTION

This chapter reviews core physical and molecular principles that underlie nanotechnology, with emphasis on how size, surface chemistry, and quantum effects translate into functional behaviors in materials and biological systems. It covers (a) length scale and common classes of nanomaterials (metals, carbon allotropes, quantum dots, lipids, polymeric nanoparticles (NPs); (b) synthesis and surface functionalization strategies that control reactivity and biodistribution; (c) molecular-level mechanism at interfaces (protein corona, membrane interactions) into products – notably lipid nanoparticles (LNPs)-based mRNA vaccines and RNAi therapeutics. Recent clinical/commercial milestones are used to link foundational mechanisms with the real-world outcomes [1].

"Nanotechnology" refers to design, characterization, and application of structures with at least one dimension in the ~1–100 nm range, where properties deviate from bulk due to high surface-to-volume ratio and quantum confinement. For perspective, a typical atom is ~0.1 nm, a DNA helix ≈2 nm, and a human hair is about ≈80,000–100,000 nm. So nanoscale engineering operates between single molecules and visible microstructures. Size-dependent phenomena include plasmonic resonance in metal NPs, discretized electronic states in quantum dots, and dramatically altered solubility/clearance for drug carriers [2].

The COVID-19 mRNA vaccines – delivered by LNPs – are the clearest example of nanotechnology's translational power, spawning an active clinical pipeline of LNP-based vaccines and

DOI: 10.1201/9781003598657-3

therapeutics. Regulators have also approved RNAi and LNP-based therapies (e.g., siRNA drugs), demonstrating clinical viability of nanoscale delivery. Market estimates vary by source, but recent reports place the global nanotechnology market in the single-digit to low-double-digit billions in 2024 with projections of fast growth over next decade, underscoring both scientific and commercial momenta [3].

3.2 HISTORICAL PERSPECTIVE

The conceptual roots of nanotechnology are commonly traced to Richard Feynman's lecture "There's Plenty of Room at the Bottom" in 1959, which articulated the possibility of manipulating matter at atomic dimensions. Practical progress accelerated decades later with enabling tools; scanning tunneling microscope (STM, 1981) and atomic force microscope (AFM, 1986) allowed visualization and manipulation of surface nanometer-scale for the first time. The 1980s–1990s saw landmark material discoveries, including fullerenes (C60), carbon nanotubes, and later graphene, each revealing extraordinary mechanical, electrical, and thermal properties unavailable in bulk matter [4, 5].

In the early 2000s, nanotechnology transitioned from laboratories curiosity to applied science. Gold NPs entered diagnostics and photothermal therapy; quantum dots revolutionized bioimaging with size-tunable fluorescence; and polymeric NPs enabled controlled drug delivery. A defining recent milestone was the worldwide use of LNP-based mRNA vaccines against COVID-19, which validated nanoscale delivery systems at unprecedented scale and speed. By 2023–2025, LNP platforms expanded into oncology, gene editing, and personalized vaccines, marking a mature translational phase for nanotechnology [6].

Two paradigms have shaped nanotechnology's evolution. The first is the shift from top-down miniaturization (etching and lithography from bulk materials) to a bottom-up assembly, where atoms, molecules, and polymers self-organize into functional nanostructures. The second paradigm recognizes that function at the nanoscale is dominated by interfaces rather than bulk composition. Surface chemistry, charge, and molecular adsorption (such as protein corona formation in biological media) often determine performance more than core materials identity [7].

Modern nanotechnology increasingly follows a convergence paradigm, integrating materials sciences, biology, computation, and artificial intelligence. This mechanism-aware, data-driven methodology now guides rational NPs design, moving the field from empirical formulation toward predictive, scalable nanomedicine and nanoengineering [8].

3.3 PHYSICAL PRINCIPLES

Figure 3.1 shows a schematic illustration of size-dependent physical phenomena in nanomaterials. As particle size decreases in the range of 1–100 nm, quantum confinement effects emerge in semiconductors, surface-to-volume ratio increases dramatically, and bulk material properties transition to interface-dominated behavior, governing optical, electronic, and biological responses.

3.3.1 Size-Dependent Properties

At the nanoscale, materials exhibit properties that differ fundamentally from their bulk counterparts because characteristic dimensions approach intrinsic physical length scale such as electron mean free path, exciton Bohr radius, or magnetic domain size. As particle size decreases below ~100 nm, optical, electrical, mechanical, and magnetic properties become size-dependent rather than composition-dependent. For instance, bulk gold is inert and opaque, whereas gold NPs display intense colors due to localized surface plasmon resonance (LSPR), enabling applications in biosensing and photothermal therapy. Similarly, iron oxide NPs below a critical size (~20 nm) exhibit superparamagnetism, a property that is exploited in magnetic resonance imaging contrast agents

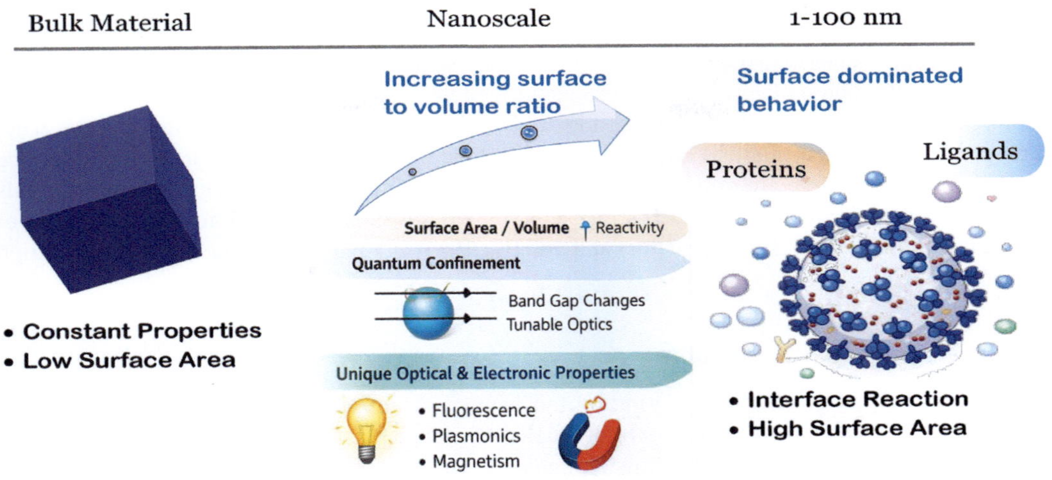

FIGURE 3.1 Size-dependent properties and surface dominance at the nanoscale.

and targeted delivery. In energy storage, nano-sized electrode materials shorten ion diffusion and enhance rate capability, explaining widespread adoption of nanostructured silicon, metal oxides, and carbons in next generation lithium-ion and sodium-ion batteries [9].

3.3.2 Quantum Confinement

Quantum confinement arises when one or more dimensions of a material become comparable to the de Broglie wavelength of charge carriers, typically less than 10 nm. Under this condition, electronic energy levels become discrete rather than continuous, leading to profound changes in optical and electronic properties. Semiconductor quantum dots are the most significant example: decreasing particle size increases band gap energy, shifting fluorescence emission shades from red to blue. This tunability underpins their use in high-resolution bioimaging, displays, and photovoltaics. Recent cadmium-free quantum dots, (e.g., InP or carbon-based dots) have gained attention due to improved safety profiles, reflecting how quantum principles now guided sustainable nanomaterial design. Quantum confinement also influences a catalytic activity, where altered electronic density of states in ultrasmall clusters enhances reaction selectivity and efficiency, as observed in sub-2 nm metal nanoclusters used for green catalysis and electrochemical reactions [10, 11].

3.3.3 Surface-to-Volume Effects

One of the most dominant physical principles in nanotechnology is the dramatic increase in surface-to-volume ratio as size decreases. For a 10-nm particle, a significant portion of atoms reside at or near the surface, making surface energy, defects, and functional groups decisive factors in materials behavior. This explains the increased chemical reactivity of NPs and their sensitivity to surface modification. In nanomedicine, surface coatings such as polyethylene glycol or zwitterionic polymers can alter circulation time, cellular uptake, and immune recognition without drug colloids, without altering the particle core. In catalysis, high surface area translates directly into more active sites, enabling lower catalyst loading and higher efficiency. However, the same surface dominance brings some challenges with it, namely aggregation, instability, and unexpected biological interaction. Modern nanotechnology thus does not regard surface engineering as a step to be called for at the end of the road, but as one of basic research and new design, relating the physical behavior to the real-world performance [12].

3.4 MATERIALS OF NANOTECHNOLOGY

Nanotechnology relies on a diverse set of materials whose properties emerge or are enhanced at the nanometer scale. These materials are often categorized into metals and metal oxides, carbon-based nanomaterials, semiconductors/quantum dots, polymeric or hybrid systems, having unique structure–property–function relation. Fundamental nanoscale parameters such as particle size, surface area, and surface charge are of decisive importance in determining the behavior of nanomaterials in biological and technological systems (Table 3.1). Size threshold below 10 nm creates effects of quantum confinement in semiconductors and greatly affects in vivo biodistribution and elimination outcomes [13].

3.4.1 Metals and Metal Oxides

Metal NPs such as gold, silver, platinum, and iron oxide are among the most widely studied nanomaterials. Gold and silver NPs exhibit localized surface plasmon resonance, enabling highly sensitive optical biosensors, lateral flow diagnostics, and photothermal treatments. Recent clinical and preclinical research continues to exploit gold NPs for cancer imaging and hyperthermia due to their biocompatibility and tunable optical absorption. Metal oxides, including titanium dioxide, zinc oxide, and iron oxide NPs, are widely use in catalysis, electronics, and biomedicine. Iron oxide NPs, typically 5–20 nm in size, are approved for clinical use as MRI contrast agents and iron-replacement therapies, demonstrating regulatory acceptance of inorganic nanomaterials. Titanium dioxide and zinc oxide NPs remain integral part of sunscreen and photocatalysis, although recent studies emphasize surface modification to mitigate oxidative stress and environmental concerns [14].

3.4.2 Carbon-Based Nanomaterials

Carbon nanomaterials encompass fullerenes, carbon nanotubes (CNTs), graphene, and carbon dots. Graphene and CNTs have excellent electrical conductivity, mechanical strength, and high surface area, driving application in flexible electronics, sensors, and energy storage. In biomedical research, functionalized CNTs and graphene oxide are explored for drug delivery and biosensing, although long-term safety and biodegradation remain active research areas. Carbon dots, typically <10 nm, have gained prominence in the last decade due to their fluorescence, water solubility, and relatively low toxicity, making them attractive for bioimaging and diagnostics [15].

TABLE 3.1
Key Nanoscale Parameters Governing Nanomaterial Behavior and Applications

Parameter	Typical Nanoscale Range	Dominant Effect	Representative Application
Particle size	1–100 nm	Size-dependent optical electronic, and biological properties	Quantum dots for imaging; NPs for drug delivery
Surface area	>10–1000 m^2/g (material dependent)	Enhanced reactivity and adsorption	Heterogeneous catalysis; biosensing
Surface charge (zeta potential)	±20–±40 mV (stable colloids)	Colloidal stability and cellular interaction	Injectable nanomedicines
Quantum confinement threshold	<10 nm (semiconductors)	Bandgap tuning and fluorescence	Displays; bioimaging
Biological clearance cutoff	<~10 nm	Renal clearance vs. organ accumulation	Design of biodegradable nanocarriers

3.4.3 Semiconductors and Quantum Dots

Semiconductor nanomaterials, particularly quantum dots, exhibit size-dependent electronic and optical properties governed by quantum confinement. Traditional cadmium-based quantum dots for breakthroughs in imaging and display technology vs. recent advancements in cadmium-free alternatives (e.g., indium phosphide, silicon). Quantum dots are now being central to high-efficiency displays and are increasingly researched for photovoltaics and photocatalysis, where nanoscale tuning of the band gap can lead to enhanced light harvesting and charge separation [16].

3.4.4 Polymers and Hybrid Materials

Polymeric NPs, micelles, dendrimers, and nanogels form the backbone of many clinically advanced nanomedicines. Their advantages include tunable size, biodegradability, and precise control over drug release. Lipid-polymer hybrids and inorganic-organic composites combine the stability or functionality of inorganic core with the biocompatibility of polymers. The most visible recent instance is LNP-based mRNA delivery systems, which validate polymer-lipid nanomaterial as scalable and clinically transformative platforms. Collectively, these materials classes illustrate how nanotechnology integrates chemistry, physics, and biology to engineer function from the bottom up [17].

3.5 SYNTHESIS AND FABRICATION

The performance and safety of nanomaterials are greatly determined by the way they are synthesized and made. Contemporary nanotechnology uses a combination of three strategies – top-down, bottom-up, and self-assembly/templating – that provide different levels of control, scalability, and cost-effectiveness.

3.5.1 Top-Down Methods

Top-down methods begin with bulk materials that are progressively miniaturized into nanoscale structures through physical or lithographic processes. Common techniques include photolithography, electron-beam lithography, focused ion-beam milling, and mechanical attrition (ball milling). These methods dominant the semiconductor and microelectronics industries, where nanoscale features are patterned with nanometer precision. As of the early 2020s, advanced semiconductor manufacturing routinely produces features below 10 nm, enabling high-performance logic and memory devices. The major advantages of top-down fabrication are precise spatial control and reproducibility. However, it is energy-intensive, costly, and often introduces surface defects or crystal damage, which can degrade functional performance. For biomedical nanomaterials, top-down methods are less common but are still used to fabricate nanochannels, nanoporous membranes, and lab-on-chip platforms for diagnostics and biosensing [18].

3.5.2 Bottom-Up Methods

Bottom-up synthesis builds nanostructures atom-by-atom or molecule-by-molecule through chemical reactions and controlled nucleation-growth processes. Wet-chemical routes such as sol–gel synthesis, co-precipitation, microemulsion, and hydrothermal methods are widely employed to produce metals and metal oxides NPs with tunable size and crystallinity. Chemical vapor deposition (CVD) is a cornerstone technique for producing high-quality graphene, CNTs, and semiconductor nanowires. Bottom-up approaches dominate nanomedicine and catalysis because they enable fine control over particle size (often 5–100 nm), morphology, and surface chemistry. Recent advances emphasize greener synthesis using plant extracts, biopolymers, or microwave-assisted processes to reduce toxic solvents and energy consumption. Such methods align with sustainability goals while maintaining reproducibility and scalability [19].

3.5.3 Self-Assembly and Templating

Self-assembly represents a refined bottom-up paradigm in which nanostructures form through non-covalent interactions such as hydrogen bonding, electrostatic attraction, hydrophobic forces, and van der Waals interactions. Block copolymers can self-organize into well-defined nanodomains, while lipids and amphiphiles form micelles, vesicles, and LNPs. These principles underpin modern drug delivery systems, including LNP platforms used for mRNA vaccines and RNA therapeutics. Templating strategies further enhance control by guiding material growth within predefined nanoscale molds, such as porous anodic alumina, silica templates, or biological scaffolds. DNA origami is a notable recent example, enabling programmable nanostructures, with near-atomic precision for sensing and nanorobotics [20].

Together, these synthesis and fabrication strategies form the technological backbone of nanotechnology, allowing researchers to balance precision, scalability, cost, and sustainability while tailoring nanomaterials for specific applications.

3.6 SURFACE CHEMISTRY AND FUNCTIONALIZATION

Surface chemistry is a defining determinant of nanomaterials behavior because, at the nanoscale, interfaces outweigh bulk composition. Functionalization strategies control colloidal stability, biology-interactions, targeting specificity, and ultimately safety and efficacy, especially in biomedical and environmental applications.

3.6.1 Ligand Exchange and Grafting

Ligand exchange is one of the most widely used strategies to tailor NP surface. Synthesized NPs often carry weakly bound ligands (e.g., citrate on gold NPs or oleic acid on metal oxides) that are unsuitable for biological or aqueous environments. Ligand exchange replaces them with functional molecules such as thiols, silanes, polymers, peptides, or antibodies, enabling solubility and biofunctionality. For instance, thiol-gold chemistry remains a gold standard for attaching biomolecules to gold NPs used in diagnostics and biosensing. Grafting techniques, including "grafting-to" and "grafting-from" polymerization, allow dense and stable polymer brushes to be grown directly from NPs' surfaces. Recent studies increasingly employ controlled radical polymerization (e.g., atom transfer radical polymerization [ATRP] or reversible addition-fragmentation chain transfer [RAFT]) to achieve precise chain length and functionality, improving reproducibility and regulatory acceptability [21].

3.6.2 Surface Charge and Stability of Colloidal

Surface charge strongly influences NP dispersion, aggregation, and interaction with biological media. The electrostatic repulsion between similarly charged particles stabilizes colloids, while near-neutral or oppositely charged surfaces are prone to aggregation. Zeta potential measurements are routinely used to predict colloidal stability, where their values above ±30 mV generally indicate stable suspensions. In physiological fluids, however, ionic strength and proteins adsorption can rapidly screen surface charge, leading to aggregation or corona formation. Recent work emphasizes charge-balanced or "zwitterionic" surfaces that maintain stability in high-salt and protein-rich environments. Such strategies are now common in nanomedicine formulations intended for intravenous administration [22].

3.6.3 Targeting Moieties and Stealth Coating

Surface functionalization also enables active targeting and immune evasion. Targeting ligands such as folic acid, transferrin, peptides, or antibodies can promote receptor-mediated uptake in specific tissues or cells, especially in cancer and inflammatory diseases. At the same time, "stealth" coatings are critical to minimize nonspecific proteins adsorption and rapid clearance by the mononuclear phagocyte system. Polyethylene glycol (PEG) remains the most widely used stealth polymer and is central to clinically approved LNP and polymeric NP systems. However, concerns about anti-PEG antibodies have driven the recent exploration of alternatives such as polysarcosine and zwitterionic polymers. These developments emphasize how surface chemistry has evolved from a supporting modification to a central design parameter that governs nanomaterial performance from bench to clinic [23].

3.7 CHARACTERIZATION TECHNIQUES

Reliable characterization is pivotal for understanding nanomaterial structure – property relationships as well as reproducibility, safety, and regulatory compliance. Modern nanotechnology therefore uses a complimentary collection of structural, spectroscopic, and surface analytical techniques rather than a single method.

3.7.1 Structural Probes (TEM, AFM, and XRD)

Transmission electron microscopy (TEM) remains the gold standard for direct visualization of NPs, routinely resolving features below 1 nm. TEM provides accurate information on particle size, shape, crystallinity, and core-shell architecture, which is crucial for metallic and semiconductor NPs. Atomic force microscopy (AFM) complements TEM by enabling three-dimensional surface topography measurements under ambient or liquid conditions, making it especially valuable for soft nanomaterials such as polymeric NPs, nanogels, and biomolecular assemblies. X-ray diffraction (XRD) is widely used to determine the crystalline phase, lattice parameters, and average crystallite size. In recent studies, XRD has been essential for distinguishing amorphous and crystalline drug-loaded NPs, directly linking solid-state structure to dissolution rate and bioavailability [24].

3.7.2 Spectroscopic Probes (UV-Visible, FTIR, Raman)

Spectroscopic techniques provide chemical and optical fingerprints of nanomaterials. UV-visible spectroscopy is commonly used to monitor NPs formation, concentration, and stability. For instance, the localized surface plasmon resonance peak of gold NPs is highly sensitive to its size and aggregation, making UV-Vis a rapid-quality control tool in the development of biosensors and nanomedicines. Fourier-transform infrared spectroscopy (FTIR) identifies surface functional groups and confirms successful ligand exchange or polymer grafting. Raman spectroscopy, including surface-enhanced Raman scattering (SERS), offers molecular-level insight with high sensitivity. Recent advances leverage SERS-active substrates for ultra-trace detection of biomarkers, environmental pollutants, and pathogens, demonstrating analytical power of nanoscale plasmonic systems [25].

3.7.3 Size and Surface Analysis (DLS, BET, Zeta Potential)

Dynamic light scattering (DLS) is widely used to measure hydrodynamic diameter and polydispersity of NPs in suspension, providing information relevant to biological and industrial formulations. While DLS is susceptible to aggregation, it is incomparable for batch-to-batch comparison and stability testing. Brunauer-Emmett-Teller (BET) analysis quantifies specific area, a critical parameter for catalysts, adsorbents, and porous nanomaterials, where higher surface area often correlates with high performance. Zeta potential measurements provide surface charge and electrostatic stability, offering predictive insight into dispersion behavior in different media. Together, these techniques form a robust characterization toolkit that underpins rational nanomaterials design and translational success [26].

3.8 MOLECULAR MECHANISMS IN SOLUTION AND INTERFACE

Understanding how nanomaterials behave in solution and at biological interfaces is central to predicting their function, safety, and translational success. At the nanoscale, molecular interactions at interfaces often dominate over bulk material properties, particularly complex biological environments. NPs' behavior in biological systems is governed by dynamic interfacial processes, including protein corona formation, membrane interaction, and intracellular trafficking pathways (Figure 3.2).

3.8.1 Nano–Bio Interface Basics

When NPs enter an aqueous or biological milieu, they are instantly surrounded by solvent molecules, ions, and biomolecules. This dynamic environment characterizes the nano–bio interface, where surface chemistry, size, shape, and charge govern interaction with proteins, membranes, and cells. Unlike small molecules, NPs present multivalent surfaces that can simultaneously engage multiple biomolecular partners. Recent studies show that even subtle changes in surface functionalization, such as replacing an anionic ligand with a zwitterinoic one, can markedly alter circulation time, biodistribution, and cellular uptake. In nanomedicine, this principle underlies the design of LNPs and polymeric carriers optimized for stability in blood while remaining responsive inside target cells [27].

3.8.2 Protein Corona Formation

A defining molecular mechanism at the nano–bio interface is protein corona formation. Within seconds of exposure to biological fluids such as plasma or interstitial fluid, proteins adsorb onto the NP surfaces, creating a corona that effectively defines particle's biological identity. The corona is often described as comprising a "hard" layer of tightly bound proteins and a more dynamic "soft" layer. Proteomic analyses over the past decade have shown that corona composition depends on NPs' size, surface charge, hydrophobicity, and the biological medium. Importantly, recent data indicate that the protein corona can either mask or enhance targeting ligands and strongly influence immune recognition. For example, apolipoproteins enriched in the corona of certain LNP formulations have been linked to preferential uptake by hepatocytes, a mechanism exploiting clinically approved RNA-based therapies. Consequently, modern nanotechnology increasingly designs surfaces not to eliminate the corona, but to control its composition and biological fate [28].

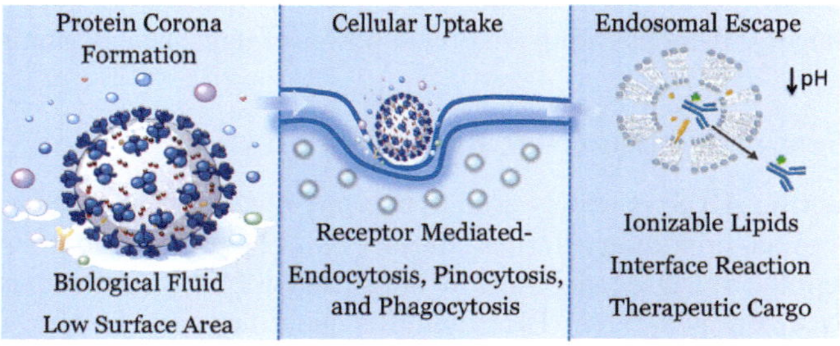

FIGURE 3.2 Molecular mechanism at the nano–bio interface.

3.8.3 Membrane Interaction and Uptake Pathways

NP interactions with cellular membranes represent the next critical interface. Depending on the size and surface properties, NPs may adsorb to the membrane, insert into the lipid bilayer, or be internalized via endocytic pathways. Clathrin-mediated endocytosis, caveolae-mediated uptake, and macropinocytosis are the most common mechanisms reported. Particles in the 20–100 nm range are particularly efficient at receptor-mediated endocytosis when decorated with the targeting ligands. For nucleic acid delivery, successful endosomes escape is a key molecular barrier. Recent LNP systems address this challenge through ionizable lipids that remain neutral in circulation but become positively charged in acidic endosomes, destabilizing the membrane and enabling cytosolic release [29].

Collectively, these molecular mechanisms illustrate that the function of NPs in biological systems emerges from dynamic, context-related interactions at interfaces. A mechanistic understanding of these processes is now required for rational nanomaterials design, replacing earlier trial-and-error approaches.

3.9 MECHANISM OF ACTION (APPLICATION-FOCUSED)

The practical value of nanotechnology emerging from nanoscale materials can translate physical and molecular properties into specific mechanisms of action. In applied systems, these mechanisms are tightly coupled to size, surface chemistry, and interface-driven phenomena.

3.9.1 Drug Delivery and Controlled Release

NPs act as carriers that enhance drug solubility, stability, and biodistribution while enabling controlled release. Polymeric NPs, LNPs, and nanogels protect therapeutic payloads from premature degradation and pharmacokinetics modulation. Controlled release is achieved through diffusion, polymer degradation, or stimulus-responsive mechanisms triggered by pH, enzymes, redox potential, or temperature. Recent clinical success of LNP-based nucleic acid delivery has demonstrated how ionizable lipids facilitate endosomal escape, enabling efficient cytosolic release of mRNA and siRNA. In oncology and inflammatory diseases, NP delivery has been demonstrated to decrease systemic toxicity by concentrating drugs at the target site, lowering the required doses [30].

3.9.2 Photothermal and Photodynamic Effects

Photothermal and photodynamic mechanisms exploit NP-light interaction for therapy and diagnostics. Metallic NPs, especially gold nanostructures, efficiently convert absorbed near-infrared light into localized heat through plasmonic effects, leading to targeted destruction of diseased tissue while sparing surrounding healthy cells. Photodynamic therapy relies on photosensitizers-loaded NPs that produce reactive oxygen species upon light activation, inducing cell death. Recent advances focus on improving tissue penetration, oxygen-independent mechanisms, and combination therapies that integrate photothermal effects with chemotherapy or immunotherapies. These approaches are increasingly explored for cancer treatment and antimicrobial applications [31].

3.9.3 Catalysis and Electron Transfer

Nanomaterials play a central role in catalysis due to their large surface area, variable electronic structure, and abundance of active sites. Metal and metal oxide NPs enhance reaction rates and selectivity in chemical synthesis, environmental remediation, and energy conversion. At the nanoscale, altered electron density and shortened charge-transfer distances improve catalytic efficiency. In electrochemical systems, nanostructured catalysts facilitate rapid electron transfer in fuel cells, batteries, and sensors. Recent work focuses on earth-abundant nanocatalysts and single-atom catalysts to lower the cost and enhance sustainability [32].

Together, these mechanisms illustrate how nanoscale design enables precise control over transport, energy conversion, and chemical reactivity, forming the foundation for real-world nanotechnology applications.

3.10 SAFETY, TOXICOLOGY, AND RISK

As nanotechnology advances toward widespread clinical, industrial, and environmental use, safety and risk assessment have become central to responsible development. Unlike conventional chemicals, nanomaterials exhibit size, shape, and surface-dependent behaviors that complicate tradition toxicological paradigms.

3.10.1 Dose, Persistence, and Biodistribution

At the nanoscale, dose cannot be defined solely by mass; surface area, particle number, and reactivity often correlate more closely with biological effects. Biodistribution shows that NPs' size and surface chemistry strongly influence organ accumulation and clearance. For example, particles below ~10 nm are more likely to undergo rapid renal clearance, whereas larger NPs tend to accumulate in the liver and spleen via mononuclear phagocyte system. Persistence is another critical factor: biodegradable polymeric NPs and LNPs are generally cleared within days to weeks, while some inorganic NPs may persist longer depending on solubility and surface modification. Recent in vivo research focuses on designing nanomaterials with predictable degradation pathways to minimize long-term accumulation [33].

3.10.2 Mechanisms of Nanotoxicity

Nanotoxicity occurs by a variety of mechanisms – oftentimes interwoven together. These include oxidative stress mediated by reactive oxygen species production, membrane disruption, protein misfolding, inflammation, and genotoxicity. Metal and metal oxide NPs have the potential of catalyzing the redox reactions, and materials with high aspect ratios could cause physical stress in the cells. Importantly, the toxicity is not an intrinsic property of all nanomaterials, but rather it is a function of physicochemical properties such as size, surface charge, solubility, and aggregation state. Recent studies have pointed to the importance of the protein corona in the modulation of toxicity through the alteration of cellular recognition and uptake pathways. Consequently, surface engineering is becoming a widely used risk mitigation strategy [34].

3.10.3 Testing Frameworks

To address these complexities, modern testing frameworks combine in vitro, in vivo, and computational approaches. Advanced cell models, such as organoids and organ-on-chip models, provide more physiologically relevant information than traditional 2D culture models. Regulatory agencies are increasingly using tiered approaches to testing using a combination of physicochemical characterization, standardized biological characterization, and life cycle analysis. International guidelines have now focused on "safe-by-design" principles, where the considerations of safety include thinking about it at the initial stages of nanomaterial development. Together, these frameworks are designed to bring innovation while preserving protection of human health and the environment in order to ensure sustainable innovations of nanotechnology [35].

3.11 REGULATION, ETHICS, AND TRANSLATION

The successful implementation of nanotechnology relies not only on scientific workings but also on good regulatory oversight, ethical responsibility, and feasible translation pathways from laboratory to market.

3.11.1 Regulatory Landscape

Regulation of nanomaterials has evolved toward a case-by-case, risk-based approach rather than treating nanotechnology as a single category. Regulatory agencies now emphasize detailed physicochemical characterization, manufacturing consistency, and biological safety data. In nanomedicine, regulatory approval pathways increasingly align with those for conventional drugs and biologics, but with added scrutiny of size distribution, surface chemistry, and stability. Recent approvals of LNP-based therapeutics prove that well-characterized nanoplatforms could meet the stringent regulatory standards when supported by robust quality control and toxicological evidence [36].

3.11.2 Ethical Considerations

Ethical concerns in nanotechnology center on safety, equity, transparency, and the environment. Uncertainties surrounding long-term exposure, environmental persistence, and unintended biological effects necessitate precautionary design and open risk communication. Ethical frameworks increasingly promote responsible innovation, ensuring that benefits such as advanced diagnostics or targeted therapies are accessible and do not exacerbate health or technological disparities. Public trust is closely tied to clear labeling, informed consent in clinical applications, and responsible data use in nano-enabled diagnostics [37].

3.11.3 Pathway Commercialization

Translation from research to commercialization requires scalable manufacturing, reproducibility, and economics viability. Industry-academia partnerships, standardized production methods, and early engagement with regulators are now recognized as critical success factors. Platforms with modular design, such as NPs delivery systems adaptable to multiple payloads, have shown particular commercial promise. Collectively, these strategies bridge discovery and deployment, enabling nanotechnology to progress from innovation to societal impact [38].

3.12 EMERGING TRENDS AND FUTURE DIRECTIONS

Nanotechnology is entering a phase defined by data-driven design, clinical personalization, and sustainability, reshaping how nanomaterials are discovered, evaluated, and deployed.

3.12.1 AI-Driven Design and Nanoinformatics

Artificial intelligence (AI) and nanoinformatics are transforming nanomaterial development from empirical trial-and-error to predictive engineering. Machine learning models now integrate physicochemical descriptors (size, shape, surface charge, composition) with biological outcomes (toxicity, uptake, and efficacy) to forecast performance before synthesis. Recent studies accelerated optimization of NP formulations for nucleic acid delivery and catalysis by screening thousands of virtual candidates – decreasing cost and development time. Standardized databases and findable, accessible, interoperable, and reusable (FAIR) data practices are enabling cross-study learning, while generative models are beginning to propose entirely new nanostructures tailored to a specific function [39].

3.12.2 Precision Medicine and Theranostics

Precision medicine is a major growth driver for nanotechnology. Nanocarriers are increasingly designed to match patient-specific molecular profiles, diseases states, and dosing requirements. Theranostics NPs – combining diagnostic imaging and therapy in a single platform – enable real-time monitoring of drug distribution and treatment response. Recent examples include stimuli-responsive systems that activate only in disease-specific microenvironments (i.e., acidic tumors or inflamed tissues), improving efficacy while reducing off-target effects. Integration with molecular imaging and omics data is bringing nanomedicine nearer to truly personalized type of interventions [40].

3.12.3 Sustainable and Green Nanotechnology

Sustainability considerations are reshaping synthesis, materials choice, and life-cycle evaluation. Green nanotechnology emphasizes renewable feedstock, low-energy fabrication, and reduced reliance on toxic solvents and rare elements. Biogenic synthesis using plant extracts, enzymes, or microorganisms has gained momentum, offering scalable and environmentally benign routes to metal and metal oxide NPs. Concurrently, biodegradable polymers and earth-abundant nanomaterials are replacing persistent or hazardous alternatives. Future success in nanotechnology will increasingly be measured not only by the performance but also by environmental compatibility and social responsibility [41].

3.13 CONCLUSION

Nanotechnology has evolved into a mature, interdisciplinary field grounded in well-defined physical principles and molecular mechanisms. By exploiting size-dependent properties, surface-dominated interactions, and controlled interfaces, nanomaterials enable functionalities unattainable with bulk materials. Advances in synthesis, characterization, and surface engineering have translated fundamental concepts into clinically and industrially useful applications, especially in medicine, energy, and catalysis. At the same time, increasing focus on safety, regulation, and sustainability reflects a shift toward responsible innovation. As data-driven design, precision medicine, and green fabrication continue to advance, nanotechnology is poised to deliver increasingly predictive, scalable, and socially impactful solutions in the coming decade.

REFERENCES

1. Khan Y, Sadia H, Ali Shah SZ, Khan MN, Shah AA, Ullah N, Ullah MF, Bibi H, Bafakeeh OT, Khedher NB, Eldin SM. Classification, synthetic, and characterization approaches to nanoparticles, and their applications in various fields of nanotechnology: A review. Catalysts. 2022;12(11):1386.
2. Chupradit S, Kavitha M, Suksatan W, Ansari MJ, Al Mashhadani ZI, Kadhim MM, Mustafa YF, Kianfar SSS. Morphological control: Properties and applications of metal nanostructures. Advances in Materials Science and Engineering. 2022;2022(1):1971891.
3. Schoenmaker L, Witzigmann D, Kulkarni JA, Verbeke R, Kersten G, Jiskoot W, Crommelin DJ. mRNA-lipid nanoparticle COVID-19 vaccines: Structure and stability. International Journal of Pharmaceutics. 2021;601:120586.
4. Raghav S, Yadav PK, Kumar D. Nanotechnology for a Sustainable Future. In Handbook of Nanomaterials for Manufacturing Applications (pp. 465–492). Elsevier; 2020.
5. Junk A, Riess F. From an idea to a vision: There's plenty of room at the bottom. American Journal of Physics. 2006;74(9):825–30.
6. Siddique S, Chow JC. Application of nanomaterials in biomedical imaging and cancer therapy. Nanomaterials. 2020;10(9):1700.
7. Koontz TM, Newig J. From planning to implementation: Top-down and bottom-up approaches for collaborative watershed management. Policy Studies Journal. 2014;42(3):416–42.

8. Roco MC. Nanotechnology: Convergence with modern biology and medicine. Current Opinion in Biotechnology. 2003;14(3):337–46.
9. Prasad RD, Sarvalkar PD, Prasad N, Prasad RS, Prasad RB, Prasad RR, Prasad S, Gour B, Barade SU, Deshmukh RN, Karhu BG. Emerging trends of bioactive nano-materials in modern veterinary science and animal husbandry. ES Food and Agroforestry. 2024;18:1144.
10. Goyal RK, Maharaj S, Kumar P, Chandrasekhar M. Exploring quantum materials and applications: A review. Journal of Materials Science: Materials in Engineering. 2025;20(1):4.
11. Jones AP. Quantum confinement and carbon nanodots: A conceptual view of the origin of diffuse interstellar bands. Astronomy & Astrophysics. 2025;699:A16.
12. Chavali MS, Nikolova MP. Metal oxide nanoparticles and their applications in nanotechnology. SN Applied Sciences. 2019;1(6):607.
13. Elzein B. Nano revolution: Tiny tech, big impact: How nanotechnology is driving SDGs progress. Heliyon. 2024;10(10):1–26.
14. Truong TT, Mondal S, Doan VH, Tak S, Choi J, Oh H, Nguyen TD, Misra M, Lee B, Oh J. Precision-engineered metal and metal-oxide nanoparticles for biomedical imaging and healthcare applications. Advances in Colloid and Interface Science. 2024;332:103263.
15. Yücer S, Sarac B, Ciftci F. Tissue engineering and biosensing applications of carbon-based nanomaterials. Biomedical Engineering Advances. 2025;9:100145.
16. Feng D, Zhang G, Yang L. Semiconductor quantum dots: Synthesis, properties and applications. Nanomaterials. 2024;14(22):1825.
17. Begines B, Ortiz T, Pérez-Aranda M, Martínez G, Merinero M, Argüelles-Arias F, Alcudia A. Polymeric nanoparticles for drug delivery: Recent developments and future prospects. Nanomaterials. 2020;10(7):1403.
18. Yu HD, Regulacio MD, Ye E, Han MY. Chemical routes to top-down nanofabrication. Chemical Society Reviews. 2013;42(14):6006–18.
19. Wolfgang L Bottom-up methods for making nanotechnology products. Erişim: http://www.azonano.com/details.asp. 2007.
20. Tang X, Xie R, Zeng B, Yi C, Su H, Chen C, Zhou L, Xia X, Zeng J, Yang J. Self-assembled nanoparticles: Overcoming limitations of conventional nanomedicines for enhanced tumor therapy. International Journal of Nanomedicine. 2025;31:15185–211.
21. Lombardo D, Calandra P, Pasqua L, Magazù S. Self-assembly of organic nanomaterials and biomaterials: The bottom-up approach for functional nanostructures formation and advanced applications. Materials. 2020;13(5):1048.
22. Oncsik T, Trefalt G, Csendes Z, Szilagyi I, Borkovec M. Aggregation of negatively charged colloidal particles in the presence of multivalent cations. Langmuir. 2014;30(3):733–41.
23. Parvin N, Aslam M, Alam MN, Mandal TK. Nanotechnology driven innovations in modern pharmaceutics: Therapeutics, imaging, and regeneration. Nanomaterials. 2025;15(22):1733.
24. Kaur M, Ebadi A, Chen CY, Stach EA, Liu Q. Semi-supervised and temporally-aware segmentation of transmission electron microscopy image sequences. Materials Today Physics. 2026;61:102033.
25. Manoto SL, El-Hussein A, Malabi R, Thobakgale L, Ombinda-Lemboumba S, Attia YA, Kasem MA, Mthunzi-Kufa P. Exploring optical spectroscopic techniques and nanomaterials for virus detection. Saudi Journal of Biological Sciences. 2021;28(1):78–89.
26. Lim J, Yeap SP, Che HX, Low SC. Characterization of magnetic nanoparticle by dynamic light scattering. Nanoscale Research Letters. 2013;8(1):381.
27. Tian X, Chong Y, Ge C. Understanding the nano–bio interactions and the corresponding biological responses. Frontiers in Chemistry. 2020;8:446.
28. Liu N, Tang M, Ding J. The interaction between nanoparticles-protein corona complex and cells and its toxic effect on cells. Chemosphere. 2020;245:125624.
29. Zhang S, Gao H, Bao G. Physical principles of nanoparticle cellular endocytosis. ACS Nano. 2015; 9(9):8655–71.
30. Mehta M, Bui TA, Yang X, Aksoy Y, Goldys EM, Deng W. Lipid-based nanoparticles for drug/gene delivery: An overview of the production techniques and difficulties encountered in their industrial development. ACS Materials Au. 2023;3(6):600–19.
31. Amaral MN, Kumar P, Faísca P, Ferreira HA, Coelho JM, Gaspar MM, Reis CP. Gold nanoparticle-mediated photothermal therapy: Expanding the frontiers of cancer treatment and theragnostics. Biomedicine & Pharmacotherapy. 2025;190:118399.
32. Baruwa A, Gbadeyan OJ, Permaul K. Revolutionizing biotechnology: The impact of nanocatalysts and nanomaterials—a comprehensive review. Discover Materials. 2025;5(1):89.

33. Dolai J, Mandal K, Jana NR. Nanoparticle size effects in biomedical applications. ACS Applied Nano Materials. 2021;4(7):6471–96.
34. Fu PP, Xia Q, Hwang HM, Ray PC, Yu H. Mechanisms of nanotoxicity: Generation of reactive oxygen species. Journal of Food and Drug Analysis. 2014;22(1):64–75.
35. Kimura H, Nishikawa M, Kutsuzawa N, Tokito F, Kobayashi T, Kurniawan DA, Shioda H, Cao W, Shinha K, Nakamura H, Doi K. Advancements in microphysiological systems: Exploring organoids and organ-on-a-chip technologies in drug development-focus on pharmacokinetics related organs. Drug Metabolism and Pharmacokinetics. 2025;60:101046.
36. Gujjar S, Kukal S, Jayabal P, Balaji N, Sainger S, Roy S, Rallapalli S, Mahadevappa R, Minocha S, Kumar S, Mathapati S. Nanomaterials for biomedical applications: Addressing regulatory hurdles and strategic solutions. Nano Trends. 2025;11:100127.
37. Sargent JF. Nanotechnology and Environmental Health and Safety: Issues for Consideration. DIANE Publishing; 2008.
38. Domokos A, Nagy B, Szilágyi B, Marosi G, Nagy ZK. Integrated continuous pharmaceutical technologies—a review. Organic Process Research & Development. 2021;25(4):721–39.
39. Mim JJ, Al Mamun A, Nayem MH, Mahmud S, Nath A, Rahman SM, Fidal SA, Hossain N. Machine learning-driven advances in nanotechnology: From materials design to process optimization-a review. Materials Today Communications. 2025:114485.
40. Mura S, Couvreur P. Nanotheranostics for personalized medicine. Advanced Drug Delivery Reviews. 2012;64(13):1394–416.
41. Abuzeid HM, Julien CM, Zhu L, Hashem AM. Green synthesis of nanoparticles and their energy storage, environmental, and biomedical applications. Crystals. 2023;13(11):1576.

4 Nanotechnology for Diabetes Complications

Nephropathy, Retinopathy, and Cardiovascular Disease

Muthukumaran Mylasalam
School of Pharmacy, SBV Karaikal, Sri Balaji Vidyapeeth, Karaikal, India

Jeevanandham Somasundaram
Sri Shanmugha College of Pharmacy (affiliated to The Tamil Nadu Dr. M.G.R. Medical University), Salem, India

M. V. Saranya
J.K.K. Munirajah Institute of Health Sciences College of Pharmacy (affiliated to The Tamil Nadu DR. M.G.R Medical University), Erode, India

Sharad Sharma
Noida Institute of Engineering and Technology (Pharmacy Institute), Greater Noida, India

Naidu Narapusetty
Bellamkonda Institute of Technology and Science, Podili, India

Suresh V. Chinni
Faculty of Medicine, Bioscience, and Nursing, MAHSA University, Jenjarom, Malaysia

K. Gayathiri
SRM College of Pharmacy, SRM Institute of Science and Technology, Chengalpattu, India

4.1 INTRODUCTION

Diabetes mellitus is a rapidly growing global health crisis: recent global estimates place adult diabetes prevalence near or above one in nine adults and suggest that >800 million adults were living with diabetes globally in 2022, with large treatment gaps in low- and middle-income countries. The scale of the disease translates directly into a massive burden of chronic microvascular and macrovascular complications that drive morbidity, mortality, and health-system costs worldwide [1].

Among the chronic complications are diabetic nephropathy (DN), diabetic retinopathy (DR), and cardiovascular disease (CVD), which are principal drivers of long-term disability and death. Global analyses estimate tens of millions of people living with DN (estimates of prevalent cases exceed

DOI: 10.1201/9781003598657-4

100 million in recent global assessments), and DN-attributed deaths have grown substantially over recent decades [2]. Meta-analytic efforts and regional surveys place DR prevalence in treated diabetes populations from ~24% to >50% depending on the study setting and case definitions (pooled estimates frequently fall near 20–30% for any DR). CVD remains the leading cause of mortality in people with diabetes; large reviews report markedly elevated rates of coronary artery disease, stroke, and heart failure in diabetic cohorts, with regional prevalence of CVD among people with type 2 diabetes often exceeding >30–40% [2, 3].

These complications have distinct clinical trajectories yet overlapping pathobiology. DN progresses from albuminuria and glomerular injury to progressive loss of renal function and end-stage kidney disease, necessitating dialysis or transplantation and incurring very high costs. DR is a leading cause of vision loss in working-age adults; the development of proliferative DR or diabetic macular edema (DME) causes permanent visual impairment if not treated promptly. CVD yields the greatest mortality burden – many patients with diabetes die of a cardiac or cerebrovascular event rather than microvascular sequelae – making cardiovascular risk reduction central to diabetes care [4].

Current standards – glycemic, blood-pressure, and lipid control; intravitreal anti-vascular endothelial growth factor (VEGF) for sight-threatening DR; renin-angiotensin blockade for nephropathy; and guideline-directed pharmacotherapy for CVD – reduce but do not eliminate risk. Therapeutic gaps include poor drug bioavailability to target tissues (retina, glomerulus, and atherosclerotic plaque), short intra-tissue half-lives requiring frequent dosing (e.g., repeated intravitreal injections), systemic side effects, and inadequate targeting of complex processes such as chronic inflammation, oxidative stress, and fibrosis [5]. Nanotechnology offers potential solutions: engineered nanocarriers can improve tissue targeting, enable sustained local release, co-deliver multiple cargoes (drug + gene), and combine imaging with therapy (theranostics) – features highlighted in recent reviews of nanotherapies for diabetic complications [6].

4.2 NANOTECHNOLOGY: CONCEPTS AND PLATFORMS FOR DIABETES COMPLICATIONS

Nanotechnology has emerged as a versatile enabling strategy for addressing the complex pathophysiology and delivery challenges associated with chronic diabetic complications. At the nanoscale (typically 1–200 nm), materials exhibit distinct physicochemical and biological properties that can be exploited to improve drug solubility, stability, tissue targeting, and therapeutic efficacy. Over the last decade, rapid advances in materials science and biomedical engineering have resulted in disease-specific nanoplatforms tailored for renal, ocular, and cardiovascular applications in diabetes [7]. A comparative overview of delivery routes and translational status for nano-enabled strategies for DN, retinopathy, and CVD is summarized in Table 4.1.

4.2.1 Basic Principles: Size, Surface Properties, and Biological Interactions

NP size is a primary determinant of biodistribution and cellular uptake. Particles below ~10 nm are rapidly cleared by the kidneys, whereas those between ~50 and 200 nm exhibit prolonged circulation and improved tissue interaction. In DN, size-tuned NPs (~30–80 nm) have been shown to preferentially interact with glomerular and tubular structures, while avoiding rapid systemic clearance. Surface charge and hydrophilicity further influence biological interactions; neutral or slightly negative surfaces reduce nonspecific protein adsorption, whereas positively charged NPs increase cellular internalization but may increase toxicity [17].

Surface functionalization, including polyethylene glycol (PEGylation), zwitterionic coatings, and biomimetic membranes, is widely used to modulate immune recognition and prolong circulation time. In the case of diabetes, where inflammation and endothelial dysfunction alter vascular permeability, NP-protein corona formation and interactions with activated immune cells play

TABLE 4.1
Comparison of Delivery Routes, Advantages, and Clinical Status of Nano-Enabled Strategies for Major Diabetic Complications

Diabetic Complication	Delivery Route	Key Advantages (Nano-Enabled)	Limitations	Current Clinical Status	References
DN	Intravenous (systemic)	Kidney-targeted nanoparticles (NPs) enable improved renal accumulation; reduced systemic toxicity: co-delivery of drugs/genes	Rapid renal clearance; off-target RES uptake	Preclinical (rodent DN models)	[8, 9]
	Oral (emerging)	Potential for chronic administration; improved stability of labile agents	Poor intestinal absorption; limited kidney specificity	Early preclinical	[10, 11]
DR	Intravitreal	High local drug concentration; sustained-release NPs reduce injection frequency	Invasive; risk of infection and inflammation	Clinically established route (nano-formulations)	[12]
	Periocular / suprachoroidal	Less invasive than intravitreal; prolonged posterior segment exposure	Variable bioavailability	Preclinical-early translational	[13]
	Topical (nano-enabled)	Non-invasive patient-friendly	Limited retinal penetration	Preclinical	[14]
CVD	Intravenous (systemic)	Targeted plaque accumulation; theranostic imaging + therapy	Liver/spleen accumulation; immune clearance	Preclinical-early clinical (non-diabetes specific)	[15]
	Local (stent-based)	Controlled drug release; reduced restenosis and thrombosis	Device-dependent; limited to focal disease	Clinically established (nano-coatings)	[16]

a crucial role in therapeutic performance. Recent in vivo studies confirm that surface chemistry strongly influences NP accumulation in inflamed renal and vascular tissues [18].

4.2.2 Common Nanocarriers and Materials

A broad range of nanocarriers have been explored for diabetic complications. Liposomes remain among the most clinically mature platforms due to their biocompatibility and ability to encapsulate both hydrophilic and lipophilic drugs. Liposomal formulations have been adapted for sustained intraocular delivery of anti-VEGF agents in DR and for targeted anti-inflammatory therapy in atherosclerosis [10, 19].

Polymeric NPs, particularly those based on poly(lactic-co-glycolic) acid (PLGA), chitosan, and polyethylene glycols (PEG)-based copolymers, dominate preclinical studies owing to tunable degradation rates and controlled drug release. In DN models, polymeric NPs have successfully delivered antioxidants, anti-fibrotic agents, and nucleic acids to renal tissue, reducing albuminuria and fibrosis [20].

Dendrimers, characterized by highly branched architectures and precise molecular weights, offer high drug-loading capacity and surface functionality. Hydroxyl- and amine-terminated dendrimers have demonstrated preferential uptake by activated microglia and retinal cells, making them attractive for neurovascular targeting in DR [21].

Metallic NPs, such as gold, iron oxide, and cerium oxide NPs, provide unique optical, magnetic, and redox properties. Cerium oxide NPs, in particular, have shown reactive oxygen species (ROS)-scavenging activity in diabetic kidney and retinal injury models. Nanofibers and hydrogels, often fabricated from biodegradable polymers, are increasingly explored for localized and sustained drug delivery, particularly in ocular and cardiovascular tissue engineering applications [22].

4.2.3 Stimuli-Responsive and "Smart" Nanosystems

Stimuli-responsive nanocarriers represent a major advance in precision therapy. These systems are engineered to release their payload in response to disease-specific triggers such as pH changes, elevated ROS, and enzymatic activity or glucose levels. Diabetic tissues are characterized by oxidative stress, inflammatory enzymes, and altered metabolic microenvironments, making them ideal targets for such "smart" systems [23].

ROS-responsive NPs incorporating thioketal or boronic ester linkages have demonstrated selective drug release in diabetic kidneys and atherosclerotic plaques. Enzyme-responsive systems sensitive to matrix metalloproteinases or esterases have been applied in diabetic vascular disease. Glucose-responsive nanosystems, initially developed for insulin delivery, are now being adapted for complications-specific therapies, with potential for self-regulated drug release linked to glycemic status [24].

4.2.4 Targeting Strategies: Passive and Active Delivery

Passive targeting relies on enhanced vascular permeability and inflammatory remodeling in diabetic tissues, allowing NPs to accumulate preferentially in diseased sites. Although the classical enhanced permeability and retention (EPR) effect is less pronounced than in cancer, EPR-like behavior has been documented in inflamed kidneys, retina, and atherosclerotic lesions [25].

Active targeting further improves specificity through surface conjugation of ligands, peptides, antibodies, or aptamers. Examples include NPs functionalized with peptides targeting renal proximal tubules, antibodies against vascular adhesion molecules in diabetic vasculature, and hyaluronic acid-based systems targeting CD44-expressing inflammatory cells. Cell-specific delivery strategies are increasingly emphasized to minimize off-target effects in chronic diseases such as diabetes [26].

4.2.5 Imaging and Theranostic Platforms

Nanotechnology also enables theranostic platforms that integrate diagnostic imaging and therapy within a single system. Iron oxide NPs serve as MRI contrast agents while simultaneously delivering anti-inflammatory drugs to atherosclerotic plaques. Gold NPs (AuNPs) have been explored for combined optical imaging and photothermal or drug-based therapy. In DR, NP-based contrast agents are under investigation for improved visualization of microvascular damage, coupled with localized drug release [27]. Organ-specific NP targeting strategies for the kidney, retina, and vasculature are schematically illustrated in Figure 4.1.

4.3 DIABETIC NEPHROPATHY (DN) – NANOTECHNOLOGY APPROACHES

DN is one of the most severe and prevalent microvascular complications of diabetes and remains the leading cause of end-stage kidney disease worldwide. Despite advances in glycemic control and renoprotective pharmacotherapy, DN continues to progress in a substantial proportion of patients,

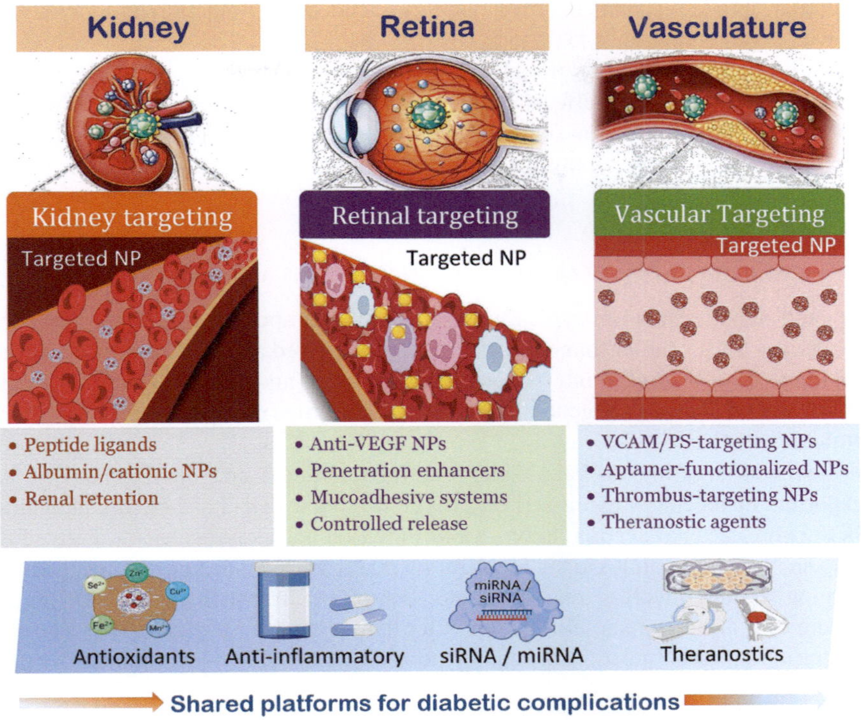

FIGURE 4.1 Schematic of NP targeting strategies for the kidney, retina, and vasculature.

highlighting the need for more precise, mechanism-driven therapeutic strategies. Nanotechnology has gained increasing attention as a promising approach to overcome biological delivery barriers and to target multiple pathogenic pathways involved in DN [28].

4.3.1 Pathophysiology Recap: Glomerular Injury, Podocyte Dysfunction, Fibrosis, and Inflammation

DN is driven by a complex interplay of metabolic, hemodynamic, and inflammatory mechanisms. Chronic hyperglycemia induces oxidative stress, advanced glycation end-product (AGE) formation, and activation of pro-fibrotic signaling pathways such as transforming growth factor-β (TGF-β). At the glomerular level, mesangial expansion, basement membrane thickening, and endothelial dysfunction disrupt the filtration barrier. Podocyte injury and loss are now recognized as central events driving albuminuria and disease progression [29].

Inflammation plays a critical role throughout DN development, with increased infiltration of macrophages and upregulation of cytokines such as TNF-α, IL-1β, and MCP-1. Persistent activation of these pathways promotes extracellular matrix (ECM) accumulation, interstitial fibrosis, and irreversible nephron loss. Importantly, these pathogenic processes often coexist spatially and temporally, making DN an ideal candidate for multi-targeted nanotherapeutic interventions [30].

4.3.2 Delivery Challenges for the Kidney

Effective renal drug delivery is particularly challenging due to the kidney's unique anatomy and filtration function. The glomerular filtration barrier restricts the passage of large or highly charged molecules, while smaller molecules are rapidly cleared, resulting in insufficient renal retention.

Proximal tubular uptake mechanisms may cause unintended accumulation and toxicity, especially for positively charged compounds [31].

Systemically administered drugs often fail to achieve therapeutic concentrations in diseased renal compartments without off-target effects in the liver, spleen, or immune system. These challenges are amplified in chronic conditions such as DN, where repeated dosing is required. Nanocarriers offer opportunities to modulate size, surface charge, and circulation time to balance renal access with systemic safety [32].

4.3.3 Kidney-Directed Nanocarriers: Design Principles and Examples

Kidney-targeted nanocarriers are typically designed within specific size ranges to exploit renal handling pathways. NPs smaller than ~10 nm are rapidly filtered and excreted, whereas those in the ~30–80 nm range show enhanced interaction with glomerular and tubular structures. Slightly negative or neutral surface charges are generally favored to minimize nonspecific protein adsorption and reduce cytotoxicity [33].

Ligand-mediated targeting has been widely explored. Peptides and small molecules that bind to renal transporters or receptors expressed on proximal tubular cells have been conjugated to polymeric NPs to enhance renal accumulation. Albumin-based and polysaccharide-derived nanocarriers have also shown preferential kidney localization due to endogenous uptake mechanisms [34].

An emerging strategy involves renal-clearable NPs, often ultrasmall inorganic or polymeric systems engineered for efficient renal elimination after delivering their payload. These systems aim to reduce long-term tissue accumulation and chronic toxicity, a critical consideration for DN therapy [35].

4.3.4 Therapeutic Cargoes for Nanodelivery

Nanotechnology enables the delivery of a broad spectrum of therapeutic cargoes relevant to DN pathophysiology. Anti-inflammatory agents, including corticosteroids and small-molecule cytokine inhibitors, have been encapsulated in polymeric NPs to reduce systemic exposure while suppressing renal inflammation [36].

Anti-fibrotic therapies targeting TGF-β signaling, connective tissue growth factor, or downstream Smad pathways have shown enhanced efficacy when delivered via nanocarriers in experimental DN models. Gene-based therapies, including small interfering RNA (siRNA) and micro-RNA (miRNA) modulators, represent a rapidly growing area. NP-mediated delivery of siRNA against pro-fibrotic or pro-inflammatory genes has demonstrated reduced renal fibrosis and improved functional outcomes in diabetic rodents [37].

Antioxidant nanotherapies are another major focus. NPs loaded with natural antioxidants or constructed from redox-active materials such as cerium oxide have shown the ability to scavenge ROS, attenuate oxidative stress, and protect podocytes and tubular cells. Growth factor modulation, either through controlled delivery or through inhibition of pathological signaling, further illustrates the versatility of nanocarrier platforms in DN [38]. As summarized in Figure 4.2, a wide range of nanocarriers can be engineered to deliver diverse therapeutic cargos relevant to diabetic complications.

4.3.5 Preclinical Evidence and Promising in Vivo Studies

A growing body of preclinical literature supports the potential of nanotechnology in DN. In streptozotocin-induced and genetically diabetic rodent models, polymeric NPs delivering anti-inflammatory or anti-fibrotic agents consistently reduce albuminuria, glomerulosclerosis, and interstitial fibrosis compared with free drug controls. Several studies report improved podocyte preservation and decreased inflammatory cell infiltration [39].

Gene-silencing approaches using NP-encapsulated siRNA have demonstrated significant downregulation of target genes in renal tissue, with corresponding functional and histological improvement.

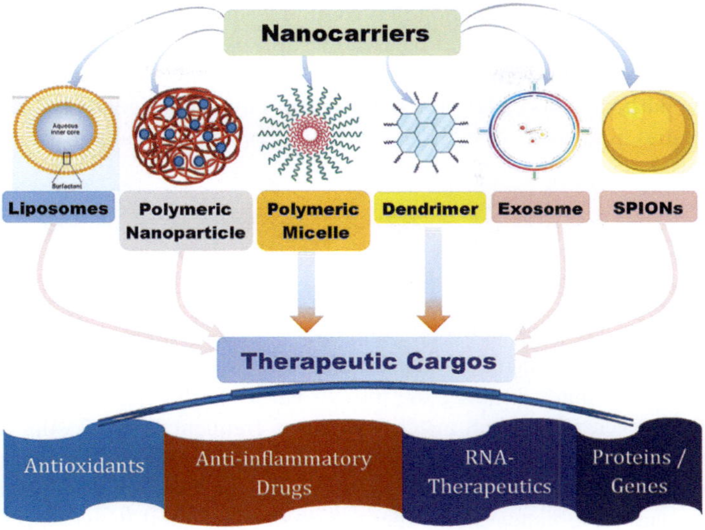

FIGURE 4.2 Summary of representative nanocarriers and cargos.

Antioxidant NPs have shown reductions in oxidative biomarkers and improvements in renal function parameters such as serum creatinine and urinary albumin excretion. Although most studies remain at the proof-of-concept or early preclinical stage, the consistency of beneficial outcomes across different platforms and disease models suggests that nanotechnology can meaningfully address multiple pathogenic mechanisms of DN simultaneously [40].

4.3.6 Translational Challenges and Future Considerations

Despite the encouraging preclinical data, several translational barriers remain. Biodistribution and long-term fate of NPs in renal and extra-renal tissues must be carefully characterized, particularly for chronic administration. Renal toxicity, immunogenicity, and unintended accumulation in the reticuloendothelial system remain key safety concerns [41].

Manufacturing challenges include reproducible large-scale synthesis, batch-to-batch consistency, and compliance with regulatory standards for complex nanomedicines. Additionally, most DN nanotherapies have yet to be evaluated in large animal models or advanced toward clinical trials, highlighting a significant gap between laboratory success and clinical translation [42].

4.4 DIABETIC RETINOPATHY (DR) – OCULAR NANOMEDICINE

Ocular nanomedicine DR remains a leading cause of vision loss among working-age adults worldwide. Over the past decade, nanotechnology-driven drug delivery and imaging approaches have been developed specifically to overcome the anatomical and physiological barriers of the eye, prolong therapeutic exposure in the posterior segment, reduce systemic exposure from repeated intravitreal dosing, and add diagnostic capabilities for earlier detection of microvascular injury [43].

4.4.1 Pathogenesis Recap: Microvascular Damage, VEGF-Driven Neovascularization, Inflammation

DR is driven by chronic hyperglycemia-induced microvascular injury. Early stages (non-proliferative DR) show microaneurysms, capillary dropout, and retinal ischemia; progression to proliferative

DR involves hypoxia-induced upregulation of VEGF and subsequent pathological neovascularization. DME is mediated by blood-retinal barrier disruption and inflammatory cytokines (TNF-α, IL-6, MCP-1), causing fluid accumulation and dysfunction. These overlapping angiogenic and inflammatory pathways make DR amenable to both anti-angiogenic and anti-inflammatory therapeutic strategies and explain why combination or multi-mechanistic nanosystems are attractive [44].

4.4.2 Ocular Barriers and Delivery Routes (Topical, Intravitreal, Periocular, Systemic)

The eye's anatomy imposes steep delivery challenges. The corneal/scleral epithelium, conjunctival lymphatics, vitreous gel, and inner/outer blood/retinal system barriers limit drug penetration from topical or systemic routes, making the intravitreal route the clinical standard for posterior-segment therapy. However, intravitreal injections require frequent repeat dosing (anti-VEGF every 4–8 weeks), increasing procedural risk and patient burden. Periocular and suprachoroidal routes offer alternatives for sustained posterior exposure; topical approaches remain limited but are being explored with mucoadhesive nanosystems that enhance transscleral delivery. NPs and hydrogels aim to extend intraocular residence and reduce injection frequency [45].

4.4.3 Nanocarrier Strategies for Retina Targeting (Mucoadhesive Systems, Nanoparticle-Based Sustained Release, Implants)

Multiple platform strategies have been tailored for retinal targeting:

- Mucoadhesive and surface-modified NPs (e.g., hyaluronic acid-coated albumin) enhance scleral/transscleral penetration and target CD44 on retinal cells, offering potential for non-invasive or less-frequent dosing.
- Sustained-release NPs and depot hydrogels (thermo- or shear-responsive hydrogels) are designed for intravitreal delivery to slowly release anti-VEGF or anti-inflammatory agents over months, thereby reducing injection frequency.
- Nano-enabled implants and microparticle depots combine mechanical residence with controlled release; while some are already used clinically for corticosteroids (e.g., non-nano implants), nanoformulations aim for finer control and combination delivery. Recent preclinical work shows that polymeric NP formulations of antibodies or small molecules maintain therapeutic retinal concentrations far longer than free drug [46].

4.4.4 Anti-Angiogenic Delivery, Anti-Inflammatory, and Neuroprotective Cargos

Anti-VEGF biologics (bevacizumab, ranibizumab, aflibercept) are effective but require repeated dosing. Encapsulation of anti-VEGF agents into biodegradable polymeric NPs or albumin-based carriers yields prolonged retinal retention and preserved biological activity in animal models; early preclinical studies demonstrate an equivalent anti-angiogenic effect with fewer administrations. Parallel strategies deliver small-molecule VEGFR inhibitors (e.g., apatinib) via hyaluronic acid-coated albumin NPs for sustained, targeted suppression of neovascularization [47].

Anti-inflammatory cargos (steroids, NSAIDs, cytokine inhibitors) and neuroprotective agents (melatonin, growth factors, antioxidant nanocerium) have been packaged into NPs to reduce retinal inflammation, prevent neuronal loss, and stabilize the blood-retinal barrier. Cerium oxide (CeO_2) NPs show intrinsic ROS-scavenging and neuroprotective effects in retinal models of diabetic injury, reducing oxidative stress and vascular leakage in vascular leakage in several preclinical studies [48].

4.4.5 Imaging and Diagnostics

NPs are also being developed as contrast enhancers for retinal imaging modalities (optical coherence tomography [OCT], fundus imaging, MRI). AuNPs and lanthanide/iron-based nanocontrast agents enhance optical or magnetic contrast and can be functionalized to bind angiogenic markers and inflammatory epitopes, enabling molecularly targeted imaging of early microvascular changes before gross structural damage. Theranostic NPs combine imaging reporters with drug payloads to image delivery and therapeutic response in the same agent [49].

4.4.6 Safety for Intraocular Use and Steps toward Clinical Translation

Intraocular safety is paramount. Key concerns include acute retinal toxicity, inflammation, impairment of intraocular pressure, and long-term NP retention in ocular tissues. Biocompatible carriers (albumin, PLGA, PEGylated polymers) and degradable hydrogels have favorable safety profiles in short-term animal studies; inorganic materials (gold, ceria) require careful surface modification and dose-finding to avoid aggregation or persistent tissue deposition. Regulatory translation demands standardized ocular toxicity testing (electroretinography, histology, IOP monitoring), scalable Good Manufacturing Practice (GMP), sterility assurance, and well-designed early-phase clinical trials that measure both safety and extended dosing intervals. Several recent studies emphasize these translational milestones and call for rigorous comparative studies with current anti-VEGF regimens [50].

4.5 CARDIOVASCULAR DISEASE (CVD) DIABETES NANOAPPROACHES

CVD is the leading cause of morbidity and mortality among individuals with diabetes, accounting for the majority of diabetes-related deaths worldwide. The diabetic cardiovascular phenotype is characterized by accelerated atherosclerosis, endothelial dysfunction, heightened inflammatory activation, and a pro-thrombotic state [51].

Conventional pharmacotherapy reduces cardiovascular risk but does not fully prevent disease progression, particularly in patients with long-standing diabetes or established vascular damage. Nanotechnology-based diagnostic and therapeutic strategies have thus appeared as potential means to better target molecules, detect early lesions, and increase the efficacy and safety of cardiovascular procedures in diabetes [52].

4.5.1 CVD in Diabetes: Mechanistic Overview

Chronic hyperglycemia promotes oxidative stress, AGE formation, and dysregulated lipid metabolism, leading to endothelial injury and impaired nitric oxide bioavailability. These changes accelerate atherogenesis through increased vascular permeability, macrophage infiltration, and foam cell formation. In diabetes, atherosclerotic plaques tend to be more diffuse, lipid-rich, and inflammation-prone, increasing the risk of rupture [53].

Endothelial dysfunction is a key early event, characterized by impaired vasodilation, increased expression of adhesion molecules (vascular cell adhesion molecule-1 [VCAM-1], intercellular adhesion molecule-1 [ICAM-1]), and enhanced leukocyte recruitment. Concurrently, diabetes induces a pro-thrombotic milieu via platelet hyperreactivity, elevated fibrinogen levels, and impaired fibrinolysis. These interlinked mechanisms explain why patients with diabetes experience higher rates of myocardial infarction, stroke, and restenosis after vascular interventions [54].

4.5.2 Nanotechnology for Imaging Atherosclerotic Plaques and Molecular Markers

NP-based imaging platforms aim to detect vulnerable plaques and molecular markers of inflammation before clinical events occur. Iron oxide NPs have been extensively studied as MRI contrast agents for imaging macrophage-rich atherosclerotic plaques, enabling visualization of inflammatory activity rather than luminal narrowing alone. Surface functionalization with ligands targeting scavenger receptors or adhesion molecules enhances plaque specificity [55].

AuNPs and liposomal contrast agents have been explored for CT and optical imaging agents, providing high signal intensity and tunable surface chemistry. In diabetic atherosclerosis models, targeted NPs binding to VCAM-1, oxidized LDL, or fibrin have shown better detection of early lesions and thrombus formation. More recent work focuses on theranostics NPs that combine imaging reporters with therapeutic payloads, allowing simultaneous plaque visualization and local drug delivery [56].

4.5.3 Nanotherapeutic: Anti-Inflammatory, Anti-Atherosclerotic Delivery, Targeted Thrombolysis

Nanotherapeutic approaches for diabetic CVD primarily target inflammation, lipid accumulation, and thrombosis. Liposomal and polymeric NPs encapsulating statins or anti-inflammatory agents have demonstrated enhanced accumulation within atherosclerotic plaques, leading to reduced macrophage content and plaque stabilization in diabetic rodent models. By concentrating drugs at disease sites, these systems reduce systemic exposure and associated adverse effects [57].

Targeted delivery of nucleic acid therapeutics has also gained momentum. NP-mediated delivery of siRNA or miRNA modulators targeting inflammatory pathways (e.g., NF-kB signaling) has shown reduced vascular inflammation and enhanced endothelial function in experimental diabetes. Antioxidant NPs, including cerium oxide and polymer-based ROS-scavenging systems, attenuate oxidative stress and preserve endothelial integrity [57, 58].

For thrombotic complications, fibrin- or platelet-targeted NPs carrying thrombolytic agents (e.g., tissue plasminogen activator) have been developed to enable site-specific clot dissolution. Preclinical studies demonstrate that NP-mediated thrombolysis achieves effective clot resolution at lower doses, reducing hemorrhage risk, an important consideration in patients with diabetes with fragile vasculature [58].

4.5.4 Nanomaterials for Endothelium Repair and Stent Coatings

Nanotechnology also plays a critical role in vascular repair and interventional cardiology. Nanostructured stent coatings incorporating biodegradable polymers, nitric oxide-releasing materials, or anti-proliferative drugs aim to reduce restenosis and late thrombosis, both of which are more common in patients with diabetes. Compared with conventional drug-eluting stents, nano-engineered coatings can allow more uniform drug distribution and controlled release kinetics [58].

Endothelium-targeted nanomaterials are being explored to promote re-endothelialization after vascular injury. Nanofiber scaffolds and NP-functionalized surfaces that mimic ECM cues enhance endothelial cell adhesion and migration while inhibiting smooth muscle cell proliferation. In diabetic animal models, such strategies have demonstrated improved endothelial recovery and reduced neointimal hyperplasia [59].

4.5.5 Preclinical and Early Clinical Studies

A substantial body of preclinical evidence supports the efficacy of NP-based imaging and therapy for diabetic CVD. However, translation to clinical practice remains limited. While several NP contrast agents and nano-based stent coatings have entered clinical evaluation in broader cardiovascular populations, diabetes-specific trials are scarce.

Key barriers include incomplete understanding of long-term NP biodistribution, potential immunogenicity, and altered pharmacokinetics in patients with diabetes. Additional challenges include manufacturing complexity, regulatory uncertainty, and the necessity for large-scale reproducible synthesis. Importantly, most studies focus on surrogate endpoints (plaque size, inflammatory markers) rather than hard cardiovascular outcomes [60].

4.6 SHARED MECHANISTIC TARGETS ACROSS DIABETIC COMPLICATIONS

Despite organ-specific manifestations, DN, retinopathy, and CVD share several core pathological mechanisms driven by chronic hyperglycemia. These common pathways – oxidative stress, inflammation, dysregulated angiogenesis, and ECM remodeling – provide a strong rationale for platform nanotechnologies capable of addressing multiple complications simultaneously [61].

4.6.1 Oxidative Stress and ROS: Nanoparticle Antioxidant Strategies

Excessive production of ROS is a unifying feature of diabetic tissue injury, contributing to podocyte loss in the kidney, endothelial dysfunction in the vasculature, and neurovascular damage in the retina. NP-based antioxidant strategies aim to overcome the poor stability and bioavailability of conventional antioxidants. Cerium oxide (CeO_2) NPs, which exhibit regenerative redox cycling between Ce^{3+}/Ce^{4+} states, have shown prolonged ROS-scavenging activity in diabetic kidney, retinal, and cardiovascular models. Polymeric NPs loaded with natural antioxidants (e.g., curcumin, resveratrol) similarly show enhanced tissue retention and reduced oxidative biomarkers compared with free compounds, supporting a shared therapeutic role across complications [62].

4.6.2 Chronic Inflammation: Targeted Immune Modulation via Nanosystems

Low-grade chronic inflammation underlies disease progression in all major diabetic complications, characterized by macrophage infiltration, cytokine release, and activation of NF-κB-dependent signaling. Nanocarriers targeting inflammatory cells or adhesion molecules enable localized immune modulation while limiting systemic immunosuppression. Liposomal and polymeric NPs delivering corticosteroids, anti-TNF agents, or siRNA against inflammatory mediators have reduced renal fibrosis, retinal vascular leakage, and atherosclerotic plaque inflammation in preclinical diabetes models. These results support inflammation-targeted nanotherapy as a cross-cutting strategy [63].

4.6.3 Angiogenesis Dysregulation: Balancing between Inhibition and Regeneration

Angiogenesis in diabetes is paradoxical – excessive and pathological in the retina, yet insufficient or dysfunctional in the ischemic myocardium and peripheral vasculature. Nanodelivery systems enable spatial and temporal control over angiogenic signaling. Anti-VEGF NP formulations inhibit aberrant retinal neovascularization, whereas pro-angiogenic growth factor-loaded NP or nanofibrous scaffolds stimulate functional neovascularization in ischemic cardiovascular tissue. This context-dependent modulation is difficult to achieve with conventional therapies but is well suited to engineered nanosystems [64].

4.6.4 Glycation and ECM Remodeling: Nano-Enabled Modulation

AGEs, and ECM remodeling drive fibrosis and stiffness in the kidney, retina, and vasculature. NPs for AGE inhibitors, anti-fibrotic, or gene modulators against TGF-v/Smad pathways have shown less accumulation of ECM and better tissue structure in diabetic models. Such methodologies thus emphasize opportunities to intervene upstream in structural tissue disease [65].

4.7 SAFETY, TOXICOLOGY, AND REGULATORY CONSIDERATIONS

While nanotechnology offers clear advantages for targeted therapy and diagnostics in diabetic complications, its clinical translation depends critically on rigorous evaluation of safety, toxicology, and regulatory compliance. Diabetes is a lifelong condition that needs chronic or repeated treatment; hence, issues of long-term safety are especially important compared to short-term therapy used in oncology or acute disease [66].

4.7.1 Nano-Toxicology: Bio-Distribution, Long-Term Accumulation, and Immunogenicity

NP biodistribution is controlled by size, shape, surface charge, and protein corona formation. Numerous in vivo studies show preferential accumulation of many NPs in the liver, spleen, and kidneys via the reticuloendothelial system. In diabetic settings, altered vascular permeability and chronic inflammation may further modify NP distribution and clearance profiles. Long-term accumulation is a special concern for inorganic NPs (e.g., gold, iron oxide, cerium oxide), which may remain for prolonged periods (months) in tissues [67].

Immunogenicity and unintended immune activation represent additional risks. Surface chemistry and contaminants during synthesis can trigger complement activation, macrophage uptake, or cytokine release. PEGylation and biomimetic coatings (albumin, cell membranes) have been found to diminish immune recognition but repeated administration can cause anti-PEG antibodies and altered clearance. For ocular and renal applications, even mild inflammation reactions may have important functional consequences and therefore require close toxicological evaluation [68].

4.7.2 Standardization and Characterization Challenges

Reproducible physicochemical characterization remains a major bottleneck for regulatory approval. Critical quality attributes include particle size distribution, polydispersity index, zeta potential, surface chemistry, drug loading, and release kinetics. Small changes in synthesis conditions can significantly alter biological behavior. Recent interlaboratory studies highlight discrepancies between dynamic light scattering, electron microscopy, and NP tracking analysis, underscoring the need for standardized measurement protocols. Surface functionalization adds further complexity: ligand density, orientation, and stability must be controlled. For chronic indications such as diabetes, batch-to-batch variability poses unacceptable risks, as long-term exposure magnifies the effects of subtle formulation differences [69].

4.7.3 Regulatory Pathways and Manufacturing Hurdles

Regulatory agencies generally evaluate nanomedicines within existing drug or device frameworks, but require additional data on nano-specific properties. Preclinical requirements normally include prolonged biodistribution studies, chronic toxicity studies, immunotoxicity studies, and degradation or clearance profiles. For ocular and renal nanomedicines, organ-specific toxicity endpoints (e.g., retinal function, glomerular integrity) are gaining more focus [70].

GMP production presents practical challenges, including scalable synthesis, sterile processing, endotoxin control, and long-term stability. Complex multifunctional NPs, especially theranostic systems, face higher regulatory scrutiny due to their combined drug-device properties. These hurdles have delayed the transition from promising preclinical studies to first-in-human trials for diabetic complications [70].

4.7.4 Risk-Benefit Considerations for Chronic Diseases

In diabetes, acceptable risk thresholds are lower than in life-threatening malignancies. Nanotechnologies must therefore demonstrate not only superior efficacy but also long-term safety and clinical advantage over established therapies. Strategies such as biodegradable carriers, renal-clearable NPs, and locally administered sustained-release systems aim to improve the risk-benefit balance. Ultimately, careful patient selection, dosing strategies, and post-marketing surveillance will be essential for successful adoption [71].

4.8 MANUFACTURING, SCALE-UP AND COMMERCIALIZATION PATHWAYS

The successful translation of nanotechnology-based therapies for diabetic complications depends not only on biological efficacy, but also on robust manufacturing, cost-effectiveness, and viable commercialization strategies. Many nano-enabled platforms demonstrating strong preclinical performance face significant challenges when transitioning from laboratory-scale synthesis to industrial production.

4.8.1 Reproducible Production and Quality Control as Scale

Scalable manufacturing requires reproducible control over critical quality attributes, including particle size distribution, surface chemistry, drug loading, and release kinetics. Batch-to-batch variability remains a major obstacle, particularly for complex multifunctional NPs. Continuous manufacturing approaches, such as microfluidic-assisted NPs and in-line quality monitoring, are increasingly adopted to improve reproducibility and regulatory compliance. Implementation of standardized analytical procedures for physicochemical characterization is required to satisfy the GMP requirements in the case of products for chronic administration in diabetes [72].

4.8.2 Cost, Stability, Cold-Chain Issues, and Formulation Optimization

Cost considerations strongly influence commercial feasibility, particularly in diabetes, where long-term treatment and large patient populations are expected. Expensive raw materials, multi-step synthesis, and sterile processing can substantially increase production costs. Formulation stability during storage and transport is another key factor; many NP systems require cold chains to certify physicochemical stability and drug potency. Efforts are being made to enhance stability using lyophilization, polymer choice, and surface modification in an effort to mitigate logistical challenges and increase accessibility on a global scale [73].

4.8.3 Intellectual Property (IP) and Partnership Models

IP protection for nanomedicines often spans material composition, fabrication methods, and therapeutic application, creating complex patent landscapes. Effective commercialization increasingly relies on early partnerships between academic innovators, biotechnology companies, and pharmaceutical manufacturers. Industry-academia collaborations enable access to GMP facilities, regulatory expertise, and clinical trial infrastructure, accelerating translation from proof-of-concept to market. Public-private partnerships and licensing models have emerged as key drivers of advancing nano-enabled nanotherapies for diabetic complications toward clinical and commercial realization [74].

4.9 FUTURE DIRECTIONS AND RESEARCH PRIORITIES

Continued advances in nanotechnology are expected to reshape the prevention and management of diabetic complications; however, progress will depend on strategic alignment of innovation with clinical and societal needs. Future research must prioritize multifunctionality, personalization, robust clinical evaluation, and equitable access.

4.9.1 Multi-Functional and Combination Nanotherapies

Next-generation nanosystems are increasingly designed to co-deliver multiple therapeutic modalities, such as small-molecule drugs, nucleic acids, and imaging agents within a single platform. For DN, retinopathy, and CVD, combination strategies targeting inflammation, oxidative stress, and fibrosis simultaneously may offer superior efficacy compared with monotherapies. Theranostic NPs that integrate diagnostic imaging with controlled drug release could enable real-time monitoring of therapeutic response and disease progression, allowing adaptive treatment strategies in chronic disease settings [75].

4.9.2 Accuracy and Personalized Nanomedicine

Heterogeneity in disease progression and treatment response among patients with diabetes underscores the need for precision nanomedicine. Biomarker-guided targeting, using molecular signatures such as inflammatory markers, angiogenic factors, or genetic risk profiles, can inform NP design and patient selection. Advances in omics technologies and machine learning procedures are anticipated to facilitate the transition from 'blanket' therapeutic paradigms to address the aim of patient subgroups most likely to benefit from certain nano-enabled interventions being evaluated [76].

4.9.3 Clinical Trial Design for Chronic Diabetic Complications

Clinical translation of nanotherapies requires trial designs adapted to chronic, slowly progressive complications. Future trials should incorporate longer follow-up periods, clinically meaningful endpoints (e.g., renal function decline, vision preservation, cardiovascular events) and comparative effectiveness against standard-of-care treatments. Adaptive trial designs and biomarker-based stratification may increase efficiency and take into account safety issues faced by long-term exposure to NPs [77].

4.9.4 Ethical and Equity Considerations

Ethical considerations include long-term safety, informed consent for novel technologies, and post-marketing surveillance. Equity is also a very important issue, as diabetes disproportionately impacts low- and middle-income countries. High production costs and the cold chain required may restrict the availability of advanced nanomedicines. Research priorities should therefore include cost-effective and scalable platforms and policies to promote global accessibility [78].

4.10 CONCLUSIONS

Nanotechnology represents a transformative approach for addressing the complex and interrelated complications of diabetes, including nephropathy, retinopathy, and CVDs. By enabling precise control over drug delivery, tissue targeting, and releasing kinetics, nano-enabled platforms offer solutions to many limitations of conventional therapies, such as poor bioavailability, off-target effects, and the need for frequent dosing. Preclinical evidence increasingly supports the potential of nanocarriers to modulate shared pathogenic mechanisms – oxidative stress, inflammation, angiogenesis dysregulation, and fibrosis – across multiple organ systems. However, the translation of these advances into clinical practices depends on rigorous evaluation of long-term safety, standardized manufacturing, and carefully designed clinical trials tailored to chronic disease setting. Equally important are considerations of cost, accessibility, and regulatory clarity to ensure broad and equitable impact. With further interdisciplinary collaboration and a focus on clinically meaningful outcomes, nanotechnology has the potential to play a major role in the prevention, diagnosis, and management of diabetes-related complications.

ACKNOWLEDGMENTS

The authors express special thanks to the editors for providing necessary support and guidance.

REFERENCES

1. Hossain MJ, Al-Mamun M, Islam MR. Diabetes mellitus, the fastest growing global public health concern: Early detection should be focused. Health Science Reports. 2024;7(3):e2004.
2. Crasto W, Patel V, Davies MJ, Khunti K. Prevention of microvascular complications of diabetes. Endocrinology and Metabolism Clinics of North America. 2021;50(3):431–55.
3. Pradeepa R, Mohan V. Epidemiology of Chronic Complications of Diabetes: A Global Perspective. In Chronic Complications of Diabetes Mellitus 2024 (pp. 11–23). Academic Press.
4. White KC, Serpa-Neto A, Hurford R, Clement P, Laupland KB, See E, McCullough J, White H, Shekar K, Tabah A, Ramanan M. Sepsis-associated acute kidney injury in the intensive care unit: Incidence, patient characteristics, timing, trajectory, treatment, and associated outcomes. A multicenter, observational study. Intensive Care Medicine. 2023;49(9):1079–89.
5. Sharma S, Venkatesh P, Kalra S, Verma H, Kapoor N, Nagendra L, Unnikrishnan AG, Prakash S, Sahay M, Hada M, Kumawat D. Evidence-based guidelines for intravitreal anti-VEGF therapy for diabetic retinopathy in chronic kidney disease. Diabetes Therapy. 2025;16(11):2073–82.
6. Islam S, Ahmed MM, Islam MA, Hossain N, Chowdhury MA. Advances in nanoparticles in targeted drug delivery-a review. Results in Surfaces and Interfaces. 2025;19:100529.
7. Nasiruddin M, Neyaz MK, Das S. Nanotechnology-based approach in tuberculosis treatment. Tuberculosis Research and Treatment. 2017;2017(1):4920209.
8. Desai N, Koppisetti H, Pande S, Shukla H, Sirsat B, Ditani AS, Mallick PP, Kathar U, Kalia K, Tekade RK. Nanomedicine in the treatment of diabetic nephropathy. Future Medicinal Chemistry. 2021;13(7):663–86.
9. Chen X, Dai W, Li H, Yan Z, Liu Z, He L. Targeted drug delivery strategy: A bridge to the therapy of diabetic kidney disease. Drug Delivery. 2023;30(1):2160518.
10. Sarkhel S, Shuvo SM, Ansari MA, Mondal S, Kapat P, Ghosh A, Sarkar T, Biswas R, Atanase LI, Carauleanu A. Nanotechnology-based approaches for the management of diabetes mellitus: An innovative solution to long-lasting challenges in antidiabetic drug delivery. Pharmaceutics. 2024;16(12):1572.
11. Zucaro L, Longobardi C, Miele A, Villanova A, Suzumoto Y. Nanocarrier-based drug delivery systems targeting kidney diseases. Kidney and Blood Pressure Research. 2024;49(1):884–97.
12. Dang M, Shoichet MS. Long-acting ocular injectables: Are we looking in the right direction?. Advanced Science. 2024;11(8):2306463.
13. Patel SR, Berezovsky DE, McCarey BE, Zarnitsyn V, Edelhauser HF, Prausnitz MR. Targeted administration into the suprachoroidal space using a microneedle for drug delivery to the posterior segment of the eye. Investigative Ophthalmology & Visual Science. 2012;53(8):4433–41.
14. Kompella UB, Amrite AC, Ravi RP, Durazo SA. Nanomedicines for back of the eye drug delivery, gene delivery, and imaging. Progress in Retinal and Eye Research. 2013;36:172–98.
15. Wang S, He H, Mao Y, Zhang Y, Gu N. Advances in atherosclerosis theranostics harnessing iron oxide-based nanoparticles. Advanced Science. 2024;11(17):2308298.
16. Kommineni N, Saka R, Khan W, Domb AJ. Non-polymer drug-eluting coronary stents. Drug Delivery and Translational Research. 2018;8(4):903–17.
17. Huang Y, Wang J, Jiang K, Chung EJ. Improving kidney targeting: The influence of nanoparticle physicochemical properties on kidney interactions. Journal of Controlled Release. 2021;334:127–37.
18. Jafari M, Heidari D, Ebrahimnejad P. Synthesizing and characterizing functionalized short multiwall carbon nanotubes with folate, magnetite and polyethylene glycol as multi-targeted nanocarrier of anti-cancer drugs. Iranian Journal of Pharmaceutical Research: IJPR. 2016;15(2):449.
19. Mohsen AM. Nanotechnology advanced strategies for the management of diabetes mellitus. Current Drug Targets. 2019;20(10):995–1007.
20. Iminova R, Berganayeva G, Shepilov D, Almabekova A, Zhurtbayeva A, Abdurakhmanova L, Vassilina G, Nurmahanova A, Kairalapova G, Dyusebaeva M. From PEGylation to next-generation polymers: Overcoming biological barriers–a review. Molecules. 2026;31:675. https://doi.org/10.3390/molecules31040675.
21. Alnasser Y, Kambhampati SP, Nance E, Rajbhandari L, Shrestha S, Venkatesan A, Kannan RM, Kannan S. Preferential and increased uptake of hydroxyl-terminated PAMAM dendrimers by activated microglia in rabbit brain mixed glial culture. Molecules. 2018;23(5):1025.
22. Vazirov RA, Sokovnin SY, Ilves VG, Bazhukova IN, Pizurova N, Kuznetsov MV. Physicochemical characterization and antioxidant properties of cerium oxide nanoparticles. Journal of Physics: Conference Series. 2018;1115(3):032094.
23. Das SS, Bharadwaj P, Bilal M, Barani M, Rahdar A, Taboada P, Bungau S, Kyzas GZ. Stimuli-responsive polymeric nanocarriers for drug delivery, imaging, and theragnosis. Polymers. 2020;12(6):1397.

24. Rinaldi A, Caraffi R, Grazioli MV, Oddone N, Giardino L, Tosi G, Vandelli MA, Calzà L, Ruozi B, Duskey JT. Applications of the ROS-responsive thioketal linker for the production of smart nanomedicines. Polymers. 2022;14(4):687.
25. Vagena IA, Malapani C, Gatou MA, Lagopati N, Pavlatou EA. Enhancement of EPR effect for passive tumor targeting: Current status and future perspectives. Applied Sciences. 2025;15(6):3189.
26. Wang Z, Zhang C. Nanomaterials for targeted therapy of kidney diseases: Strategies and advances. Materials Today Bio. 2025;31:101534.
27. Aboushoushah SF. Iron oxide nanoparticles enhancing magnetic resonance imaging: A review of the latest advancements. Journal of Science: Advanced Materials and Devices. 2025;10(2):100875.
28. Xue R, Gui D, Zheng L, Zhai R, Wang F, Wang N. Mechanistic insight and management of diabetic nephropathy: Recent progress and future perspective. Journal of Diabetes Research. 2017;2017(1):1839809.
29. Ratan Y, Rajput A, Pareek A, Pareek A, Singh G. Comprehending the role of metabolic and hemodynamic factors alongside different signaling pathways in the pathogenesis of diabetic nephropathy. International Journal of Molecular Sciences. 2025;26(7):3330.
30. Rispoli RM, Popolo A, De Fabrizio V, d'Emmanuele di Villa Bianca R, Autore G, Dalli J, Marzocco S. Targeting inflammatory imbalance in chronic kidney disease: Focus on anti-inflammatory and resolution mediators. International Journal of Molecular Sciences. 2025;26(7):3072.
31. Naren T, Lv W, Aazmi A, Wang Y, Yu H, Lee JY, Yang H, Yu M, Jiang X, Yang H, Ma L. Construction, evaluation, and applications of renal barrier-on-a-chip system. Bioactive Materials. 2026;59:421–49.
32. Vignesh A, Menaka C, Amal TC, Selvakumar S, Vasanth K. Exploring the dual impact of nanoparticles on human well-being: A comprehensive review of risks and benefits. Next Nanotechnology. 2025;8:100223.
33. Shang S, Li X, Wang H, Zhou Y, Pang K, Li P, Liu X, Zhang M, Li W, Li Q, Chen X. Targeted therapy of kidney disease with nanoparticle drug delivery materials. Bioactive Materials. 2024;37:206–21.
34. Wang J, Masehi-Lano JJ, Chung EJ. Peptide and antibody ligands for renal targeting: Nanomedicine strategies for kidney disease. Biomaterials Science. 2017;5(8):1450–59.
35. Peng C, Huang Y, Zheng J. Renal clearable nanocarriers: Overcoming the physiological barriers for precise drug delivery and clearance. Journal of Controlled Release. 2020;322:64–80.
36. Parvin N, Joo SW, Mandal TK. Biodegradable and stimuli-responsive nanomaterials for targeted drug delivery in autoimmune diseases. Journal of Functional Biomaterials. 2025;16(1):24.
37. Zou Y, Dai J, Li J, Liu M, Li R, Li G, Lai J, Wang L. Role of the TGF-β/Smad signaling pathway in the transition from acute kidney injury to chronic kidney disease. International Journal of Molecular Medicine. 2025;56(4):162.
38. Li CW, Li LL, Chen S, Zhang JX, Lu WL. Antioxidant nanotherapies for the treatment of inflammatory diseases. Frontiers in Bioengineering and Biotechnology. 2020;8:200.
39. Wang Y, Shu H, Cheng G, Zhou X, Gao H, Qi Z, Ma X, Zhang W, Wang J. A novel treatment for diabetic nephropathy: Folate receptor-targeted delivery of Tlr4 siRNA via functionalized PLGA nanoparticles in streptozotocin-induced diabetic murine models. 2025;SSRN 5289782.
40. Wang X, Huang X, Yang B. siRNA-mediated therapeutic approaches improve acute kidney injury and limit its worsening. Frontiers in Pharmacology. 2025;16:1697460.
41. Bourquin J, Milosevic A, Hauser D, Lehner R, Blank F, Petri-Fink A, Rothen-Rutishauser B. Biodistribution, clearance, and long-term fate of clinically relevant nanomaterials. Advanced Materials. 2018;30(19):1704307.
42. Paliwal R, Babu RJ, Palakurthi S. Nanomedicine scale-up technologies: Feasibilities and challenges. AAPS PharmSciTech. 2014;15(6):1527–34.
43. Lin X, Zhou Y, Lv K, Wu W, Chen C. Nanomedicine-based ophthalmic drug delivery systems for the treatment of ocular diseases. International Journal of Nanomedicine. 2025;31:9221–49.
44. Ciftci, SN. Epidemiology and pathophysiology of diabetic retinopathy; 2025.
45. Patel A, Cholkar K, Agrahari V, Mitra AK. Ocular drug delivery systems: An overview. World Journal of Pharmacology. 2013;2(2):47.
46. Sahu A, Patel AR, Shetty KH, Shah DO, Willcox MD, Maulvi FA, Desai DT. Revolutionizing age-related macular degeneration treatment: Advances and future directions in non-invasive retinal drug delivery systems. International Journal of Pharmaceutics. 2025:126009.
47. Iyer S, Lee C, Amiji MM. Biodegradable polymeric microsphere formulations of full-length anti-VEGF antibody bevacizumab for sustained intraocular delivery. Drug Delivery and Translational Research. 2025:1–2.
48. Yang C, Song S, Zhou X, Li D, Xu C, Yu C, Sun G, Lin K, Xie Y. Controlled releasing melatonin nanoparticles promote restoration of nucleus pulposus cell homeostasis for alleviating intervertebral disc degeneration. Materials Today Bio. 2025:101994.

49. Kavalaraki A, Spyratou E, Kouri MA, Efstathopoulos EP. Gold nanoparticles as contrast agents in ophthalmic imaging. Optics. 2023;4(1):74–99.
50. Xia B, Sun X, Yu L, Shi J, Zhang Z, He Z, Sun J, Luo C, Zhang S. Nanogel-Engineered drug delivery systems for enhanced ocular therapeutics. Advanced Healthcare Materials. 2025;14(32):e01730.
51. Panozzo CA, Curtis LH, Marshall J, Fine L, Wells BL, Brown JS, Haynes K, Pawloski PA, Hernandez AF, Malek S, Syat B. Incidence of statin use in older adults with and without cardiovascular disease and diabetes mellitus, January 2008–March 2018. PLoS One. 2019;14(12):e0223515.
52. Yang C, Mo L, Zhang G, Dai Y, Li B, Tan Z, Guo Y, Lu S, Hong Y, He H, Yang H. Advancements in dual-targeting nanoparticle strategies for enhanced atherosclerosis therapy: Overcoming limitations of single-targeting approaches. Bioactive Materials. 2026;55:302–33.
53. Alam S, Aijaz M. Complications of cardiovascular disease: The impact of diabetes, dyslipidemia, and metabolic disorders. World Journal of Pharmaceutical Research. 2024;13:321–56.
54. Młynarska E, Bojdo K, Frankenstein H, Krawiranda K, Kustosik N, Lisińska W, Rysz J, Franczyk B. Endothelial dysfunction as the common pathway linking obesity, hypertension and atherosclerosis. International Journal of Molecular Sciences. 2025;26(20):10096.
55. Qin J, Peng C, Zhao B, Ye K, Yuan F, Peng Z, Yang X, Huang L, Jiang M, Zhao Q, Tang G. Noninvasive detection of macrophages in atherosclerotic lesions by computed tomography enhanced with PEGylated gold nanoparticles. International Journal of Nanomedicine. 2014:5575–90.
56. Connor DM, Broome AM. Gold nanoparticles for the delivery of cancer therapeutics. Advances in Cancer Research. 2018;139:163–84.
57. Mukhtar M, Ali H, Ahmed N, Munir R, Talib S, Khan AS, Ambrus R. Drug delivery to macrophages: A review of nano-therapeutics targeted approach for inflammatory disorders and cancer. Expert Opinion on Drug Delivery. 2020;17(9):1239–57.
58. Sun M, Pontius MH, Yang S, Pendekanti T, Raghunathan S, Shavit JA, Gupta AS. Direct delivery of plasmin using clot-anchoring thrombin-responsive nanoparticles for targeted fibrinolytic therapy. Journal of Thrombosis and Haemostasis. 2023;21(4):983–94.
59. Zhuang Y, Zhang C, Cheng M, Huang J, Liu Q, Yuan G, Lin K, Yu H. Challenges and strategies for in situ endothelialization and long-term lumen patency of vascular grafts. Bioactive Materials. 2021;6(6):1791–809.
60. Jha G, Sharma RB, Sridhar S, Hayagreev D, Sinha T, Kaur H, Das A, Bollineni RL, Brijbhushankishor Nanoparticle-based therapies for cardiovascular diseases: A literature review of recent advances and clinical potential. Cureus. 2024;16(10): e72808. https://doi.org/10.7759/cureus.72808.
61. Zhao L, Yuan J, Yang Q, Ma J, Yang F, Zou Y, Liu K, Liu F. Diabetes and its complications: Molecular mechanisms, prevention and treatment. Signal Transduction and Targeted Therapy. 2026;11(1):22.
62. Rohowetz LJ, Kraus JG, Koulen P. Reactive oxygen species-mediated damage of retinal neurons: Drug development targets for therapies of chronic neurodegeneration of the retina. International Journal of Molecular Sciences. 2018;19(11):3362.
63. Cao L, Ding L, Xia Q, Zhang Z, Li M, Song S, Yin K, Li Z, Li X, Wang Z, Zhao D. Macrophage polarization in diabetic vascular complications: Mechanistic insights and therapeutic targets. Journal of Translational Medicine. 2025;23(1):1050.
64. Jia G, Martinez-Lemus LA, Sowers JR. Interaction of adipogenesis and angiogenesis in dietary-induced obesity. Diabetes. 2015;64(7):2326.
65. Zhou G, Li C, Cai L. Advanced glycation end-products induce connective tissue growth factor-mediated renal fibrosis predominantly through transforming growth factor β-independent pathway. The American Journal of Pathology. 2004;165(6):2033–43.
66. He Y, Al-Mureish A, Wu N. Nanotechnology in the treatment of diabetic complications: A comprehensive narrative review. Journal of Diabetes Research. 2021;2021(1):6612063.
67. Murali S, Thomas J, Abraham J, Kanna V, Ramachandiran S, Suruthi SS. Nanodiagnostics and nanotoxicology: A systematic review and meta-analysis on nanoparticle applications and safety in metabolic organs. OpenNano. 2025;27:100266.
68. Pondman K, Le Gac S, Kishore U. Nanoparticle-induced immune response: Health risk versus treatment opportunity?. Immunobiology. 2023;228(2):152317.
69. Hussain S, Malik NS, Tulain UR, Erum A, Mahmood A, Akram S, Javaid A, Jabeen A, Shao C, Wang S, Younas A. Itraconazole-loaded polycaprolactone nanoparticle gel for enhanced transdermal delivery: Development, characterization, and ex vivo evaluation. International Journal of Nanomedicine. 2025; 20:15655–81.
70. Stucchi F, Li M, Castellano G, Cellesi F. Regulatory framework for polymer-based nanotherapeutics in clinical translation. Frontiers in Bioengineering and Biotechnology. 2026;14:1735885.

71. Ma X, Tian Y, Yang R, Wang H, Allahou LW, Chang J, Williams G, Knowles JC, Poma A. Nanotechnology in healthcare, and its safety and environmental risks. Journal of Nanobiotechnology. 2024;22(1):715.
72. Shepherd SJ, Issadore D, Mitchell MJ. Microfluidic formulation of nanoparticles for biomedical applications. Biomaterials. 2021;274:120826.
73. Yadav PS, Singh M, Vinayagam R, Shukla P. Therapies and delivery systems for diabetic wound care: Current insights and future directions. Frontiers in Pharmacology. 2025;16:1628252.
74. Desai N, Rana D, Patel M, Bajwa N, Prasad R, Vora LK. Nanoparticle therapeutics in clinical perspective: Classification, marketed products, and regulatory landscape. Small. 2025;21:e2502315.
75. Paul P, Chacko L, Dua TK, Chakraborty P, Paul U, Phulchand VV, Jha NK, Jha SK, Kandimalla R, Dewanjee S. Nanomedicines for the management of diabetic nephropathy: Present progress and prospects. Frontiers in Endocrinology. 2023;14:1236686.
76. Franks PW, Rich SS, Linder B, Zaghloul NA, Cefalu WT. A research roadmap to address the heterogeneity of diabetes and advance precision medicine. The Journal of Clinical Endocrinology & Metabolism. 2025;110(3):601–10.
77. Zhang P, Xiao Y, Sun X, Lin X, Koo S, Yaremenko AV, Qin D, Kong N, Farokhzad OC, Tao W. Cancer nanomedicine toward clinical translation: Obstacles, opportunities, and future prospects. Med. 2023;4(3):147–67.
78. Mathur R, Swaminathan S. National ethical guidelines for biomedical & health research involving human participants, 2017: A commentary. Indian Journal of Medical Research. 2018;148(3):279–83.

5 Nano-Biosensors for Glucose Monitoring

K. Venkateswarlu
Aditya College of Pharmacy, Peddapuram, India

Rashmi Sharma
Saraswathi College of Pharmacy, Hapur, India

Muggu Murali Krishna
A.M. Reddy Memorial College of Pharmacy, Petlurivaripalem, India

Varsha Deva
Glocal University Pharmacy College, Glocal University, Saharanpur, India

Snehal Dilip Kank
Shree Santkrupa College of Pharmacy, Karad, India

Iftikhar Ahmed
College of Health Sciences, Abu Dhabi University, Abu Dhabi, United Arab Emirates

S. Manodhini Elakkiya
Karpagam College of Pharmacy, Coimbatore, India

5.1 INTRODUCTION

The global burden of diabetes is rising rapidly: recent estimates indicate that roughly 589 million adults (aged 20–79 years) are living with diabetes worldwide, with projections to exceed 800–850 million by 2050 if the current trends continue. This rising prevalence, together with substantial gaps in diagnosis and treatment in many regions, is driving an urgent demand for improved tools to detect and manage dysglycemia [1].

Continuous glucose monitoring (CGM) has transformed diabetes care by providing near-real-time glucose profiles that support tighter glycemic control and enable advanced closed-loop insulin therapy. Market analyses show excellent clinical uptake and investment in CGM technologies: the CGM device market was estimated to be the multibillion-dollar range in the early 2020s and is expected to see rapid growth in the next decade, while CGMs are being extended to people at risk beyond type 1 diabetes [2].

Despite these advances, current sensor technologies face persistent challenges that limit adoption: sensor lifetime, biocompatibility and fouling, analytical interference, calibration drift, and minimally invasive, wearable, or implantable formats. Nanotechnology offers promising routes to address many of these limitations because nanomaterials offer exceptionally high surface area, tunable surface chemistry, special electrochemical/optical properties, and the ability to integrate

DOI: 10.1201/9781003598657-5

recognition elements at molecular scales. Recent reviews document how nano-enabled transducers – including carbon nanomaterials (CNTs), noble metal nanoparticles, metal oxides, metal-organic frameworks, and engineered polymeric assemblies – have improved sensitivity, lowered detection limits, and enabled new transduction modes for glucose sensing [2, 3].

Current research trends emphasize several converging priorities for nano-biosensors: (1) moving from enzyme-based to robust non-enzymatic or biomimetic recognition to enhance long-term stability; (2) integrating flexible, printed, or microfluidic platforms for wearable continuous monitoring; and (3) combining advanced signal processing and machine learning (ML) to correct drift and interference in real-world environments. These directions aim to bridge bench-scale performance gains with clinical requirements for accuracy, safety, and manufacturability [4].

This chapter reviews the state of nano-biosensor technologies for glucose monitoring, including material platforms, recognition chemistry, transduction strategies, device integration, and translational challenges – all focused to identify realistic near-term opportunities to translate nano-biosensor technologies innovated in the laboratory into clinically viable nano-biosensor glucose sensors.

5.2 CLINICAL REQUIREMENTS

For nano-biosensors to be clinically relevant in glucose monitoring, their performance must align with stringent medical, physiological, and regulatory requirements. Unlike laboratory assays, in vivo or wearable glucose sensors operate in complex biological environments and must deliver reliable data that directly informs therapeutic decisions [5].

5.2.1 Accuracy and Clinical Targets

Accuracy is the most important clinical requirement, as glucose readings directly influence insulin dosing and the prevention of hypoglycemia. Current international standards for glucose monitoring systems emphasize high analytical performance. For self-monitoring and CGM devices, mean absolute relative difference (MARD) values of under 10% are generally considered indicative of high clinical accuracy, although next-generation CGM devices are increasingly reporting MARD values in the 7–9% range. In addition, ≥95% of measurements are expected to fall within clinically acceptable error zones when evaluated using consensus error grid analyses. Nano-biosensors must therefore have high accuracy over a broad glucose range (hypoglycemia to hyperglycemia) with little interference from endogenous electroactive species such as ascorbic acid, uric acid, and acetaminophen [6].

5.2.2 Response Time and Sampling Frequency

Physiological glucose levels change dynamically through meals, physical activity, stress, and insulin administration. Clinically useful sensors therefore need rapid response times, typically ranging from seconds to a few minutes, together with and high-frequency sampling (e.g., every 1–5 minutes) for CGM applications. Excessive sensor lag may result in rapid glucose excursions being masked and/or therapeutic response being delayed. Nano-enabled transducers, internationally dissolved diffusion routes, and high transceiver reactivity are especially adapted for quick signal generation in addition to real-time tracing of the kinetics of glucose [7].

5.2.3 Biocompatibility and Safety

Long-term biocompatibility is essential, especially for implantable or minimally invasive sensors. Clinical deployment requires materials that do not induce significant inflammation, fibrosis, or immune rejection, as these responses can impair sensor accuracy through biofouling and signal drift. Nanomaterials must also demonstrate low cytotoxicity, controlled degradation, and low systemic exposure. Importantly, regulatory evaluation increasingly focuses on chronic safety, emphasizing stable performance over days to weeks rather than short-term analytical excellence. Addressing these biological limitations is just as important as optimizing sensor sensitivity for the successful clinical translation of nano-biosensors [8].

5.3 CONVENTIONAL GLUCOSE SENSORS

Conventional glucose monitoring technologies form the clinical and technological foundation upon which nano-biosensor innovations are built. Understanding their operating principles and limitations is essential for contextualizing the need for the next generation of nano-enabled systems.

5.3.1 Strip/Electrochemical Sensors Enzymes

Disposable electrochemical test strips remain the most widely used method of self-monitoring of blood glucose (SMBG). These sensors are predominantly based on enzyme-catalyzed electrochemical detection, using glucose oxidase (GOx) or glucose dehydrogenase (GDH) immobilized on electrode surfaces. Upon glucose oxidation, electrons are transferred via mediators to generate a current proportional to glucose concentration. Modern strip-based sensors provide high analytical accuracy and rapid readout, usually within 5–10 seconds, and meet international performance standards for clinical use [9].

However, strip-based monitoring provides only intermittent glucose measurements, requiring finger-prick blood sampling multiple times per day. This approach fails to capture rapid glycemic excursions, nocturnal hypoglycemia, or postprandial variability. In addition, enzymatic instability, hematocrit effects, and interference from endogenous electro-active compounds remain inherent limitations. These constraints have driven the transition toward continuous sensing modalities [10].

5.3.2 Commercial CGM Overview

CGM systems represent a major advancement in diabetes management. Current CGMs generally use subcutaneous enzymatic electrochemical sensors that measure interstitial glucose at 1–5 minute intervals, and the resulting glucose concentrations are used to display current glucose trends, glucose alerts, and time-in-range measurements. Recent generations of CGM devices show sensor longevity of 7–14 days, manufacturer calibration (or limited calibration), and MARD values that are often less than 10% [10].

Despite their success, existing CGMs still have limitations, including sensor lag between blood and interstitial glucose, foreign body responses causing signal drift, limited sensor longevity, and enzyme-based chemistry. These unresolved issues highlight the need for alternative materials, architectures, and transduction strategies and present a clear opportunity for nano-biosensor technologies to go well beyond the performance of current commercial CGM systems [11].

5.4 WHY NANOTECHNOLOGY?

Nanotechnology has become a powerful enabler for next-generation glucose biosensors because it directly addresses many of the analytical and biological limitations of conventional sensing platforms. By engineering materials and interfaces at the nanometer scale, it is then possible to increase sensitivity, speed, and device integration in ways that cannot be easily achieved with bulk materials [4, 12].

5.4.1 Advantages at the Nanoscale

At the nanoscale, materials exhibit an exceptionally high surface-to-volume ratio, which significantly increases the density of active sites available for glucose recognition and signal transduction.

This property enables improved sensitivity and lower limits of detection, supporting accurate glucose measurement even in dilute biofluids, such as interstitial fluid, sweat, or tears. Nanomaterials also exhibit unique electronic, optical, and catalytic properties – for example, enhanced electron transfer in CNTs, localized surface plasmon resonance (LSPR) in noble metal nanoparticles, and intrinsic electrocatalytic activity in metal oxides. These characteristics have enabled the creation of both sophisticated enzymatic sensors with faster kinetics and non-enzymatic glucose sensors that avoid enzyme instability [13].

Nanotechnology further supports miniaturization and integration, allowing sensors to be embedded into flexible, wearable, or implantable platforms compatible with CGM. Nanoscale architectures reduce diffusion distances and thus reduce response time and allow for multiplexed or multimodal sensing in combination with microelectronics and wireless systems. Importantly, on the nanoscale, surface functionalization allows precise control over biomolecule immobilization, antifouling coatings, and selective glucose recognition [14].

5.4.2 Challenges Specific to Nanoapproaches

Despite these advantages, nano-enabled glucose sensors face distinct challenges that complicate clinical translation. Reproducibility and batch-to-batch variability remain significant issues, as small changes in nanomaterial size, shape, or surface chemistry can markedly affect sensor performance. Long-term biocompatibility and stability are also critical concerns, particularly for implantable devices, where nanoparticle leaching, degradation, and immune responses may compromise safety and accuracy. In addition, nanosensors may be more vulnerable to biofouling and signal drift in complex biological environments. Finally, scalable manufacturing and regulatory validation of nanomaterial-based devices remain nontrivial, underscoring the need to balance nanoscale innovation with practical clinical requirements [15].

5.5 NANOMATERIAL PLATFORMS

The performance of nano-biosensors for glucose monitoring is largely determined by the choice of nanomaterial platform, as its material properties govern sensitivity, selectivity, stability, and compatibility with device architectures. Recent advances have focused on tailoring nanoscale interfaces to optimize electron transfer, catalytic activity, and biological interactions [16]. The key nanomaterial platforms used in glucose biosensing, along with their principal advantages, limitations, and representative applications, are summarized in Table 5.1

5.5.1 Gold Nanoparticles and Plasmonics

Gold nanoparticles (AuNPs) are among the most widely reported nanomaterials in glucose biosensing due to their excellent electrical conductivity, chemical stability, and biocompatibility. AuNPs improve electron transfer between GOx and electrode surfaces, improving signal amplification in enzymatic sensors. Their surfaces are readily functionalized with thiolated enzymes, polymers, or antifouling layers, enabling controlled biointerfaces. Beyond electrochemical sensing, AuNPs support plasmonic transduction, where LSPR enables optical glucose detection through refractive index changes or enzyme-mediated reactions. Recent work has emphasized plasmonic nanostructures that enable label-free, real-time glucose monitoring with high sensitivity, although integration into compact wearable devices remains challenging [23].

5.5.2 Carbon Nanomaterials (Graphene)

Carbon nanotubes (CNTs) and graphene-based materials are central to nano-biosensor development because of their exceptional electrical conductivity, mechanical flexibility, and large surface area.

TABLE 5.1
Comparison of Nanomaterial Platforms for Glucose Biosensing

Nanomaterial Platform	Key Advantages	Main Limitations	Applications	References
Gold nanoparticles	High conductivity, easy biofunctionalization, plasmonic effects	Cost, limited flexibility	Enzymatic electrochemical sensors, plasmonic optical glucose sensors	[17]
CNTs, graphene	Large surface area, fast electron transfer, mechanically flexible	Aggregation batch variability	Wearable and flexible CGM electrodes	[16, 18]
Quantum dots/ semiconductor NPs	Strong fluorescence, high photostability	Potential toxicity regulatory hurdles	Optical and fluorescence-based glucose sensing	[19]
Metal oxides (NiO, CuO, ZnO)	Intrinsic electrocatalytic activity, enzyme-free detection	Limited selectivity fouling	Non-enzymatic electrochemical glucose sensors	[20]
Metal-organic framework (MOFs) and porous materials	High porosity, tunable chemistry, enzyme protection	Aqueous stability concerns	Enzyme immobilization and hybrid sensing platforms	[21]
Conductive polymers and hybrids	Flexible, biocompatible, scalable processing	Long-term electrical drift	Skin-mounted and implantable glucose sensors	[17, 22]

CNTs provide efficient pathways for electron transport, reducing over-potential and enabling rapid electrochemical response. Graphene and its derivatives (graphene oxide and reduced graphene oxide) offer tunable surface chemistry for enzyme immobilization and antifouling modification. These materials have been widely applied in flexible and wearable glucose sensors, including epidermal and textile-based devices. Importantly, CNTs have also enabled non-enzymatic glucose sensing through catalytic surface reactions, although selectivity in complex biofluids remains an area of research [24].

5.5.3 Quantum Dots and Semiconductor Nanoparticles

Quantum dots (QDs) and other semiconductor nanoparticles introduce unique size-dependent optical and electronic properties that are attractive for glucose sensing. Fluorescent QDs have been used in optical biosensors where glucose-dependent enzymatic reactions modulate fluorescence intensity, wavelength, or lifetime. Compared to traditional dyes, QDs exhibit high photostability and tunable emission spectra. Semiconductor nanomaterials such as ZnS, CdSe, and silicon nanoparticles have also been explored for photoelectrochemical glucose sensing. However, concerns regarding long-term toxicity, heavy metal content, and regulatory acceptance have limited clinical translation, motivating the design of heavy-metal-free and biodegradable alternatives [25].

5.5.4 Metal Oxides and Catalytic Nanoparticles

Metal oxide nanomaterials, including nickel oxide, copper oxide, cobalt oxide, and zinc oxide, are widely investigated for non-enzymatic glucose sensing due to their intrinsic electrocatalytic activity. These materials catalyze glucose oxidation directly at the electrode surface, eliminating enzyme-related instability and extending sensor life. Nanostructured metal oxides offer high surface reactivity and fast electron transfer, leading to rapid response times and high sensitivity. Recent studies have focused on hierarchical nanostructures and doped metal oxides to enhance catalytic efficiency and mitigate interference. Despite promising analytical performance, obstacles associated with selectivity, surface fouling, and operation under physiological conditions persist [22, 26].

5.5.5 Metal-Organic Frameworks (MOFs) and Porous Materials

MOFs and related porous materials represent a rapidly growing class of nanoplatforms for glucose biosensing. MOFs combine high surface area, tunable pore size, and versatile chemical functionality, making them ideal scaffolds for enzyme immobilization or catalytic glucose detection. Recent nano-biosensors leverage MOFs to protect enzymes from denaturation, improve mass transport, and enable multi-functional sensing architecture. Some MOFs also exhibit intrinsic catalytic activity, supporting enzyme-free glucose detection. However, issues related to long-term stability in aqueous environments and scalable fabrication must be overcome before clinical adoption [27].

5.5.6 Conductive Polymers and Hybrid Systems

Conductive polymers such as polyaniline, polypyrrole, and PEDOT: PSS offer attractive properties for glucose sensing, including mechanical flexibility, biocompatibility, and compatibility with low-cost fabrication techniques. These polymers facilitate efficient electron transfer while supporting enzyme immobilization and antifouling modifications. Recent trends emphasize hybrid nanomaterials, where conductive polymers are combined with nanoparticles, carbon nanostructures, or MOFs to synergistically enhance sensitivity, stability, and device integration. Such hybrid systems are especially promising for wearable and implantable glucose sensors, bridging the gap between high-performance nanomaterials and clinically practical device formats [28].

5.6 RECOGNITION ELEMENTS

The recognition element is the core component that confers specificity to glucose biosensors. In nano-enabled systems, recognition chemistry must be compatible with nanoscale interfaces, maintain stability under physiological conditions, and support continuous or long-term monitoring. Recent research has concentrated on biological and non-biological recognition strategies to balance between sensitivity, selectivity, and durability [29].

5.6.1 Enzymatic (GOx, PQQ-GDH) Approaches

Enzyme-based recognition remains the clinical gold standard for glucose sensing due to its high specificity. GOx is the most widely used enzyme, catalyzing the oxidation of glucose to gluconic acid with concomitant hydrogen peroxide generation. In nano-biosensors, immobilization of GOx onto nanomaterials such as AuNPs, carbon nanostructures, or MOFs improves electron transfer efficiency and reduces response time. However, GOx activity depends on oxygen availability and is sensitive to temperature and pH fluctuations, which can affect long-term stability [30].

Pyrroloquinoline quinone-dependent glucose dehydrogenase (PQQ-GDH) has gained increasing attention as an alternative enzyme. Unlike GOx, PQQ-GDH is oxygen-independent, reducing signal variability in hypoxic tissue environments typical of subcutaneous sensing. Recent reports have shown improved operational stability and compatibility with CGM when PQQ-GDH is integrated with nano-engineered electrodes. Nonetheless, enzymatic approaches remain susceptible to denaturation, leaching, and biofouling in long-term use [31].

5.6.2 Aptamers and Nucleic Acid Sensors

Aptamers – short, single-stranded DNA or RNA sequences selected for high-affinity binding – offer a promising non-enzymatic biological alternative. Glucose-responsive aptamers change conformation upon binding, which can be transduced electrochemically or optically at nanostructured interfaces. Nano-enabled aptamer sensors benefit from improved surface density, signal amplification, and reduced reagent consumption. While aptamers demonstrate excellent stability compared to enzymes, achieving high selectivity for small molecules like glucose in complex biofluids remains challenging, and their clinical maturity is still limited [32].

5.6.3 Molecularly Impressed Polymers (MIPs)

Molecularly imprinted polymers provide a synthetic recognition strategy that mimics biological binding sites. MIPs are fabricated by polymerizing functional monomers around a glucose template, which is subsequently removed to leave complementary binding cavities. When integrated with nanomaterials, MIPs offer enhanced binding kinetics, mechanical robustness, and resistance to harsh environments. Recent advances include nano-MIPs and surface-imprinted films that improve sensitivity and response time. Importantly, MIPs are appealing for long-term and implantable sensors due to their chemical stability and low cost, although their selectivity can be compromised by structurally similar saccharides [33].

5.6.4 Non-Biological/Catalytic Recognition

Non-biological recognition relies on direct catalytic oxidation of glucose at nanostructured surfaces, typically using metal or metal oxide nanoparticles. These systems eliminate biological components entirely, offering superior stability and simplified fabrication. Nano-engineered catalytic interfaces provide rapid response and high sensitivity, but selectivity remains a key limitation, as other electroactive species can produce competing signals. Current research focuses on surface engineering and hybrid materials to improve specificity under physiological conditions [34].

5.7 TRANSDUCTION MECHANISMS

Transduction mechanisms convert glucose recognition events into quantifiable electrical, optical, or mechanical signals. In nano-biosensors, the transducer is often the key factor of sensitivity, response time, and suitability for continuous monitoring. Advances over the past decade have focused on leveraging nanoscale effects to enhance signal amplification while maintaining clinical relevance. A schematic overview of common nanocarrier-transducer configurations used in glucose biosensors is presented in Figure 5.1, highlighting electrochemical, field-effect transistor (FET)-based, optical, and mechanical sensing strategies.

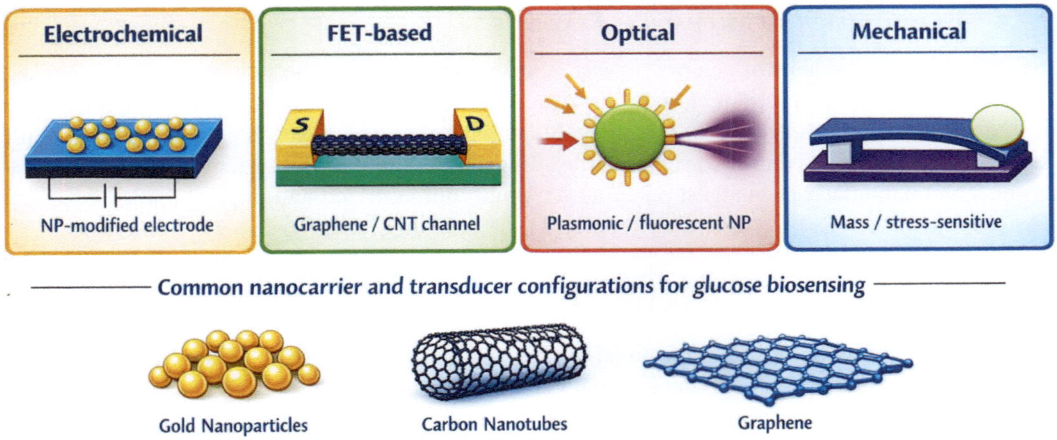

FIGURE 5.1 Schematic of common nanocarrier/transducer type.

5.7.1 Electrochemical Transduction

Electrochemical sensing remains the most mature and clinically validated transduction strategy for glucose sensing. Amperometric sensors, which measure current generated by glucose oxidation reactions, dominate both SMBG and CGM technologies. Nano-engineered electrodes incorporating nanoparticles, carbon nanostructures, or porous structures greatly improve electron transfer kinetics and lower detection limits. Potentiometric sensors, which measure changes in potential related to glucose-induced ionic or pH changes, provide low-power operation but are more prone to drift. Impedimetric sensors track changes in interfacial resistance or capacitance upon glucose binding, enabling label-free detection. Recent nano-biosensors combine glucose impedimetric readouts with antifouling nanocoatings to improve long-term stability in biological fluids [30, 35].

5.7.2 Field-Effect Transistor (FET) Sensor

FET-based glucose sensors translate surface charge or potential changes into modulations of channel conductivity. Nanomaterials such as graphene, carbon nanotubes, and silicon nanowires are widely used as FET channels because of their high carrier mobility and sensitivity to interfacial events. In enzyme-functionalized FETs, glucose oxidation alters the local charge distribution, producing rapid, real-time responses. FET sensors offer ultra-low detection limits and fast response times, often within seconds. However, Debye screening in physiological media and sensitivity to nonspecific adsorption represent major challenges. Recent strategies, such as nanogap engineering, surface functionalization and operation in low ionic strength microenvironments, attempt to overcome these shortcomings [36].

5.7.3 Optical Transduction

Optical glucose sensing exploits nanoscale interactions between light and matter to generate analyte-specific signals. Surface plasmon resonance (SPR) and LSPR enable label-free glucose detection through refractive index changes near plasmonic nanostructures. Fluorescence-based sensors, including QD and dye-coupled systems, offer high sensitivity and multiplexing capability. Surface-enhanced Raman scattering provides molecular fingerprinting with exceptional sensitivity supported by plasmonic "hot spots" generated by metallic nanostructures. Although optical approaches deliver high analytical performance, integration into compact, wearable CGM devices remains challenging due to optical alignment, power requirements, and cost [37].

5.7.4 Piezoelectric and Mechanical Readouts

Piezoelectric and mechanical glucose sensors detect mass or viscoelastic changes related to glucose binding or enzymatic reactions. Quartz crystal microbalance and microcantilever-based devices have demonstrated high sensitivity when combined with nanostructured recognition layers. While these methods are mostly utilized in research settings, recent advances in micro-electromechanical systems and nanomaterials suggest potential for future miniaturized and implantable glucose sensors [38].

5.8 DEVICE DESIGN AND INTEGRATION

The translation of nano-biosensors from laboratory prototypes to clinically viable glucose monitoring systems depends critically on device- and system-level integration. Recent advances emphasize scalable fabrication, efficient sample handling, and user-friendly form factors compatible with continuous and wearable monitoring. Representative wearable and implantable device architectures for nano-enabled glucose monitoring are shown in Figure 5.2.

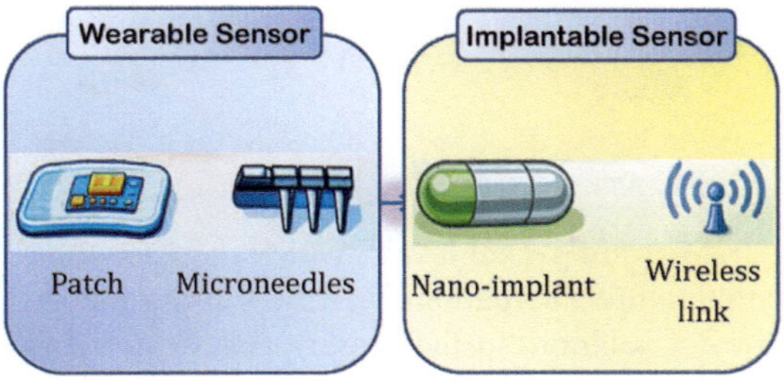

FIGURE 5.2 Representative device architectures (wearable/implant).

5.8.1 Microfabrication and Printing Techniques

Modern glucose biosensors increasingly rely on microfabrication technologies adapted from the semiconductor and microelectronics industry. Photolithography, thin-film deposition, and etching enable precise patterning of electrodes, transducer channels, and interconnects at the micrometer and nanometer scales. These techniques support high device reproducibility and integration with on-chip electronics. To overcome cost and scalability constraints, additive manufacturing and printing approaches including screen printing, inkjet printing, and aerosol jet printing have gained prominence. Nano-inks incorporating metallic nanoparticles, CNTs, or conductive polymers allow rapid fabrication of disposable electrodes and flexible sensor platforms. Recent studies demonstrate that printed nano-enabled glucose sensors can achieve analytical performance comparable to that of lithographically fabricated devices while enabling high-throughput manufacturing [39].

5.8.2 Microfluidics and Sample Handling

Effective sample handling is essential for accurate glucose measurement, especially when targeting alternative biofluids such as interstitial fluid, sweat, or tears. Microfluidic integration enables precise control over fluid transport, minimizes sample volume, and reduces contamination or evaporation. In nano-biosensor systems, microfluidic channels are often combined with capillary-driven flow, osmotic pumping, or minimally invasive microneedles to extract interstitial fluid without active pumping. Recent microfluidic designs also include on-chip filtration and dilution to reduce interference and stabilize sensor response. The convergence of microfluidics and nanomaterials has allowed faster response times and improved correlation between glucose measurements and systemic levels [40].

5.8.3 Flexible, Stretchable, and Wearable Form Factors

Wearability is a defining requirement for next-generation glucose monitoring. Recent advancements in flexible, skin-conformal sensors allow devices to tolerate the mechanical deformation associated with daily activities. Elastomeric substrates, such as silicone and thermoplastic polymers, are widely used to host nano-engineered sensing elements without compromising electrical performance. Recent wearable glucose sensors integrate nanomaterials with textiles, patches, or microneedle arrays to enable continuous monitoring with minimal discomfort. Importantly, flexible platforms support wireless data transmission, energy-efficient operation, and compatibility with mobile health ecosystems. While these designs show great promise, offering long-term adhesion, signal stability, and user compliance remains a key focus of ongoing research [41].

5.9 SIGNAL PROCESSING AND DATA

Robust signal processing is essential for transforming raw nano-biosensor outputs into clinically reliable glucose readings. In continuous and wearable systems, sensor signals are influenced by biological variability, environmental factors, and material aging, making data handling just as critical as sensor design.

5.9.1 Noise, Baseline Drift, and Filtering

Nano-biosensors often operate at low signal levels, which increase their vulnerability to electrical noise, motion artifacts, temperature fluctuations, and biofouling-induced drift. In CGM, baseline drift can arise from enzyme degradation, surface passivation by proteins, or gradual changes in the sensor-tissue interface. Modern systems use digital filtering techniques, such as moving average filters, adaptive filters, and Kalman filters, to suppress high-frequency noise while preserving physiologically relevant glucose trends. Recent studies focus on adaptive filtering concepts to dynamically adjust the filter to changing signal characteristics during daily activities to improve stability without increasing latency [42].

5.9.2 Calibration Strategies and Algorithms

Calibration is a major issue for glucose sensors, especially for long-lasting and minimally invasive sensors. Traditional SMBG and early CGM systems required frequent finger-stick calibration. However, an increasing number of commercial CGMs are actually based on a factory calibration and calculation of correction factors (algorithms). Nano-biosensors attempt to further reduce calibration requirements by using such stable materials, reference electrodes, or internal standards. Algorithmic calibration methods such as sensor redundancy, temperature compensation, and physiological models correct systematic bias and drift. Recent studies have also been made with self-calibrating systems that use multi-parametric sensing (e.g., pH, oxygen, impedance) to infer and correct sensor deviations in real time [3, 10].

5.9.3 AI/ML for Pattern Recognition and Prediction

Artificial intelligence (AI) and ML are rapidly transforming glucose data interpretation. Data-driven models are increasingly used to identify patterns in glucose traces, detect sensor anomalies, and predict future glucose excursions. ML techniques – including regression models, neural networks, and recurrent architectures – have demonstrated improved accuracy in glucose trend prediction and hypoglycemia forecasting compared to rule-based approaches. When integrated with nano-enabled sensors, AI-oriented analytics support personalized glucose management, improve robustness under real-world conditions, and facilitate closed-loop insulin delivery. As sensor datasets grow, AI/ML approaches are expected to play an expanding role in bridging nanoscale sensing and clinical decision-making [43].

5.10 Performance Metrics

Standardized performance metrics are essential for evaluating nano-biosensors and benchmarking their readiness for clinical glucose monitoring. While laboratory demonstrations often emphasize analytical sensitivity, clinical applicability requires a balanced assessment of several interdependent parameters. Typical calibration behavior and major the key performance metrics used to evaluate glucose biosensors are schematically shown in Figure 5.3.

5.10.1 Sensitivity, Limit of Detection, and Linear Range

Sensitivity defines the change in sensor signal per unit glucose concentration and is directly affected by nanomaterial surface area, catalytic activity, and transduction efficiency. Nano-biosensors commonly achieve high sensitivities that enable detection of glucose at the micromolar or even

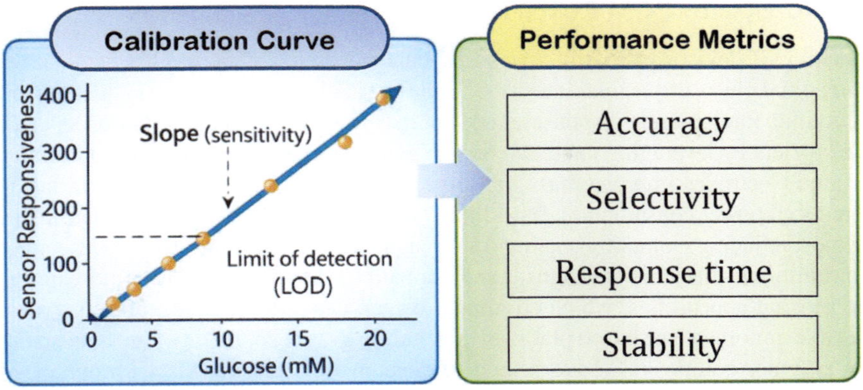

FIGURE 5.3 Example calibration curve and performance metrics.

nanomolar level under controlled conditions. However, for clinical relevance, sensors must maintain a linear dynamic range that spans physiologically meaningful glucose concentrations, typically from hypoglycemic to hyperglycemic levels. The limit of detection should be sufficiently low to accurately detect rapid drops in glucose, while avoiding signal saturation at high concentrations. Recent research increasingly emphasizes analytical performance in clinically relevant ranges rather than maximizing sensitivity alone [34].

5.10.2 Selectivity and Interference

Selectivity is an important requirement in complex biological matrices where electroactive and chemically related species coexist. Common interferents in glucose sensing include acetaminophen, ascorbic acid, and uric acid, which can produce false signals in electrochemical systems. Nano-biosensors overcome these problems through selective recognition elements, size-exclusion membranes, permselective coatings, and surface charge engineering. Recent studies show that carefully engineered nanostructured interfaces can significantly suppress interference effects while preserving response times. However, selectivity must be validated under realistic physiological conditions rather than idealized buffer systems [34].

5.10.3 Stability, Lifetime, and Replicability

Long-term operational stability is essential for CGM applications. Sensor lifetime is affected by enzyme degradation, nanomaterial corrosion, biofouling, and mechanical stress. Clinically viable systems must maintain consistent performance over days to weeks with minimal recalibration. Reproducibility, both within a single device and across manufacturing batches, is equally important for regulatory approval and large-scale deployment. Recent advances in surface passivation, encapsulation strategies, and standardized fabrication protocols have improved stability and reproducibility, but achieving reliable long-term performance remains a major obstacle to the clinical translation of nano-biosensors [44].

5.11 CONTINUOUS GLUCOSE MONITORING (CGM)

CGM has become a cornerstone of modern diabetes management, enabling real-time tracking of glucose dynamics and supporting data-driven therapeutic decisions. Nano-biosensor technologies offer an evolving solution to persistent limitations of current CGM systems and enable next-generation closed-loop solutions.

5.11.1 Nano-Enabled CGM Concepts

Conventional CGM devices primarily rely on subcutaneous enzymatic electrochemical sensors that measure interstitial glucose at regular intervals. While clinically effective, these systems are constrained by sensor lifetime, foreign-body responses, and signal drift. Nano-enabled CGM concepts aim to overcome these barriers by leveraging nanomaterials to enhance sensitivity, stability, and miniaturization. Nanostructured electrodes improve mass transport and electron transfer, resulting in faster response times and reduced power consumption. In addition, nanoscale surface engineering permits more stable immobilization, reducing biofouling and improving signal consistency over extended wear periods [45].

Beyond traditional enzymatic designs, nano-enabled CGMs increasingly explore non-enzymatic and hybrid sensing approaches, which eliminate oxygen dependence and reduce enzymatic degradation. Flexible nanomaterial-based platforms, including graphene, metal oxide nanostructures, and conductive polymer composites, have helped to develop wearable CGMs with enhanced comfort and mechanical robustness. Emerging designs also target alternative sampling strategies, such as microneedle-assisted interstitial fluid extraction or minimally invasive epidermal sensors, to further reduce user burden [46].

5.11.2 Closed-Loop Compatibility

Closed-loop insulin delivery systems, often referred to as artificial pancreas technologies, require CGMs that provide accurate, low-latency glucose data. Nano-enabled sensors are particularly well suited for closed-loop integration due to their fast response kinetics and potential for continuous operation with minimal drift. High-frequency data acquisition supports predictive control algorithms that adjust insulin delivery in real time, reducing hyperglycemia and hypoglycemia risk [47].

Recent research emphasizes the co-design of nano-biosensors with control algorithms, ensuring compatibility with automated insulin pumps and decision-support systems. As regulatory standards evolve, nano-enabled CGMs that demonstrate consistent accuracy, safety, and interoperability are expected to play a key role in advancing fully autonomous glucose management [48].

5.12 PRECLINICAL AND CLINICAL CONSIDERATIONS

Successful translation of nano-biosensors for glucose monitoring requires rigorous evaluation beyond analytical performance. Preclinical and clinical considerations focus on biological interactions, safety, and the relevance of testing models to the real world.

5.12.1 Biocompatibility, Immune Response, and Fouling

Biocompatibility is an important factor in sensor performance, especially for implantable or prolonged CGM devices. Upon implantation, nano-biosensors interact with complex biological environments that can induce foreign-body responses, including protein adsorption, inflammation, and fibrotic encapsulation. These processes contribute to biofouling and signal drift by hindering analyte diffusion and changing interfacial properties. Nanomaterials must therefore be designed to be non-cytotoxic, non-inflammatory, and non-disruptive to tissues during long-term implantation. Recent strategies include surface passivation with hydrophilic polymers, antifouling coatings, and controlled nanostructured morphology to minimize immune activation. Regulatory evaluation increasingly emphasizes chronic exposure and stability rather than short-term compatibility alone [49].

5.12.2 Animal Models and Human Trials

Preclinical validation typically relies on rodent models to assess sensor accuracy, biocompatibility, and temporal correlation between sensor output and blood glucose levels. While these models are useful for preliminary screening, physiological differences in skin structure, immune response, and glucose kinetics mean that findings from these models cannot be estimated or extrapolated to humans directly. Larger animal models, such as pigs, offer more clinically pertinent data for wearable and implantable sensors, but have lower use because of cost and ethical issues [50].

Human clinical trials remain the definitive benchmark for glucose sensor validation. Recent trials emphasize metrics such as accuracy over extended wear, sensor longevity, safety, and user compliance. For nano-enabled sensors, demonstrating equivalence or superiority to existing CGM technologies under real-world conditions is essential for regulatory approval and clinical adoption [51].

5.13 Manufacturing and Scalability

For nano-biosensors to achieve widespread clinical adoption, laboratory-scale innovations must be translated into manufacturing processes that are reproducible, scalable, and compliant with regulatory standards. Manufacturing is very often a bottleneck in the commercialization of nano-enabled glucose monitoring technologies.

5.13.1 Batch and Reproducibility and Quality Control

Batch-to-batch reproducibility is especially difficult for nanomaterial-based sensors, as small variations in particle size, morphology, and surface chemistry can significantly impact sensor performance. Scalable fabrication methods must incorporate robust quality control protocols to ensure consistent material properties and device function. Recent approaches emphasize standardized synthesis, in-line characterization, and process automation to reduce variability. In device manufacturing, reproducibility is also important for electrode patterning, enzyme immobilization, and encapsulation processes. Regulatory agencies are placing more demands on manufacturers to demonstrate tight control over important quality attributes throughout the production pipeline [52].

5.13.2 Cost, Regulatory, and Supply Chain Aspects

Cost-effectiveness is a key determinant of market adoption, especially for disposable or short-lifetime glucose sensors. Manufacturing strategies must balance material performance with affordability, favoring processes compatible with high-throughput production. From a regulatory perspective, nano-biosensors are evaluated as medical devices, requiring compliance with known safety, performance, and manufacturing standards. The inclusion of nanomaterials introduces additional scrutiny related to material characterization and long-term safety. Addressing these economic and regulatory factors early in development is critical for successful translation [53].

5.14 REGULATION, ETHICS, AND SAFETY

The clinical deployment of nano-biosensors for glucose monitoring must comply with regulatory frameworks that ensure patient safety, device efficacy, and ethical data use. As sensing technologies become increasingly integrated with digital health ecosystems, regulatory and ethical considerations are expanding beyond traditional device performance metrics.

5.14.1 Regulatory Pathways for Sensor Devices

Glucose monitoring systems are regulated as medical devices and must demonstrate analytical accuracy, clinical performance, and manufacturing quality. Regulatory approval typically requires staged evaluation, including preclinical testing, human clinical trials, and post-market surveillance. For nano-enabled sensors, regulators are increasingly emphasizing material characterization, long-term biocompatibility, and stability, especially for implantable or continuous-use devices.

Demonstrating equivalence to established technologies can streamline approval, but new nanomaterials may necessitate additional data. Alignment with international standards and transparent risk assessment are therefore critical for regulatory success [54].

5.14.2 Data Privacy and Clinical Responsibility

Modern glucose monitoring generates continuous, high-resolution personal health data. Ethical deployment requires robust data privacy, cybersecurity, and informed consent frameworks to protect patient information. Clinicians and manufacturers share responsibility for ensuring data accuracy, preventing misuse, and clearly communicating the limitations of sensor readings. As nano-enabled systems increasingly integrate AI-driven analytics, transparency and accountability in algorithmic decision-making process are essential to maintain patient trust and clinical integrity [55].

5.15 FUTURE DIRECTIONS

Nano-biosensor research for glucose monitoring is moving toward more integrated, intelligent, and patient-centered solutions. Several emerging directions are expected to influence the next generation of technologies.

5.15.1 Multi-Analyte Sensing and Multiplexing

Future glucose sensors are increasingly envisioned as multi-analyte platforms capable of simultaneously monitoring glucose alongside complementary biomarkers such as lactate, ketones, or inflammatory markers. Nano-enabled multiplexing can provide a more holistic metabolic profile, improving risk prediction and personalized treatment. Advances in nanomaterials patterning and signal discrimination are enabling such integrated sensing architectures [56].

5.15.2 Autonomous Implantables and Energy Harvesting

Long-term implantable glucose sensors require autonomous operation with minimal maintenance. Emerging research focuses on self-powered or energy-harvesting systems, including biofuel cells and piezoelectric nanomaterials, to reduce reliance on external batteries. Combined with stable nano-biosensors, such approaches can enable continuous monitoring for long periods of time [57].

5.15.3 Emerging Nanomaterials and Hybrid Systems

New classes of nanomaterials such as bio-derived nanostructures, two-dimensional materials, and multifunctional hybrids are expanding the design space for glucose biosensors. Hybrid systems that integrate sensing, antifouling, and signal processing functions at the nanoscale offer promising routes toward robust, clinically viable devices [34].

5.16 CONCLUSIONS

Nano-biosensors represent a transformative approach to glucose monitoring, offering enhanced sensitivity, faster response, and improved integration with wearable and implantable platforms. By leveraging nanoscale materials and architectures, these systems address key limitations of conventional sensors, including stability, miniaturization, and continuous operation. Despite considerable progress, challenges related to biocompatibility, long-term reliability, manufacturing scalability, and regulatory validation remain. Continued interdisciplinary collaboration among materials scientists, engineers, and clinicians, and regulators will be essential to translate nano-enabled glucose biosensors from experimental prototypes to clinically useful technologies. As advances continue in nanomaterials, data analytics, and device integration, nano-biosensors are poised to play a central role in the future of precision diabetes management.

ACKNOWLEDGMENTS

The authors are highly thankful to all the affiliated colleges of the authors for providing necessary support and facilities.

REFERENCES

1. Kumar A, Gangwar R, Ahmad Zargar A, Kumar R, Sharma A. Prevalence of diabetes in India: A review of IDF diabetes atlas 10th edition. Current Diabetes Reviews. 2024;20(1):105–14.
2. Kwon SY, Moon JS. Advances in continuous glucose monitoring: Clinical applications. Endocrinology and Metabolism. 2025;40(2):161–73.
3. Klonoff DC, Ahn D, Drincic A. Continuous glucose monitoring: A review of the technology and clinical use. Diabetes Research and Clinical Practice. 2017;133:178–92.
4. Madan A, Toro AU, Saini R, Akange ET, Rahimi M. Advanced nano-biosensors with multiscale applications: A comprehensive review. Sensing and Bio-Sensing Research. 2026;51:1–19.
5. Cash KJ, Clark HA. Nanosensors and nanomaterials for monitoring glucose in diabetes. Trends in Molecular Medicine. 2010;16(12):584–93.
6. Freckmann G, Pleus S, Grady M, Setford S, Levy B. Measures of accuracy for continuous glucose monitoring and blood glucose monitoring devices. Journal of Diabetes Science and Technology. 2019;13(3):575–83.
7. Sevil M, Rashid M, Hajizadeh I, Park M, Quinn L, Cinar A. Physical activity and psychological stress detection and assessment of their effects on glucose concentration predictions in diabetes management. IEEE Transactions on Biomedical Engineering. 2021;68(7):2251–60.
8. Mariello M. Reliability and stability of bioelectronic medicine: A critical and pedagogical perspective. Bioelectronic Medicine. 2025;11(1):16.
9. Yoo J, Kim IT, Park JY, Kim YR. Electrochemical glucose sensor based on a phenothiazine derivative mediator with nicotinamide adenine dinucleotide-dependent glucose dehydrogenase. Sensors and Actuators B: Chemical. 2025;422:136630.
10. Rayan MN, Reddy N, Verma N, et al. Monitoring technologies-continuous glucose monitoring, mobile technology, biomarkers of glycemic control. [Updated 2026, Apr 12]. In: Feingold KR, Adler RA, Ahmed SF, et al., editors. Endotext [Internet]. South Dartmouth (MA): MDText.com, Inc.; 2000. Available from: https://www.ncbi.nlm.nih.gov/sites/books/NBK279046/.
11. Vaddiraju S, Burgess DJ, Tomazos I, Jain FC, Papadimitrakopoulos F. Technologies for continuous glucose monitoring: Current problems and future promises. Journal of Diabetes Science and Technology. 2010;4(6):1540–62.
12. Cho Y, Choi Y, Jang Y, Seong H. Nanomaterial-Enhanced biosensing: Mechanisms and emerging applications. Advanced Healthcare Materials. 2025;14(31):2500189.
13. Darwish MA, Abd-Elaziem W, Elsheikh A, Zayed AA. Advancements in nanomaterials for nanosensors: A comprehensive review. Nanoscale Advances. 2024;6(16):4015–46.
14. Park J, Seo B, Jeong Y, Park I. A review of recent advancements in sensor-integrated medical tools. Advanced Science. 2024;11(20):e2307427.
15. Sedighi A, Kou T, Huang H, Li Y. Noninvasive on-skin biosensors for monitoring diabetes mellitus. Nano-Micro Letters. 2026;18(1):16.
16. Safarkhani M, Aldhaher A, Heidari G, Zare EN, Warkiani ME, Akhavan O, Huh Y, Rabiee N. Nanomaterial-assisted wearable glucose biosensors for noninvasive real-time monitoring: Pioneering point-of-care and beyond. Nano Materials Science. 2024;6(3):263–83.
17. Jamshidnejad-Tosaramandani T, Kashanian S, Omidfar K, Schiöth HB. The role of nanomaterials in the wearable electrochemical glucose biosensors for diabetes management. Biosensors. 2025;15(7):451.
18. Saha T, Del Caño R, Mahato K, De la Paz E, Chen C, Ding S, Yin L, Wang J. Wearable electrochemical glucose sensors in diabetes management: A comprehensive review. Chemical Reviews. 2023;123(12):7854–89.
19. Juntree N, Sangjan A, Pongchaikul P, Arjfuk P, Wanmolee W, Khemthong P, Srifa A, Posoknistakul P, Laosiripojana N, Sakdaronnarong C. Unveiling role of carbon dots for non-invasive and ultra-sensitive glucose detection in biofluids for personal preventive care testing. Green Analytical Chemistry. 2024; 11:100165.

20. Kalhoro KA, Anwar M, Zhang C, Khan A, Wu D, Rehman AU, Shokouhimehr M, Liu Z. Recent trends and prospective developments in metal oxide composites-based electrochemical nonenzymatic glucose sensors. Talanta. 2025; 295:128366. https://doi.org/10.1016/j.talanta.2025.128366.
21. Ntuli LM, Nyembwe A, Mwengula G, Munonde T, Mulopo J. Recent advances in metal oxide, bimetallic nanocomposites, metal-organic frameworks (MOFs), and non-invasive technologies for biofluid-based glucose sensors: A comprehensive review. International Journal of Electrochemical Science. 2025;20(11):101184. https://doi.org/10.1016/j.ijoes.2025.101184.
22. Harun-Or-Rashid M, Aktar MN, Preda V, Nasiri N. Advances in electrochemical sensors for real-time glucose monitoring. Sensors & Diagnostics. 2024;3(6):893–913.
23. Lee MJ, Choi JH, Shin JH, Yun J, Kim T, Kim YJ, Oh BK. Gold nanoclusters with two sets of embedded enzyme nanoparticles for applications as electrochemical sensors for glucose. ACS Applied Nano Materials. 2023;6(13):12567–77.
24. Yuwen T, Shu D, Zou H, Yang X, Wang S, Zhang S, Liu Q, Wang X, Wang G, Zhang Y, Zang G. Carbon nanotubes: A powerful bridge for conductivity and flexibility in electrochemical glucose sensors. Journal of Nanobiotechnology. 2023;21(1):320.
25. Wegner KD, Hildebrandt N. Near infrared quantum dots for biosensing and bioimaging. TrAC Trends in Analytical Chemistry. 2024;180:117922.
26. Chitare YM, Jadhav SB, Pawaskar PN, Magdum VV, Gunjakar JL, Lokhande CD. Metal oxide-based composites in nonenzymatic electrochemical glucose sensors. Industrial & Engineering Chemistry Research. 2021;60(50):18195–217.
27. Chandra DK, Kumar A, Mahapatra C. Smart nano-hybrid metal-organic frameworks: Revolutionizing advancements, applications, and challenges in biomedical therapeutics and diagnostics. Hybrid Advances. 2025;9:100406. https://doi.org/10.1016/j.hybadv.2025.100406.
28. Gamboa J, Paulo-Mirasol S, Estrany F, Torras J. Recent progress in biomedical sensors based on conducting polymer hydrogels. ACS Applied Bio Materials. 2023;6(5):1720–41.
29. Ayanda OS, Mmuoegbulam AO, Okezie O, Durumin Iya NI, Mohammed SA, James PH, Muhammad AB, Unimke AA, Alim SA, Yahaya SM, Ojo A. Recent progress in carbon-based nanomaterials: Critical review. Journal of Nanoparticle Research. 2024;26(5):106.
30. Guoqiang G, Liang Q, Yani Z, Pengyun W, Fanzhuo K, Yuyang Z, Zhiyuan L, Xing N, Xue Z, Qiongya L, Bin Z. Recent advances in glucose monitoring utilizing oxidase electrochemical biosensors integrating carbon-based nanomaterials and smart enzyme design. Frontiers in Chemistry. 2025;13:1591302.
31. Quintero-Jaime AF, Conzuelo F, Cazorla-Amorós D, Morallon E. Pyrroloquinoline quinone-dependent glucose dehydrogenase bioelectrodes based on one-step electrochemical entrapment over single-wall carbon nanotubes. Talanta. 2021;232:122386.
32. Hassibian S, Amin M, Taghdisi SM, Sameiyan E, Ghaffari R, Alibolandi M, Ramezani M, Abnous K, Dehnavi SM. Aptamers: Design, theory, and applications to diagnosis and therapy for diseases. MedComm. 2025;6(5):e70180.
33. Abdel-Hamied M, Rajpal S, Mishra P, Kranz C, Mizaikoff B. Molecularly imprinted polymers for biomarker detection: Advances in design, modeling, and sensing strategies. TrAC Trends in Analytical Chemistry. 2025;194:118487. https://doi.org/10.1016/j.trac.2025.118487.
34. Rajamohan R, Sun S. Nanostructured materials in glucose biosensing: From fundamentals to smart healthcare applications. Biosensors. 2025;15(10):658.
35. Kilic NM, Singh S, Keles G, Cinti S, Kurbanoglu S, Odaci D. Novel approaches to enzyme-based electrochemical nanobiosensors. Biosensors. 2023;13(6):622.
36. Krishnan SK, Nataraj N, Meyyappan M, Pal U. Graphene-based field-effect transistors in biosensing and neural interfacing applications: Recent advances and prospects. Analytical Chemistry. 2023; 95(5):2590–622.
37. Butt MA, Akca BI, Mateos X. Next-generation photonic sensors for single-molecule detection: Challenges overcome and horizons ahead. Chip. 2025;5(2):100174. https://doi.org/10.1016/j.chip.2025.100174.
38. Pohanka M. Piezoelectric chemosensors and biosensors in medical diagnostics. Biosensors. 2025;15(3):197.
39. Siavashy S, Soltani M, Rahimi S, Hosseinali M, Guilandokht Z, Raahemifar K. Recent advancements in microfluidic-based biosensors for detection of genes and proteins: Applications and techniques. Biosensors and Bioelectronics: X. 2024;19:100489.
40. Heikenfeld J. Continuous and minimally invasive biofluid access and biosensing: Challenges and prospects. Journal of Science and Medicine in Sport. 2022;25:S12–3.
41. Ali SM, Noghanian S, Khan ZU, Alzahrani S, Alharbi S, Alhartomi M, Alsulami R. Wearable and flexible sensor devices: Recent advances in designs, fabrication methods, and applications. Sensors. 2025;25(5):1377.

42. Maqbool Z, Raza N, Hayat A, Salem ME, Nazar MF. Functional solid–liquid interfaces for electrochemical blood glucose sensing: New insights and future prospects. Chemosensors. 2025;13(11):385.
43. Jacobs PG, Herrero P, Facchinetti A, Vehi J, Kovatchev B, Breton MD, Cinar A, Nikita KS, Doyle FJ, Bondia J, Battelino T. Artificial intelligence and machine learning for improving glycemic control in diabetes: Best Practices, pitfalls, and opportunities. IEEE Reviews in Biomedical Engineering. 2023;17:19–41.
44. Yang H, Yan S. A comprehensive review of electrochemical lactate biosensors: Principles, innovations, and future perspectives. International Journal of Electrochemical Science. 2025;22(10):101132. https://doi.org/10.1016/j.ijoes.2025.101132.
45. Teymourian H, Barfidokht A, Wang J. Electrochemical glucose sensors in diabetes management: An updated review (2010–2020). Chemical Society Reviews. 2020;49(21):7671–709.
46. Mihai DA, Stefan DS, Stegaru D, Bernea GE, Vacaroiu IA, Papacocea T, Lupuşoru MO, Nica AE, Stiru O, Dragos D, Olaru OG. Continuous glucose monitoring devices: A brief presentation. Experimental and Therapeutic Medicine. 2022;23(2):174.
47. Badini S, Regondi S, Pugliese R. Unleashing the power of artificial intelligence in materials design. Materials. 2023;16(17):5927.
48. Templer S. Closed-loop insulin delivery systems: Past, present, and future directions. Frontiers in Endocrinology. 2022;13:919942.
49. Khosravi Ardakani H, Gerami M, Chashmpoosh M, Omidifar N, Gholami A. Recent progress in nanobiosensors for precise detection of blood glucose level. Biochemistry Research International. 2022;2022(1):2964705.
50. Rodrigues D, Barbosa AI, Rebelo R, Kwon IK, Reis RL, Correlo VM. Skin-integrated wearable systems and implantable biosensors: A comprehensive review. Biosensors. 2020;10(7):79.
51. Bhatia D, Paul S, Acharjee T, Ramachairy SS. Biosensors and their widespread impact on human health. Sensors International. 2024;5:100257.
52. Bailey TS. Clinical implications of accuracy measurements of continuous glucose sensors. Diabetes Technology & Therapeutics. 2017;19(S2):S-51.
53. Ijjeh Y, Alsarayreh N, Rifai A, Abdelnabi H, Al-Mahamid S, Alqudah DA, Nsairat H, Lafi Z, Mousa MA, Al-Hiari Y, Alshaer W. Quality by digital design for accelerated sustainable nanomedicine development. European Journal of Pharmaceutical Sciences. 2025;213:107239. https://doi.org/10.1016/j.ejps.2025.107239.
54. Mallik R, Kar P, Mulder H, Krook A. The future is here: An overview of technology in diabetes. Diabetologia. 2024;67(10):2019–26.
55. Amaral C, Paiva M, Rodrigues AR, Veiga F, Bell V. Global regulatory challenges for medical devices: Impact on innovation and market access. Applied Sciences. 2024;14(20):9304.
56. Britton KE, Britton-Colonnese JD. Privacy and security issues surrounding the protection of data generated by continuous glucose monitors. Journal of Diabetes Science and Technology. 2017;11(2):216–19.
57. Lu JC, Morrison D, Halim B, Manos G, Obeyesekere V, Kannard B, Shah R, Wolfe K, Morrow B, Pagliuso B, Liang B. Accuracy and feasibility of a novel glucose/lactate continuous multi-analyte sensing platform in humans. Journal of Diabetes Science and Technology. 2024;20:87–94.

6 Fragment-Based Drug Design Meets Nanotechnology

Harigopal S. Sawarkar, Nitin B. Kohale, Abhijit S. Raut, Suraj K. Yadav, Gajanan M. Jawalkar, Akash S. Jumble, and Akshay B. Ghanmode
Dr. Rajendra Gode College of Pharmacy University, Amravati, India

6.1 INTRODUCTION

Fragment-based drug discovery (FBDD) begins with low-molecular-weight fragments (<300 Da) that have low affinity toward biological targets, which are then evolved into potent lead molecules using structure-guided chemistry. FBDD has matured into a mainstream discovery strategy because it efficiently samples chemical space and often yields high-quality leads for challenging targets, including oncology and kinase families. Modern FBDD workflows rely on sensitive biophysical readouts (nuclear magnetic resonance [NMR], X-ray crystallography, surface plasmon resonance [SPR]) and iterative medicinal chemistry to convert fragments into drug-like molecules [1].

Since its conceptual development in the early 2000s, FBDD has progressed from proof-of-concept fragments to clinical-stage and approved agents. Case studies and reviews document multiple FBDD-derived clinical candidates and several approved drugs, underscoring the approach's translational validity. Advances in fragment library, automated crystallography, and enhanced detection sensitivity have accelerated hit identification and hit-to-lead progression [2].

Nanotechnology brings new physical, chemical, and engineering tools to the fragment discovery pipeline. Nanoparticles and magnetic nanomaterials enable the sensitive capture, preconcentration, and separation of weak fragment–target complexes; nanofluidics and microfluidic reactors give precise, high-throughput fragmented screening control and nanoparticle synthesis; and DNA-based nanostructures (DNA origami) provide programmable nanoscale scaffolds for presentation and selection of fragment libraries. These nano-tools increase throughput, reduce sample consumption, and allow novel readouts that complement classical biophysical assays [3]. The synergistic integration of fragment-based drug design with nanotechnology across screening, validation, and optimization stages is schematically shown in Figure 6.1.

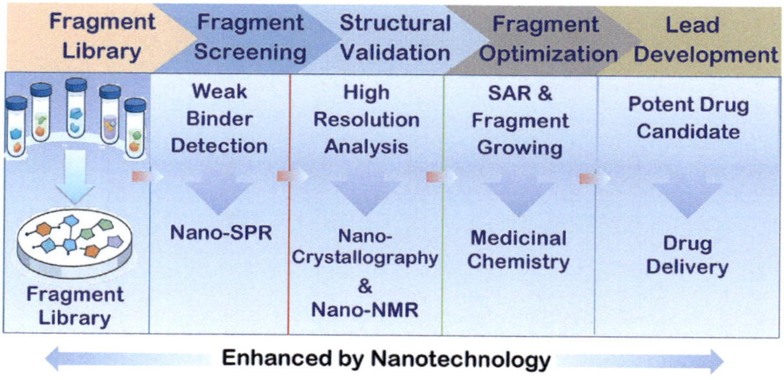

FIGURE 6.1 Conceptual integration of FBDD and nanotechnology.

DOI: 10.1201/9781003598657-6

This chapter surveys core FBDD principles, summarizes modern biophysical methods, and reviews how nanotechnology (nanoparticles, nanofluidics, nanostructured sensors, and DNA nanotech) augments fragment screening, hit validation, and optimization. Selected case studies illustrate practical synergies and translational prospects; final sections discuss limitations, safety, and future directions at the FBDD-nanotech interface.

6.2 PRINCIPLES OF FRAGMENT-BASED DRUG DESIGN

6.2.1 Essential Concepts and Definitions

FBDD is a ligand discovery approach that starts with very small, low-molecular-weight compounds ("fragments," usually ≤300 Da) that bind to biological targets with low affinity but high ligand efficiency. Unlike high-throughput screening of large, complex molecules, FBDD emphasizes efficient coverage of chemical space using relatively small libraries (from 500 to 3000 fragments). The core principle is using small, structurally mapped chemical fragments that bind to target sites, and building them into larger, high-potency drugs through fragment growing, linking, or merging. Ligand efficiency (binding energy per heavy atom) and lipophilic ligand efficiency are widely used metrics to prioritize fragment hits in modern FBDD workflows [4].

6.2.2 Fragment Libraries

Fragment libraries are intentionally programmed to be small, structurally diverse, and are physicochemically simple. Typical fragments obey modified "Rule of Three" guidelines (molecular weight ≤300, clogP ≤3, ≤3 hydrogen bond donors and acceptors), although recent libraries increasingly include three-dimensional, sp^3-rich fragments to better explore complex binding pockets. Contemporary fragment collections often integrate halogenated fragments for crystallographic detection, covalent fragments for targeting nucleophilic residues, and electrophile-focused libraries for covalent FBDD. Advances in computational chemistry and chemoinformatics have enabled rational library design based on diversity metrics, target class bias, and predicted binding hot spots – improving hit rates for challenging targets such as protein–protein interfaces [5].

6.2.3 Screening Strategies

Because fragment binding affinities are generally in the high micromolar to millimolar range, FBDD relies on sensitive biophysical screening techniques. NMR spectroscopy remains a gold standard for identifying weak fragments–target interaction in solutions. X-ray crystallography enables direct visualization of fragment binding modes and is increasingly used in high-throughput fragment soaking campaigns. SPR, thermal shift assays, microscale thermophoresis, or native mass spectrometry are widely used as orthogonal screening tools. In recent years, microfluidic and nano-enabled platforms have brought down sample consumption and increased screening throughput, supporting rapid fragment evaluation [1, 5].

6.2.4 Hit Identification and Validation

Fragment hits are defined by reproducible binding signals confirmed across at least two independent biophysical methods. Structural validation – most commonly by X-ray crystallography or NMR – is very important, as it reveals binding orientation and key interactions that guide fragment optimization. Modern FBDD programs emphasize early evaluation of developability, including solubility, chemical tractability, and absence of assay interference. Several clinically successful small-molecule drugs originated from rigorously validated fragment hits, reinforcing FBDD as a robust and industry-proven approach. Today, integrations with computational modeling, machine learning (ML), and nanotechnology-assisted assays continue to enhance hit confidence and accelerate progression from fragment to lead [6].

6.3 NANOTECHNOLOGY IN DRUG DISCOVERY

6.3.1 Nanomaterials Overview

Nanotechnology has become an essential part of modern drug discovery by enabling manipulation of matter at the 1–100 nm scale, where distinctive physicochemical properties arise. Common nanomaterials used in drug discovery include metal nanoparticles (e.g., gold and silver), carbon-based nanostructures (graphene, carbon nanotubes), polymeric nanoparticles, lipid-based nanocarriers, quantum dots, and metal-organic frameworks (MOFs). These materials have high surface-to-volume ratios, tunable surface chemistry, and unique optical, electronic, or magnetic properties. Recent studies have demonstrated that nanostructured materials can enhance molecular recognition, stabilize biomolecular interaction, and improve assay sensitivity, making them valuable tools throughout early-stage discovery pipelines, especially for challenging targets such as protein–protein interactions and membrane proteins [7].

6.3.2 Nano-Enabled Screening Platforms

Nano-enabled platforms have significantly advanced target identification and ligand screening. Nanoparticle-based assays allow immobilization of proteins or fragments in controlled orientations, facilitating the detection of weak or transient binding interactions. Nanofluidic and microfluidic systems enable ultra-low-volume screening, reducing reagent consumption while increasing throughput and reproducibility. For example, nanofluidic chips in combination with biophysical readouts such as SPR and mass spectrometry have been applied to fragment screening campaigns, enabling the detection of millimolar-affinity binders with high confidence. In parallel, DNA-encoded and nanoparticle-assisted libraries have expanded chemical diversity and facilitated rapid screening against complex biological targets [8].

6.3.3 Advantages of Nanoscale Systems

The main advantage of nanoscale systems lies in their ability to amplify weak molecular signals, a critical requirement for fragment-based and early drug discovery. Nano-enabled assays offer enhanced sensitivity, improved signal-to-noise ratios, and better control over molecular interactions compared with conventional bulk methods. Additionally, nanoscale platforms support multiplexing, real-time analysis, and integration with computational and artificial intelligence (AI)-driven workflows. Recent reports demonstrate that nano-assisted screening can shorten hit identification timelines and improve hit quality, contributing to more efficient lead optimization. Collectively, nanotechnology provides scalable, versatile, and increasingly translational solutions that reshape contemporary drug discovery [9].

6.4 NANOTECHNOLOGY PLATFORMS FOR FRAGMENT-BASED DRUG DESIGN

6.4.1 Nanoparticles-Assisted Screening

Nanoparticle-assisted screening has emerged as a powerful approach to improving the detection of weak fragment–target interactions that are characteristic of FBDD. Metallic nanoparticles, especially gold nanoparticles (AuNPs), are widely used due to their high surface area, tunable size, and ease of functionalization with proteins or small molecules. By immobilizing targets on nanoparticles surface, local concentration effects are increased, enabling improved sensitivity for low-affinity fragment binding. Recent studies have demonstrated that magnetic nanoparticles can be used to capture transient fragment–protein complexes, followed by rapid separation and identification using mass spectrometry. Such nanoparticle-based enrichment strategies reduce false negatives and improve hit confidence, especially for challenging targets such as protein–protein interfaces [10].

6.4.2 Nanofluidics and Microfluidics

Nanofluidic and microfluidic platforms provide precise control over fluids at pico- to nanoliter volumes, making them highly attractive for fragment screening with biofluids. These systems significantly reduce protein and fragment consumption while allowing parallelization and automation. Recent advances include microfluidic X-ray crystallography chips that allow fast fragment soaking and in situ data collection, accelerating structure-based hit validation. Nanofluidic devices have also been integrated with NMR and SPR readouts to monitor fragment binding in real time. Such platforms are especially useful in early discovery area, where protein availability is limited and high-throughput yet sensitive screening is required [11].

6.4.3 DNA-Encoded Libraries with Nanocarriers

DNA-encoded libraries (DELs) have expanded the chemical space accessible to drug discovery, and their integration with nanotechnology has further enhanced their applicability to FBDD. Nanocarriers such as polymeric nanoparticles and lipid-based nanostructures are used to present or protect the DNA-tagged fragments, improving stability and target accessibility. Recent work shows that nanoparticle-assisted DEL screening can improve binding signal discrimination and reduce nonspecific interactions. Additionally, nanoscale carriers facilitate multivalent presentation of fragments, enabling cooperative binding effects that are difficult to observe in traditional solution-phase assays [12].

6.4.4 Nanostructured Surfaces and Sensors

Nanostructured surfaces and sensors play a critical role in detection and validation. Techniques such as nanostructured SPR chips, nanoelectrode arrays, and graphene-based sensors offer enhanced sensitivity and lower detection limits compared to conventional platforms. These systems allow label-free, real-time monitoring of fragment–target interactions and are particularly effective for identifying low-affinity binders. Recent reports highlight the use of nanostructured biosensors to quantify fragment binding kinetics with high precision, for rational fragment optimization. Collectively, these platforms in nanotechnology bolster FBDD workflows through an improved sensitivity, efficiency, and translation. Recent developments in nano-enabled platforms have been instrumental in the improvement of fragment-based drug-design by increasing the sensitivity, throughput, and structural resolution [13]. Representative nanotechnology tools that are currently being used in FBDD and their respective roles in functioning and typical flash point of detection are summarized in Table 6.1.

6.5 BIOPHYSICAL TECHNIQUES AND NANO-TOOLS

6.5.1 NMR and Nanoprobes

NMR spectroscopy remains a cornerstone technique in FBDD because of its ability to detect weak, transient interactions typical of fragment binding. Recent advances integrate nanotechnology through the use of nanoprobes and nanoparticle-assisted NMR. For example, paramagnetic nanoparticles and nanodiscs have been employed to stabilize membrane proteins and enhance spectral quality, enabling fragments screening against previously intractable targets such as GPCRs and ion channels. In addition, fluorine-19 (^19F) NMR combined with fluorinated fragments and nanoparticles-based signal amplification has improved sensitivity and throughput, allowing reliable detection of millimolar-affinity binders in complex mixtures [17].

TABLE 6.1
Nano-Enabled Platforms Used in Fragment-Based Drug Design

Nano-Platform	Primary Role in FBDD	Typical Detection Limit	Applications	Reference
Gold nanoparticles (AuNPs)	Signal amplification, target immobilization	High μM fragments	Kinase and bromodomain fragment screening via nano-SPR	[14]
Magnetic nanoparticles	Enrichment of weak binders	High μM-mM	Fragment capture followed by native mass spectrometry (MS) in oncology targets	[15]
Nanofluidic chips	Low-volume, high throughput screening	μM	Fragment soaking and microcrystal X-ray screening	[16]
Nanostructure SPR surfaces	Kinetic and affinity analysis	100–500 μM	Protein–protein interaction fragment detection	[15, 16]
Nanodiscs/lipid nanostructures	Membrane protein stabilization	μM	G protein-coupled receptors (GPCR) and ion channel fragment screening by NMR	[15, 16]

6.5.2 X-ray Crystallography Using Nanocrystals

X-ray crystallography is the gold standard for structural validation fragment hits, and nanotechnology has expanded its applicability through nanocrystal-based approaches. Advances in micro-and nano-crystallization enable the growth of protein nanocrystals that are suitable for serial femtosecond crystallography and microfocus synchrotron beamlines. Recent fragment screening campaigns have used nanocrystal soaking methods to rapidly determine binding poses for hundreds of fragments with minimal protein consumption. These approaches have been particularly impactful in kinase and enzyme, where high-resolution fragment–protein structures directly guide fragment growing and linking strategies [18].

6.5.3 Surface Plasmon Resonance and Nano-SPR

SPR provides real-time, label-free measurement of binding kinetics and affinities. Nano-SPR platforms, which incorporate nanostructured gold surfaces or nanoparticle-enhanced plasmonic chips, offer significantly improved sensitivity compared with conventional SPR. Recent studies demonstrate that nano-SPR can reliably detect fragment interactions in the high micromolar range, a critical threshold for FBDD. For instance, nanostructured SPR sensors have been used to screen fragment libraries against protein–protein interaction targets, delivering kinetics that inform fragment prioritization and early combinatorial decisions [19].

6.5.4 Mass Spectrometry on Nano Platforms

Native MS has emerged as a powerful complementary method for fragment screening and validation. Nano-enabled MS platforms, including nano-electrospray ionization and nanoparticle-assisted ionization methods, allow preservation and detection of non-covalent fragment–protein complexes. Recent applications show that nano-MS can rapidly identify fragment binders, assess binding stoichiometry, and detect covalent fragment engagement with high specificity. Microfluidic sample handling integrated with nano-MS has also provided better throughput and reproducibility, further making it more palatable to standard FBDD processes [20]. Nano-enabled biophysical platforms have become a significant part of detection and validation of weak fragment–target interactions, as shown in Figure 6.2.

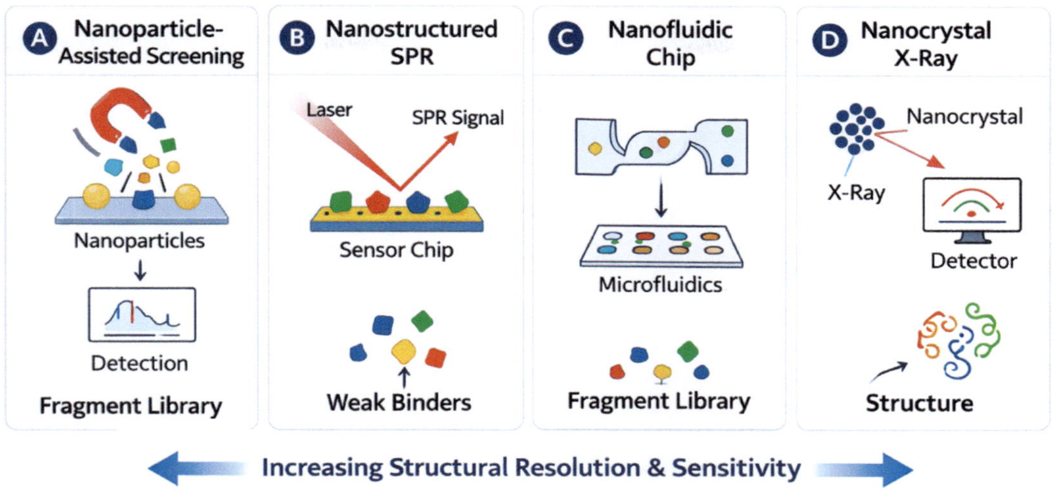

FIGURE 6.2 Nano-enabled biophysical platforms used in FBDD.

6.6 FRAGMENT OPTIMIZATION VIA NANOTECHNOLOGY

6.6.1 Fragment Linking and Growing

Fragment optimization transforms low-affinity fragments hits into potent leads by fragment growing, linking, or merging. Nanotechnology supports these approaches by enabling precise spatial control and enhanced detection of incremental affinity gains. For example, nanoparticle-immobilized targets have been used to map adjacent binding hot spots, allowing rational fragment growing based on proximity effects. Magnetic nanoparticles coupled with MS have enabled rapid evaluation of fragment linking efficiency by selectively enriching linked fragments that exhibit improved binding. Recent oncology-focused FBDD campaigns targeting kinases and epigenetic enzymes have successfully applied such nano-assisted methods guide fragment expansion while maintaining high ligand efficiency [21].

6.6.2 Nano-Guideline Structure Refinement

Nanotechnology enhances structures refinement by increasing resolution and sensitivity in structural biology workflows. Nanocrystals-based X-ray crystallography and microfocus beamlines allow visualization of subtle binding changes introduced during fragment growing. In several recent kinase and protease programs, nanocrystal-soaking experiments enabled rapid comparison of fragment analogs, revealing optimal growth vectors and water displacement patterns. Moreover, nanostructured biosensors such as graphene-based SPR and nanoelectrode arrays have been used to monitor real-time binding kinetics of optimized fragments, providing early feedback on residence time and binding mode refinement. These data-rich nano-guided insights reduce trials-and-error during medicinal chemistry [22].

6.6.3 Computational Nanodesign Aids

Calculational methods increasingly integrate nanoscale considerations into fragment optimization. Molecular dynamics simulations performed on nanostructured-to-microsecond timescales are used to predict how fragments interact with confined or nanostructured environments, such as nanoparticles-presented target or membrane-mimicking nanodiscs. ML models trained on nano-SPR and nano-MS crystallographic datasets have recently been applied to prioritize fragment modifications with the highest probability of affinity improvement. Simultaneously, in silico nanoformulation screening is becoming a technology to assess the behavior of optimized fragments upon incorporation into nanocarriers in support of the early developability. The computational nanodesign helps speed up fragment-to-lead progression by combining data on structural, kinetic, and nanoscale interactions [23].

6.7 CASE STUDIES AND APPLICATIONS

6.7.1 FBDD for Kinases Using Nanostructures

Protein kinases are among the most successful targets for FBDD, yet their conserved ATP-binding sites demand high sensitivity and structural precision. Nanostructured platforms have improved kinase-focused FBDD by improving detection of weak fragment interactions and rapid structure determination. For example, nanocrystal X-ray crystallography has been widely used to screen fragments against kinases like Bruton's tyrosine kinase (BTK) and cyclin-dependent kinases (CDK) family members, enabling rapid identification of binding poses with minimal protein consumption. Nanostructured SPR chips and nanoparticle-immobilized kinases have further kinetic discrimination between closely related fragment hits, guiding selective fragment growing strategies [24].

6.7.2 Nanoparticle-Mediated Fragment Screening in Oncology

In oncology drug discovery, nanoparticle-assisted screening has proven particularly valuable for challenging targets, including protein–protein interactions and epigenetic regulators. Oncogenic protein functionalized magnetic nanoparticles have been used to enrich low-affinity fragment binders in complex mixtures, after which those binders are identified using native MS. Recent cancer-oriented FBDD programs targeting Kirsten rat sarcoma viral oncogene homolog (KRAS) and bromodomain proteins have used nano-enrichment to enhance hit confidence and minimize false positives. These approaches have been used to complement classical biophysical assays and have helped accelerate the hit-to-lead of relatively competitive oncology pipelines [25].

6.7.3 Application in CNS Drug Discovery

Central nervous system (CNS) targets pose additional challenges due to conformational flexibility and restrictive physicochemical requirements. Nanotechnology-assisted FBDD has enabled screen against CNS-relevant targets with membrane-mimetic nanodiscs and nanoparticle-stabilized proteins. An example of a nanodisc-based NMR methodology is used to screen fragments to GPCRs and ion channels using nanodiscs, and enables weak-affinity interactions to be observed under near-native conditions. In parallel, nano-SPR and microfluidic platforms have facilitated rapid evaluation of fragment binding kinetics, helping medicinal chemists balance affinity, selectivity, and CNS drug properties early in optimization [26].

6.7.4 Emerging Targets and Novel Modalities

Beyond classical enzymes and receptors, nano-enabled FBDD is expanding into emerging target classes and modalities. Nanostructured sensors have been applied to fragment screening against RNA targets and intrinsically disordered proteins, both of which are traditionally difficult to address. Covalent fragment screening supported by nanoparticle enrichment has also gained traction for identifying ligands against previously "undruggable" targets. Moreover, integration of FBDD with nanotechnology is increasingly relevant for targeted protein degradation and molecular glues, where weak initial interaction can be amplified and characterized by nanoscale systems [27].

6.8 CHALLENGES AND LIMITATIONS

6.8.1 Sensitivity and Specificity

Despite significant progress, achieving sufficient sensitivity and specificity remains a core challenge in nano-enabled FBDD. Fragment binding affinities are inherently weak, and while nanostructured sensors and nanoparticle-assisted assays amplify signals, they can also introduce nonspecific adsorption and background noise. As an illustration, nanomaterials made of gold and carbon can be subjected to nonspecific interactions with hydrophobic fragments or protein surfaces without proper control over surface chemistry, resulting in false positives. According to recent reports, surface passivation, orthogonal validation (e.g., nano-SPR and NMR or crystallography), and close assay design are required to differentiate between true fragment binders and artifacts [28].

6.8.2 Data Complexity and Throughput

Nano-enabled platforms generate large, multidimensional datasets that combine kinetic, structural, and physicochemical information. While this richness is valuable, it also increases analytical complexity. High-throughput nanofluidic screening, nano-SPR, and nano-MS can produce thousands of binding traces or spectra in a single campaign, requiring advanced data processing and statistical filtering. Recent reports highlight that without standardized pipelines and automated analysis, data interpretation can become a bottleneck rather than an advantage. ML integration has been demonstrated to be able to manage this complexity, although it requires high-quality and well-annotated datasets, which are not available to many targets [29].

6.8.3 Nanotoxicology and Safety

The use of nanomaterials raises important safety and regulatory issues. Certain types of nanoparticles, such as quantum dots, some metal oxides, and the poorly characterized carbon nanostructures, have caused some concerns related to cytotoxicity, immunogenicity, and long-term accumulation. Although many of the nano-tools in FBDD are limited to in vitro discovery stages, growing interest in translating nano-enabled approaches for therapeutic applications requires early toxicological assessment. Recent regulatory guidance emphasizes thorough characterization of nanomaterial size, surface chemistry, and degradation behavior, underscoring that safety evaluation can add time and complexity to development pipelines [30].

6.8.4 Scalability and Cost

Scalability remains a practical limitation for widespread adoption of nanotechnology for FBDD. Fabrication of nanostructured sensor, nanofluidic devices, and high-quality nanoparticles often requires specialized equipment and expertise, which increases upfront cost. While these platforms reduce reagents consumption and can shorten discovery timelines, their cost-effectiveness depends on reuse, standardization, and integration into existing workflows. Recent industrial case studies suggest that nano-enabled methods are most impactful when selectively applied to high-value or high-risk targets rather than as universal screening solutions [31].

6.9 REGULATORY AND TRANSLATIONAL ASPECTS

6.9.1 Validation and Standards

Robust validation is essential for translating nano-enabled FBDD outputs into clinical candidates. Assays that incorporate nanomaterials must demonstrate accuracy, reproducibility, and relevance across orthogonal methods. International standards emphasize physicochemical characterization of nanomaterials (size distribution, surface charge, and composition), assay performance metrics (sensitivity and specificity), and data integrity. Recent guidance encourages method qualification early in discovery – especially for nano-SPR, nano-MS, and nanofluidics platforms – to ensure that fragment hits and structure-activity relationships are reliable and transferable across laboratories [32].

6.9.2 Regulatory Pathways for Nano-Enabled Drugs

Regulatory agencies have developed evolving frameworks for nanotechnology-enabled therapeutics. The U.S. Food and Drug Administration and the European Medicines Agency recommend complete characterization of nanomaterials, including manufacturing controls, stability, and in vivo fate, alongside conventional pharmacology and toxicology. While nano-tools used solely in discovery may not require direct regulatory review, nano-enabled drug products must address additional consideration such as batch-to-batch consistency and potential nano-specific risks. Alignment with the International Council for Harmonisation guidelines supports global development and reduces regulatory uncertainty [5].

6.9.3 Clinical Translation Considerations

Clinical translation demands early attention to developability, safety, and scalability. Nano-enabled FBDD can improve hit quality and reduce attrition by providing high-confidence structural and kinetic data; however, candidates must ultimately meet standard criteria for bioavailability, efficacy, and safety. Recent translational programs show that integrating nano-derived insights with conventional medicinal chemistry accelerates lead optimization without overhead in development. Successful translation is best achieved if nanotechnology is used strategically to improve discovery decisions and produce a final therapeutic that meets established clinical/regulatory expectations [33].

6.10 FUTURE PROSPECTS

6.10.1 AI and Machine Learning (ML) Integration

AI and ML technologies have been forecasted to be a transformative for nano-enabled FBDD. By combining measurements from nano-SPR, nanocrystallography, nano-MS, and molecular simulations, ML models can be used to discern subtle structure-affinity relationships that are hard to represent with traditional analysis. Recent advances propose the application of deep learning to fragment growth vector prioritization and binding hot spot prediction to minimize experimental cycles and accelerate fragment-to-lead optimization [34].

6.10.2 Self-Assembling Nanobio Systems

Self-assembling nanobio systems, including DNA origami, peptide nanostructures, and supramolecular assemblies, offer new possibilities for controlled fragment presentation and multivalent binding. These systems enable programmable spatial organization of fragments and targets, allowing cooperative interactions to be studied at the nanoscale. Emerging research shows that such platforms can improve detection of weak binders and support innovative screening formats for complex biological targets [35].

6.10.3 Personalized Nanotherapeutics

Personalized nanotherapeutics represents a forward-looking application of nano-enabled FBDD. By combining patient-specific molecular data with nano-assisted discovery tools, future pipelines may tailor fragment optimization toward individual genetic or proteomic profiles. This convergence supports precision medicine approaches, especially in oncology and CNS disorders, where target variability influences therapeutic response [36].

6.11 CONCLUSION

The convergence of fragment-based drug design and nanotechnology represents a significant advance in modern drug discovery. By addressing the intrinsic limitations of weak fragment binding, nano-enabled platforms improve sensitivity, structural resolution, and data-enrichment at different stages of screening and optimization. Integration with nanomaterials, nanofluidics, and nanoscale sensors has expanded the scope of FBDD to include targets and new modalities. Importantly, these technologies enable better decision-making, reduce attrition, and accelerate the progression of fragment hits into viable drug candidates. As regulatory frameworks mature and computational tools such as AI become more integrated, nano-enabled FBDD is poised to play an increasingly important role in precision and translational drug discovery, bridging innovative science with clinical impact.

ACKNOWLEDGMENTS

I am grateful to **Dr. Rajendra Gode College of Pharmacy, Amravati**, for providing the necessary facilities and support to complete this chapter.

REFERENCES

1. AlKharboush DF, Kozielski F, Wells G, Porta EO. Fragment-based drug discovery: A graphical review. Current Research in Pharmacology and Drug Discovery. 2025;10:100233.
2. Erlanson DA, Fesik SW, Hubbard RE, Jahnke W, Jhoti H. Twenty years on: The impact of fragments on drug discovery. Nature Reviews Drug Discovery. 2016;15(9):605–19.
3. Liu N. DNA nanotechnology meets nanophotonics. Nano Letters. 2020;20(12):8430–31.
4. Kennedy C, McPhie K, Rittinger K. Targeting the ubiquitin system by fragment-based drug discovery. Frontiers in Molecular Biosciences. 2022;9:1019636.
5. Kirsch P, Hartman AM, Hirsch AK, Empting M. Concepts and core principles of fragment-based drug design. Molecules. 2019;24(23):4309.
6. Begley DW, Davies DR, Hartley C, Edwards TE, Staker BL, Van Voorhis WC, Myler PJ, Stewart LJ Fragment Screening of Infectious Disease Targets in a Structural Genomics Environment. In Methods in Enzymology (Vol. 493, pp. 533–556). Academic Press; 2011.
7. Sim S, Wong NK. Nanotechnology and its use in imaging and drug delivery. Biomedical Reports. 2021; 14(5):42.
8. Strano MS, Ahn JH, Kim JH, Barone PW, Reuel NF, inventors; Massachusetts Institute of Technology, assignee. Nanotube array for optical detection of protein-protein interactions. United States patent US 10,215,752. 2019.
9. Malode SJ, Akhdar H, Alodhayb AN, Shetti NP. Bio-based nanomaterials for smart and sustainable nano-biosensing and therapeutics. Industrial Crops and Products. 2025;234:121603.
10. Amina SJ, Guo B. A review on the synthesis and functionalization of gold nanoparticles as a drug delivery vehicle. International Journal of Nanomedicine. 2020:9823–57.
11. Javid-Naderi MJ, Shaegh SA. Advanced microfluidic techniques for the preparation of solid lipid nanoparticles: Innovations and biomedical applications. International Journal of Pharmaceutics: X. 2025:100399.
12. Gironda-Martínez A, Donckele EJ, Samain F, Neri D. DNA-encoded chemical libraries: A comprehensive review with successful stories and future challenges. ACS Pharmacology & Translational Science. 2021;4(4):1265–79.
13. Goodrum R, Weldekidan H, Li H, Mohanty AK, Misra M. Graphene-based nanostructures from green processes and their applications in biomedical sensors. Advanced Industrial and Engineering Polymer Research. 2024;7(1):37–53.
14. Georgeous J, AlSawaftah N, Abuwatfa WH, Husseini GA. Review of gold nanoparticles: Synthesis, properties, shapes, cellular uptake, targeting, release mechanisms and applications in drug delivery and therapy. Pharmaceutics. 2024;16(10):1332.

15. Dong Y, Tang H, Dai H, Zhao H, Wang J. The application of nanodiscs in membrane protein drug discovery & development and drug delivery. Frontiers in Chemistry. 2024;12:1444801.
16. Acharya R, Patil TV, Dutta SD, Lee J, Ganguly K, Kim H, Randhawa A, Lim KT. Single-walled carbon nanotube-based optical nano/biosensors for biomedical applications: Role in bioimaging, disease diagnosis, and biomarkers detection. Advanced Materials Technologies. 2024;9(20):2400279.
17. Li Y, Kang C. Solution NMR spectroscopy in target-based drug discovery. Molecules. 2017;22(9):1399.
18. Garman EF. Developments in x-ray crystallographic structure determination of biological macromolecules. Science. 2014;343(6175):1102–8.
19. Basak S, Borah A, Ramchiary B. Surface plasmon resonance: A comprehensive review of principles, instrumentation, analytical procedures, and pharmaceutical applications. Journal of Preventive, Diagnostic and Treatment Strategies in Medicine. 2025;4(2):93–103.
20. Cui M, Du Y. Native mass spectrometry for characterization of proteins binding with small molecules and application in drug discovery. TrAC Trends in Analytical Chemistry. 2024;174:117701.
21. de Souza Neto LR, Moreira-Filho JT, Neves BJ, Maidana RL, Guimarães AC, Furnham N, Andrade CH, Silva Jr FP. In silico strategies to support fragment-to-lead optimization in drug discovery. Frontiers in Chemistry. 2020;8:93.
22. Kuriyan J. *Award Winners and Abstracts of the 31st Annual Symposium of The Protein Society*, Montreal, Canada, July 24–27, 2017 (Doctoral dissertation, Tsinghua University).
23. Marrink SJ, Monticelli L, Melo MN, Alessandri R, Tieleman DP, Souza PC. Two decades of martini: Better beads, broader scope. Wiley Interdisciplinary Reviews: Computational Molecular Science. 2023;13(1):e1620.
24. Wang ZZ, Shi XX, Huang GY, Hao GF, Yang GF. Fragment-based drug design facilitates selective kinase inhibitor discovery. Trends in Pharmacological Sciences. 2021;42(7):551–65.
25. Yang C, Merlin D. Nanoparticle-mediated drug delivery systems for the treatment of IBD: Current perspectives. International Journal of Nanomedicine. 2019;13:8875–89.
26. Mittal KR, Pharasi N, Sarna B, Singh M, Rachana, Haider S, Singh SK, Dua K, Jha SK, Dey A, Ojha S. Nanotechnology-based drug delivery for the treatment of CNS disorders. Translational Neuroscience. 2022;13(1):527–46.
27. Lundquist KP, Panchal V, Gotfredsen CH, Brenk R, Clausen MH. Fragment-based drug discovery for RNA targets. ChemMedChem. 2021;16(17):2588–603.
28. Scott DE, Coyne AG, Hudson SA, Abell C. Fragment-based approaches in drug discovery and chemical biology. Biochemistry. 2012;51(25):4990–5003.
29. Xu X, Valavanis D, Ciocci P, Confederat S, Marcuccio F, Lemineur JF, Actis P, Kanoufi F, Unwin PR. The new era of high-throughput nanoelectrochemistry. Analytical Chemistry. 2023;95(1):319–56.
30. Zhang N, Xiong G, Liu Z. Toxicity of metal-based nanoparticles: Challenges in the nano era. Frontiers in Bioengineering and Biotechnology. 2022;10:1001572.
31. Bi Y, Xie S, Li Z, Dong S, Teng L. Precise nanoscale fabrication technologies, the "last mile" of medicinal development. Acta Pharmaceutica Sinica B. 2025; 15(5):2372–401.
32. Abram SL, Tavernaro I, Johnston LJ, Zou S, Resch-Genger U. Nanoscale reference and test materials for the validation of characterization methods for engineered nanomaterials—Current state, limitations, and needs. Analytical and Bioanalytical Chemistry. 2025;417(12):2405–25.
33. Prabhu RH, Patravale VB, Joshi MD. Polymeric nanoparticles for targeted treatment in oncology: Current insights. International Journal of Nanomedicine. 2015;10:1001–18. https://doi.org/10.2147/IJN.S56932.
34. Ravn P, Madhurantakam C, Kunze S, Matthews E, Priest C, O'Brien S, Collinson A, Papworth M, Fritsch-Fredin M, Jermutus L, Benthem L. Structural and pharmacological characterization of novel potent and selective monoclonal antibody antagonists of glucose-dependent insulinotropic polypeptide receptor. Journal of Biological Chemistry. 2013;288(27):19760–72.
35. Chen R, Jia X, Pang W, Yang Y, Zhou H, Gao Z. Applications of DNA origami in biomedicine: Advances, challenges, and prospects. Advanced Composites and Hybrid Materials. 2025;8(5):375.
36. Alghamdi MA, Fallica AN, Virzì N, Kesharwani P, Pittalà V, Greish K. The promise of nanotechnology in personalized medicine. Journal of Personalized Medicine. 2022;12(5):673.

7 Encapsulation of Natural Antidiabetics in Nanoparticles
Advances and Applications

S. Rizwana Begum, Anjum A., Aruna G., Tasleem Tabassum A., S. Carmel Punitha, R. Ramya, and Mumtaz Begum T.A.K.
Justice Basheer Ahmed Sayeed College for Women (Autonomous), Chennai, India

7.1 INTRODUCTION

Diabetes is a growing epidemic worldwide: in 2024, an estimated 589 million adults (20–79 years) were living with diabetes. This count will see a significant increase in the coming decades. About 3.4 million deaths were caused in 2024, and diabetes is responsible for a tremendous healthcare cost in the world. These figures underline an urgent need for safer, more accessible therapies, especially in low- and middle-income regions where the disease burden and treatment gaps are largest [1].

Natural products (phytochemicals) – including polyphenols (curcumin, quercetin, resveratrol), alkaloids (berberine), terpenoids, and plant extracts (bitter melon, *Momordica charantia*) – have long shown multimodal antidiabetic activities: insulin sensitization, inhibition of carbohydrate-digesting enzymes (a-glucosidase/a-amylase), antioxidant and anti-inflammatory functions, and beta cell protection in preclinical models. These activities are attractive as being candidates for complementary or alternative intervention that may be low-cost and acceptable [2].

However, translation to clinical benefits has been limited by persistent pharmacokinetics (PKs) and formulation problems. Curcumin, a flagship example, exhibits extremely low systemic exposure after oral dosing due to poor aqueous solubility, rapid intestinal and hepatic metabolism, and instability in physiological media. Multiple reviews note that a conventional curcumin formulation produces only trace plasma levels, limiting its therapeutic effect. Similarly, berberine's absolute oral bioavailability is <1% in animal and human research, forcing high oral doses that cause gastrointestinal adverse effects and variable efficacy [3].

Nanoparticle (NP) encapsulation directly targets these weaknesses by improving aqueous dispersibility, protecting actives from enzymatic degradation and first pass-metabolism, and enabling controlled release or targeted uptake. For example, curcumin-loaded poly(lactic-co-glycolic acid) (PLGA) NPs have been reported repeatedly to increase bioavailability and tissue delivery compared with unencapsulated curcumin, while berberine micro/nanoemulsion formulations have demonstrated several-fold increase in bioavailability and enhanced hypoglycemic efficacy in preclinical models. These tangible PKs and efficacy improvements illustrate why nanoencapsulation is a primary strategy to convert promising natural antidiabetics into clinically useful therapies [4]. Figure 7.1 provides visual overview comparing the important shortcomings of free phytochemicals such as poor stability, low absorption, and off-target effects with the improved stability, targeting, and circulation achieved through nanoencapsulation.

DOI: 10.1201/9781003598657-7

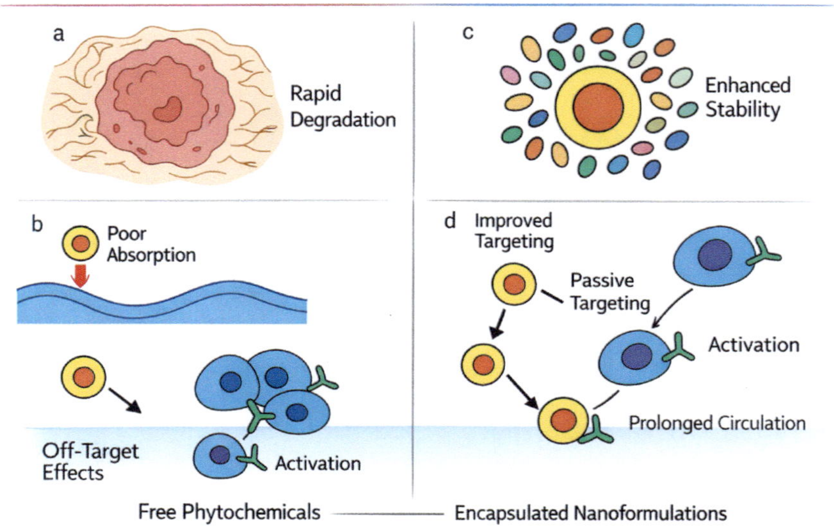

FIGURE 7.1 Comparison of free phytochemical versus encapsulated nanoformulations.

7.2 NATURAL ANTIDIABETICS: CLASSES AND EXAMPLES

7.2.1 Polyphenols

Polyphenols represent the most widely researched class of natural antidiabetics because of their antioxidant, anti-inflammatory, and insulin-sensitizing effects. Curcumin, a diarylheptanoid from *Curcuma longa*, modulates multiple glucose-regulating pathways, including activation of adenosine monophosphate-activated protein kinase (AMPK), inhibition of NF-κB-mediated inflammation, and protection of pancreatic β-cells from oxidative stress. Despite strong preclinical efficacy, curcumin shows extremely low oral bioavailability (<1%) in humans, necessitating advanced delivery approaches [5].

Quercetin, a flavonol common in onions and apples, improves insulin sensitivity by increasing GLUT4 translocation and inhibiting α-glucosidase and α-amylase. In diabetic rodent models, quercetin supplementation has been shown to significantly reduce fasting blood glucose and oxidative biomarkers. Resveratrol, a stilbene present in grapes, activates SIRT1 and AMPK signaling, improves mitochondria function, and reduces insulin resistance. Clinical studies report modest glycemic improvement, but rapid metabolism and poor stability limit sustained plasma exposure [6].

7.2.2 Alkaloids

Berberine, an isoquinoline alkaloid isolated from *Berberis* species, is one of the most promising natural antidiabetic compounds with efficacy comparable to metformin in some clinical studies. Its mechanisms include AMPK activation, suppression of hepatic gluconeogenesis, modulation of gut microbiota, and improved insulin receptor signaling. However, berberine has a very poor oral bioavailability (<1%), largely due to low intestinal permeability, P-glycoprotein efflux, and extensive first-pass metabolism. High oral doses (0.9–1.5 g/day) are often required clinically, increasing the risk of gastrointestinal side effects [7].

7.2.3 Terpenoids

Terpenoids, including triterpenes and diterpenes, exert antidiabetic effects through enzyme inhibition and insulin sensitization. Gymnemic acids from *Gymnema Sylvestre* suppress intestinal glucose absorption and promote pancreatic β-cell regeneration. Ginsenosides (triterpene saponins) from *Panax ginseng* enhance insulin signaling, decrease oxidative stress, and regulate lipid metabolism. Although potent, many terpenoids suffer from poor aqueous solubility and chemically instability, limiting their oral effectiveness [8].

7.2.4 Peptides and Plant Extracts

Polypeptide-k, isolated from *Momordica charantia* (bitter melon), is an insulin-like peptide that lowers blood glucose by enhancing peripheral glucose uptake. Bitter melon extracts also contain charantin and vicine, which together enhance insulin secretion and block gluconeogenesis. While effective in animal models and small clinical studies, peptide instability, enzymatic degradation, and batch variability in extracts restrict clinical translation without protective delivery systems [9].

7.3 LIMITATIONS OF NATIVE COMPOUNDS

7.3.1 Poor Aqueous Solubility

One major limitation of most of natural antidiabetic compounds is their poor water solubility, which directly restricts dissolution in gastrointestinal fluids and limits absorption after oral administration. Polyphenols such as curcumin, quercetin, and resveratrol are highly lipophilic and exhibit aqueous solubilities in micrograms-per-milliliter range. For example, curcumin has an intrinsic solubility of <0.01 mg/mL in water, resulting in minimal dissolution in the intestinal lumen. Low solubility causes erratic absorption, and high interindividual variability even in the case of high oral doses [10].

7.3.2 Rapid Metabolism and First-Pass Effect

Many phytochemicals undergo extensive presystemic metabolism in the intestine and liver. Polyphenols are quickly conjugated through glucuronidation and sulfation forming metabolites that are less or differently bioactive. Resveratrol, for example, is well absorbed but is quickly metabolized and very low levels of unbound parent compound are found in systemic circulation. Alkaloids such as berberine are also extensively subject to first-pass metabolism combined with active efflux by P-glycoprotein transporters leading to very low plasma exposure [11].

7.3.3 Low Oral Bioavailability

Due to the combined effects of poor solubility, low permeability, and fast metabolism, the oral bioavailability of many natural antidiabetics is extremely low. Berberine is a prominent example, with reported oral bioavailability below 1% in both preclinical and clinical studies. Consequently, high doses orally are needed to achieve therapeutic effects with a risk of gastrointestinal discomfort and poor patient compliance [12].

7.3.4 Chemical and Biological Instability

Native phytochemicals often exhibit instability under physiological and processing conditions. Curcumin degrades rapidly at neutral and alkaline pH, while peptide-based antidiabetics, like polypeptide-k are prone to being broken down by enzymes in the gastrointestinal tract. Additionally, plant extracts may suffer from batch-to-batch variability, oxidation, and photodegradation, further complicating formulation and standardization [13].

7.4 NANOCARRIERS: TYPES

7.4.1 Polymeric Nanoparticles (PLGA, Chitosan)

Polymeric NPs (PLGA, chitosan) are widely used to encapsulate lipophilic phytochemicals because they offer controlled release and protection from gastro-intestinal (GI) degradation. PLGA particles loaded with curcumin or other polyphenols demonstrate enhanced stability and several-fold higher oral exposure and delivery to tissues in preclinical studies. Chitosan acts as an effective absorption enhancer due to its mucoadhesive properties and its ability to transiently open epithelial tight junctions. This mechanism is particularly advantageous for alkaloids with poor membrane permeability, such as berberine. In vivo studies indicate that chitosan-based berberine formulations facilitate sustained drug release and exhibit enhanced hypoglycemic effects [14].

Pros: High drug-loading of hydrophobic actives, to control their degradation and functionalization of the surface for targeting.
Cons: Burst release risk, polymer residuals/toxicity issues at scale, sometimes complex manufacturing.

7.4.2 Lipid-Based Systems (Liposomes, SLN, NLC)

Lipid nanocarriers, including liposomes, solid lipid nanoparticles (SLNs), and nanostructured lipid carriers (NLCs), are extensively exploited for curcumin and related polyphenols because lipids solubilize lipophilic actives and protect labile molecules. Curcumin-loaded SLNs and NLCs have shown improved chemical stability, higher entrapment efficiency, and enhanced biological activity in vitro and in vivo [15].

Pros: Excellent biocompatibility, scalable excipients (many generally recognized as safe [GRAS] lipids), and good for oral or topical routes.
Cons: Poor long-term physical stability (aggregation), moderate loading power of drug (drugs with high lipophilic value), and polymorphic transformation of lipids.

7.4.3 Nanoemulsions

Nanoemulsions (oil-in-water, droplet size <200 nm) enhance solubilization and intestinal lymphatic uptake of phytochemicals (e.g., berberine, curcumin); and in some recent works, they enhance superior dissolution and enhancement in bioactivity also. Nanoemulsions can be prepared for food/nutraceutical applications as well [16].

Pros: Simple manufacturing, high solubilization capacity, and transparency for liquid dosing.
Cons: Thermodynamic instability (requires surfactants) and oxidative sensitivity of oils.

7.4.4 Nanocrystals

Nanocrystals reduce particle size of the pure drug to <200 nm, dramatically increasing dissolution rate and apparent solubility. These are especially attractive for poorly soluble phytochemicals. Recent reviews highlight rapid dissolution and very high release (>80–90% in minutes) for several model compounds [17].

Pros: Very high drug loading (DL) (purity of drug) and rapid onset.
Cons: Physical stability (Ostwald ripening), need for stabilizers, and difficulty in controlling the release kinetics.

7.4.5 Inorganic (Metal/Oxide) Nanoparticle

Gold, silver, and magnetic NPs have been investigated, especially in biosensing and proof-of-concept bioactivity studies, where phytochemicals are conjugated or applied in green synthesis studies. Some biosynthesized Au/Ag NPs exhibit enzyme-inhibition and glucose-lowering effects in pre-clinical models [18].

Pros: Facile optical/magnetic properties for theranostics and targeted delivery.
Cons: Long-term biopersistence regulatory safety hurdles, potential cytotoxicity at high doses.

7.4.6 Green/Biogenic Nanoparticles

"Green" NPs synthesized using plant extracts combine reduction/stabilization and may carry inherent phytochemical activity; multiple recent reports demonstrate antidiabetic enzyme inhibition and antioxidant activity for biogenic Ag/Au NPs [19].

Pros: Easy eco-friendly synthesis, combined activity from metal and plant biomolecules.
Cons: Batch variability, unclear composition, and limited translational safety data.

7.5 ENCAPSULATION STRATEGIES AND TECHNIQUES

Encapsulation strategies for natural antidiabetics are selected to address common formulation barriers – poor solubility, instability, and low oral bioavailability – while preserving biological activity. Nanoprecipitation is one of the most commonly used techniques for polymeric NPs, especially with the PLGA and related copolymers. In this technique, a water-miscible organic solvent is rapidly diffused into an aqueous phase and precipitates polymers and entraps drugs. It is particularly effective for hydrophobic polyphenols such as curcumin and resveratrol. Recent experiments have found encapsulation efficiencies (EE) usually exceeding 70% when experimenting with solvent choice, polymer concentration, and drug-to-polymer ratio. The simplicity, scalability, and low thermal stress of nanoprecipitation represents sensitivity to sensitive phytochemicals [20]. The popular nanocarrier system discussed for encapsulation of natural antidiabetics, their general materials, merits and demerits, DL capacity, and release characteristics are summarized in Table 7.1.

Emulsification-solvent evaporation and solvent evaporation methods remain standard for both polymeric and lipid systems. These approaches form oil-in-water emulsions containing dissolved phytochemicals, followed by solvent removal to yield solid particles. They are frequently applied to berberine, quercetin, and mixed plant extracts. However, encapsulation efficiency (EE) and particle size are highly dependent on emulsifier type, homogenization energy, and phase viscosity. Excessive shear can lead to drug leakage, while insufficient stabilization promotes aggregation [21].

For polysaccharide-based carriers, ionic gelation is particularly relevant. Chitosan NPs formed via electrostatic interaction with tripolyphosphate enable mild, aqueous processing conditions that preserve bioactivity of alkaloids and peptides. Ionic strength, polymer molecular weight and cross-linker ratio play a very strong role in particle stability and drug release kinetics. Sustained release from 12 to 48 hours is also commonly reported for chitosan encapsulated berberine and bitter melon actives [22].

Spray-drying is increasingly used to convert nano-dispersions into dry powders suitable for oral dosage forms or functional foods. This technique enhances shelf stability and handling; however thermal exposure can reduce EE for heat-labile polyphenols unless inlet temperatures and feed rates are carefully controlled. Self-assembly techniques, polymeric micelles, and lipid self-assembled systems use hydrophobic interactions to encapsulate phytochemicals without harsh solvents. Although

TABLE 7.1
Comparative Overview of Nanocarriers for Encapsulation of Natural Antidiabetics

Nanocarrier Type	Typical Materials	Key Advantages	Main Limitations	Typical Drug Loading	Release Profile
Polymeric NPs	PLGA, chitosan	Controlled release; protection from degradation; surface functionalization	Burst release risk; scale-up complexity	Moderate-high	Sustained (hours-days)
Liposomes	Phospholipids, cholesterol	High biocompatibility; suitable for hydrophilic and lipophilic drugs	Physical instability; leakage	Moderate	Controlled, diffusion-driven
SLNs	Solid lipids (glyceryl behenate, stearic acid)	Good stability; GRAS lipids; scalable	Limited loading; lipid crystallization	Low-moderate	Sustained
NLCs	Solid + liquid lipids	Higher loading than SLN; improved stability	Formulation complexity	Moderate-high	Sustained
Nanoemulsions	Oil, surfactants	High solubilization rapid absorption	Thermodynamic instability	High	Rapid to moderate
Nanocrystals	Pure drug + stabilizer	Very high drug content; fast dissolution	Limited release control; aggregation	Very high	Immediate-fast
Inorganic NPs	Gold, iron oxide	Targeting/diagnostic potential	Long-term toxicity concerns	Low	Variable
Green/biogenic NPs	Plant extract-derived	Eco-friendly synthesis; inherent bioactivity	Batch variability; unclear composition	Low-moderate	Variable

these systems often reach very small particle sizes (<100 nm) and improved dissolution rates, they suffer from limited stability upon dilution [23].

Beyond core encapsulation, surface functionalization such as polyethylene glycol (PEGylation), ligand binding, or mucoadhesive coating has gained attention for improving circulation time, intestinal residence, and cellular uptake. Across all methods, formulation parameters, including drugs/carriers ratio, solvent polarity, surfactant concentration, particle size, and surface charge, critically determine EE, release behavior, and biological performance. Optimizing these variables is essential for translating natural antidiabetic nanoformulations from laboratory studies toward reproducible and scalable products [24].

7.6 PHYSICOCHEMICAL CHARACTERIZATION

7.6.1 Particle Size, PDI, and Surface Charge

Particle size is a critical determinant of stability, cellular uptake, and in vivo performance of nano-encapsulated natural antidiabetics. Most oral and parenteral formulations aim for mean sizes below 200 nm to enhance dissolution and absorption. Dynamic light scattering (DLS) is routinely used to measure hydrodynamic size and polydispersity index (PDI), with PDI values below 0.3 indicating a narrow and uniform size distribution. Surface charge assessed by zeta potential provides insight into colloidal stability; values greater than ±20 usually confer electrostatic repulsion and reduced aggregation. For example, chitosan-based NPs often exhibit positive zeta potentials (+25–+40 mV), which enhance mucoadhesion and intestinal residence time, whereas PLGA and lipid NPs typically show negative surface charges due to terminal carboxyl groups [25].

7.6.2 Morphology, Encapsulation Efficiency, and Drug Loading

NP morphologies affect drug release and biological interaction. Transmission and scanning electron microscopy (TEM/SEM) are used to observe shape and surface texture and structural integrity of particles, where spherical and smooth particles are preferred to produce predictable release behavior. EE and DL are measures of the success of formulation strategies and are typically quantified using indirect approaches after separation of particles. For hydrophobic polyphenols like curcumin or quercetin, values for the EE ranging between 60% and 90% are commonly found when formulation parameters for polymeric and lipid-based systems are optimal. Higher drug loading enhances the therapeutic efficiency, but it may affect the particle stability and/or cause burst release; a balance between EE, DL, and long-term stability is needed [26].

7.6.3 Thermal and Chemical Stability

Assessment of thermal and chemical stability is essential to ensure successful encapsulation and predict storage behavior. Differential scanning calorimetry (DSC) is used to evaluate melting behavior and crystallinity; disappearing or shifting of the drug's melting peak indicates molecular dispersion within the carrier matrix. Fourier-transform infrared spectroscopy (FTIR) gives information on possible interactions such as hydrogen bonding or electrostatic interactions between the phytochemical and carrier, without chemical degradation. X-ray diffraction (XRD) distinguishes crystalline from amorphous states, with reduced crystallinity often correlating with improved solubility and dissolution. Together, these complementary techniques confirm structural integrity, drug-carrier compatibility, and enhanced stability of nanoencapsulated natural antidiabetics [27].

7.7 RELEASE, STABILITY AND IN VITRO EVALUATION

7.7.1 In Vitro Release Behavior

In vitro release studies are central to understanding how nanoencapsulated natural antidiabetics perform under physiological conditions. Release is commonly evaluated using dialysis or diffusion methods in buffered media, revealing characteristic biphasic release patterns; an initial mild burst followed by steady release over several hours. Polymeric and lipid-based carriers typically slow the diffusion of hydrophobic phytochemicals such as curcumin and quercetin, maintaining therapeutic concentrations for prolonged periods. Controlled release is especially important for antidiabetic uses, where steady plasma exposure can improve glycemic control and reduce dosing frequency [28].

7.7.2 Simulated Gastrointestinal and Biological Stability

Stability studies in a simulated gastric (pH ~1.2) and intestinal fluids (pH ~6.8) are routinely conducted to assess protection against harsh gastrointestinal environment. Free phytochemicals often degrade rapidly or precipitate under these conditions, whereas nanoencapsulation significantly enhances the chemical stability and dispersibility. Additional evaluation of biological media such as serum or simulated intestinal fluids containing bile salts helps predict colloidal stability after oral administration. Stable formulations maintain particle size and zeta potential over time, indicating resistance to aggregation and premature drug leakage [29.

7.7.3 Protection against Enzymatic Degradation

Nanoencapsulation also provides protection against enzymatic degradation, especially for peptide- or alkaloid-based antidiabetics. Encapsulated systems protect active compounds from digestive enzymes, delaying degradation and allowing greater fractions of the drug to reach absorptive sites.

This protective effect has been found to increase apparent bioavailability and prolong biological action compared with native compounds [30].

7.7.4 Enzymatic and Antioxidant Activity Assays

Functional in vitro assays are needed to ensure that biological activity is retained after encapsulation. Antioxidant tests like 2,2-diphenyl-1-picrylhydrazyl (DPPH), 2,2'-azino-bis(3-ethylbenzothiazoline-6-sulfonic acid) (ABTS), and ferric reducing antioxidant power (FRAP) are used extensively to demonstrate preserved or enhanced radical-scavenging capacity of encapsulated polyphenols. In parallel, enzyme inhibition assays targeting α-glucosidase and α-amylase are employed to determine antidiabetic potential. Numerous studies report that nanoencapsulated phytochemicals exhibit equal or superior inhibitory activity compared with free compounds, an outcome attributed to improved solubility and sustained release. Collectively, these in vitro evaluations establish the stability, functional integrity, and therapeutic relevance of nanoencapsulated natural antidiabetics before in vivo validation [31].

7.8 IN VIVO EFFICACY AND PHARMACOKINETICS

7.8.1 Glucose-Lowering Efficacy in Animal Models

In vivo studies consistently demonstrate that nanoencapsulation improves the antidiabetic effect of natural compounds compared with native compounds. In streptozotocin- or high-fat-diet-induced diabetic rodents, nanoformulated polyphenols, including curcumin, quercetin, and resveratrol, produce greater reduction in fasting blood glucose and improved glucose tolerance than doses of free compounds. For example, curcumin-loaded PLGA or lipid NPs have been reported to reduce fasting glucose by 30–50% accompanied over 2–4 weeks of oral administration, whereas free curcumin shows modest or inconsistent effects at similar doses. Improvements are frequently accompanied by reduced oxidative stress markers and inflammatory cytokines in pancreatic and hepatic tissues [32].

7.8.2 Insulin Sensitivity and Metabolic Effects

Beyond glucose lowering, nanoencapsulated natural antidiabetics can enhance insulin sensitivity and lipid metabolism. Berberine nanoformulations, including polymeric NPs and nanoemulsions, have been shown to enhance activation of the AMPK signaling, resulting in improved insulin receptor sensitivity and reduced hepatic gluconeogenesis. Animal studies frequently report that decreased homeostatic model assessment of insulin resistance (HOMA-IR) values improved lipid profiles, and partial restoration of pancreatic β-cells architecture are achieved following treatment with encapsulated formulations; these outcomes are rarely achieved with native compounds alone [33].

7.8.3 Pharmacokinetic Enhancement

Pharmacokinetic (PK) studies provide direct evidence of the benefit of nanoencapsulation. Encapsulation typically increases peak plasma concentration (Cmax), area under the curve (AUC), and elimination half-life (T1/2) of phytochemicals. Berberine NPs have shown several-fold increases in AUC and prolonged systemic exposure compared with free berberine, which is otherwise rapidly cleared due to extensive first-pass metabolism. Similarly, nanoencapsulation of curcumin exhibits delayed Tmax and prolonged T1/2, reflecting sustained release and reduced metabolic degradation. These PK improvements correlate well with improved in vivo efficacies [34].

7.8.4 Biodistribution and Tissue Targeting

Biodistribution studies using fluorescent or radiolabeled NPs reveal preferential accumulation of nanoencapsulated compounds in metabolically active organs such as the liver, pancreas, and adipose tissue. Such distribution patterns improve modulation of glucose homeostasis while potentially reducing off-target exposure [35].

7.9 CLINICAL EVIDENCE: CURRENT STATUS

Clinical data on nanoencapsulated natural antidiabetics remain limited. While conventional formulations of curcumin and berberine have shown glycemic benefits in small trials, only a few early-phase studies have explored nanoformulations, mainly focusing on safety and bioavailability, rather than efficacy. Thus, although in vivo animal data are compelling, well-designed clinical trials are still required to validate translational potential. The PK advantages of nanoencapsulation, including increased systemic exposure and prolonged circulation compared with free phytochemicals, are illustrated in Figure 7.2.

7.9.1 Mechanisms of Improved Action

Nanoencapsulated enhances the therapeutic performance of natural antidiabetics by addressing multiple biological and PK barriers simultaneously. One of the main mechanisms is increased absorption, achieved through enhanced aqueous dispersibility and dissolution of poorly soluble phytochemicals. By decreasing the particle size to the nanometer scale, encapsulated compounds present a larger surface area to gastrointestinal fluids, promoting more efficient uptake across the intestinal epithelium. In the case of mucoadhesive carriers such as chitosan NPs, prolonged intestine residence further enhances absorption [36].

Protection from metabolic degradation is another key advantage. Encapsulation shields phytochemicals from harsh gastric pH, enzymatic hydrolysis, and extensive first-pass metabolism in the liver. While polyphenols such as curcumin and resveratrol are rapidly conjugated when administered in free form, encapsulation protects these drugs from being degraded by enzymes or cleared by the mononuclear phagocyte system (MPS) [37].

Nanoformulations also enable controlled and timed release, reducing burst effects and maintaining therapeutically relevant concentrations over extended periods. This is especially important for chronic diseases like diabetes, where stable plasma levels improve glycemic control and reduce

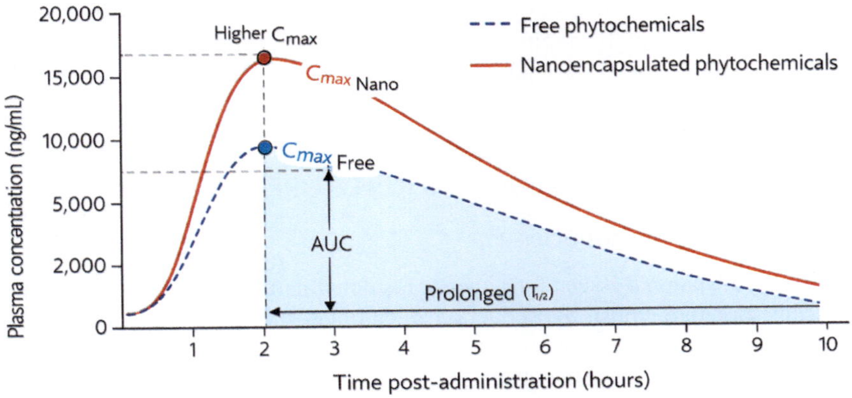

FIGURE 7.2 Representative PK profiles of free versus nanocapsulated phytochemicals illustrating enhanced bioavailability.

dosing frequency. Additionally, surface-modified NPs can facilitate improved cellular uptake via endocytosis, increasing intracellular delivery to insulin-sensitive tissues such as liver, muscle, and adipose tissue [38].

Beyond delivery advantages, encapsulation can amplify synergistic antioxidant and anti-inflammatory effects. Many nanocarriers stabilize the active compound in its bioactive form, enhancing its ability to suppress oxidative stress and inflammatory pathways implicated in insulin resistance and β-cell dysfunction. Collectively, these mechanisms explain why nanoencapsulated natural antidiabetics consistently outperform their native counterparts in preclinical models and represent a rational strategy for enhancing therapeutic outcomes [39].

7.9.2 Safety, Toxicity, and Regulatory Considerations

Safety evaluation is a critical requirement for translating nanoencapsulated natural antidiabetics from laboratory research to clinical and commercial applications. Acute and chronic toxicity studies on animal models generally indicate that well-designed polymeric and lipid-based NPs exhibit an acceptable safety profile when composed of biodegradable materials such as PLGA, chitosan, and physiological lipids. Short-term studies frequently report no significant alteration in liver and kidney function markers, hematological parameters, or histopathology at therapeutic dose levels. However, chronic exposure raises additional concerns, including possible accumulation, altered biodistribution, and metabolic effects in long term, which highlight the need for long-term toxicity and reproductive safety studies [40].

Immunogenicity and inflammatory responses represent another important consideration. NPs can interact with immune cells and plasma proteins, potentially triggering complement activation or cytokine release. Surface characteristics such as size, charge, and coating strongly influence immunogenic potential. For example, cationic NPs may induce higher inflammatory responses than neutral or PEGylated systems, necessitating careful surface optimization to minimize unintended immune activation [41].

Excipient safety is closely linked to regulatory acceptance. Many carriers used in phytochemical nanoformulations – such as PLGA, lecithin, medium-chain triglycerides, and certain surfactants – have GRAS status or prior approval for pharmaceutical or food use. Leveraging GRAS excipients significantly lowers regulatory barriers and facilitates translational development. Nonetheless, the nano-scale itself may alter toxicological behavior, requiring nano-specific safety assessment rather than only using bulk material data [42].

From a translational perspective, scale-up and manufacturing reproducibility remain major hurdles. Methods optimized at laboratory scale may face challenges in maintaining particle size, encapsulation efficiency, and batch-to-batch reproducibility during the large-scale production. Regulatory agencies increasingly emphasize robust quality control, physicochemical characterization, and stability testing for nanoformulations. Furthermore, the lack of harmonized global regulatory guidelines for nanomedicines complicates approval pathways [43].

7.10 TRANSLATIONAL CHALLENGES AND FUTURE PROSPECTS

7.10.1 Scalability and Reproducibility

One of the major translational issues for nanoencapsulated natural antidiabetics is developing the laboratory formulation into industrial production. Techniques such as nanoprecipitation or emulsification that work well on a small scale often struggle to have a consistent particle size, encapsulation efficiency, and surface characteristics at large-scale manufacture. Batch-to-batch variability is a major issue for phytochemicals because variability exists in raw plant materials. Scalable, continuous manufacturing approaches and control of critical quality attributes will have to be the focus of future efforts [44].

7.10.2 Stability in Real-World Formulations

While many nanoformulations demonstrate stability under controlled laboratory conditions, maintaining long-term stability in real dosage forms (capsules, suspensions, functional foods) remains challenging. Issues such as particle aggregation, drug leakage, oxidation of lipids, and moisture sensitivity can affect shelf life. Integration of nanoencapsulated antidiabetics into patient-friendly, commercially viable products requires robust stabilization strategies and real-time stability testing under regulatory guidelines [45].

7.10.3 Translation to Clinical Trials

Despite strong preclinical evidence, clinical translation is limited by insufficient human PK and efficacy data. Many studies focus on proof-of-concept animal models without standardized dosing or comparator formulations. Carefully designed early-phase clinical trials are needed to establish safety, enhance bioavailability, and demonstrate clinically meaningful glycemic outcomes. Standardization of formulations and transparent reporting is essential to build regulatory and clinical confidence [46].

7.10.4 Advanced and Combination Strategies

Future directions include combination therapies, where multiple natural antidiabetics or phytochemicals and conventional drugs are co-encapsulated to achieve synergistic effects. Additionally, smart and targeted nanocarriers – such as glucose-responsive systems or ligand-modified NPs targeting insulin-sensitive tissues – represent promising next-generation approaches to improve therapeutic precision [47].

7.10.5 Regulatory Pathway Considerations

Clearer regulatory pathways for phytochemical nanoformulations are needed. Aligning product development with existing pharmaceutical or nutraceutical frameworks, prioritizing GRAS excipients, and early regulatory engagement can streamline approval. Overall, bridging the gap between the promising preclinical data and clinical application will define the future impact of nanoencapsulated natural antidiabetics [48].

7.11 CONCLUSION

Nanoencapsulation has emerged as a powerful strategy to overcome the inherent PK and formulation limitations of natural antidiabetic compounds. By improving solubility, stability, bioavailability, and tissue delivery, nanocarrier systems significantly enhance the therapeutic potential of phytochemicals such as curcumin, quercetin, and berberine. Preclinical evidence consistently demonstrates superior glucose-lowering efficacy, improved insulin sensitivity, and favorable PK profiles for encapsulated formulations compared with native compounds. Despite these advances, successful clinical translation requires careful attention to safety, scalability, stability, and regulatory compliance. Continued integration of rational formulation design, standardized evaluation, and well-designed clinical studies will be essential to realize the full potential of nano-enabled natural antidiabetics in diabetes management.

ACKNOWLEDGMENTS

I wish to express my sincere appreciation to the Department of Biochemistry, Justice Basheer Ahmed Sayeed College for Women (Autonomous), Chennai, India for the excellent facilities and constant support provided during the preparation of this chapter.

REFERENCES

1. Magliano DJ, Boyko EJ, Atlas D. 3. The Global Picture of Diabetes. In Diabetes Atlas [Internet]. 11th edition. International Diabetes Federation; 2025.
2. Kim HP, Lim H, Kwon YS. Therapeutic potential of medicinal plants and their constituents on lung inflammatory disorders. Biomolecules & Therapeutics. 2016;25(2):91.
3. Smail SW, Bergsten P, Taha KO, Yashooa RK, Hawezy DJ, Abbas MA, Shekha MS. Curcumin: Biochemistry, pharmacology, advanced drug delivery systems, and its epigenetic role in combating cancer. Frontiers in Pharmacology. 2025;16:1695200.
4. Fu Y, Ge Y, Yi S, Peng Q, Jiang H, Zhou J. Smart nanoparticle delivery systems for curcumin: A targeted strategy to enhance anticancer efficacy and bioavailability. Journal of Materials Science: Materials in Medicine. 2026;37:7012–27. https://doi.org/10.1007/s10856-026-07012-7.
5. Centonze M, Aloisio Caruso E, De Nunzio V, Cofano M, Saponara I, Pinto G, Notarnicola M. The antiaging potential of dietary plant-based polyphenols: A review on their role in cellular senescence modulation. Nutrients. 2025;17(10):1716.
6. Al-Ishaq RK, Abotaleb M, Kubatka P, Kajo K, Büsselberg D. Flavonoids and their anti-diabetic effects: Cellular mechanisms and effects to improve blood sugar levels. Biomolecules. 2019;9(9):430.
7. Belwal T, Bisht A, Devkota HP, Ullah H, Khan H, Pandey A, Bhatt ID, Echeverría J. Phytopharmacology and clinical updates of *Berberis* species against diabetes and other metabolic diseases. Frontiers in Pharmacology. 2020;11:41.
8. Soni LK, Dobhal MP, Arya D, Bhagour K, Parasher P, Gupta RS. In vitro and in vivo antidiabetic activity of isolated fraction of *Prosopis cineraria* against streptozotocin-induced experimental diabetes: A mechanistic study. Biomedicine & Pharmacotherapy. 2018;108:1015–21.
9. Sirn YY, Lok LC, Weng PH, Ahmad Z, Hakim MN. Anti-diabetic activity of polypeptide-k isolated from *Momordica charantia*: A retrospective study of 142 cases. Biomedical and Pharmacology Journal. 2021;14(4):2007–16.
10. Halevas EG, Avgoulas DI, Katsipis G, Pantazaki AA. Flavonoid-liposomes formulations: Physicochemical characteristics, biological activities and therapeutic applications. European Journal of Medicinal Chemistry Reports. 2022;5:100059.
11. Peñalva R, Morales J, González-Navarro CJ, Larrañeta E, Quincoces G, Peñuelas I, Irache JM. Increased oral bioavailability of resveratrol by its encapsulation in casein nanoparticles. International Journal of Molecular Sciences. 2018;19(9):2816.
12. Khoshandam A, Imenshahidi M, Hosseinzadeh H. Pharmacokinetic of berberine, the main constituent of *Berberis vulgaris* l: A comprehensive review. Phytotherapy Research. 2022;36(11):4063–79.
13. Kuzminska J, Szyk P, Mlynarczyk DT, Bakun P, Muszalska-Kolos I, Dettlaff K, Sobczak A, Goslinski T, Jelinska A. Curcumin derivatives in medicinal chemistry: Potential applications in cancer treatment. Molecules. 2024;29(22):5321.
14. Imam SS, Alshehri S, Ghoneim MM, Zafar A, Alsaidan OA, Alruwaili NK, Gilani SJ, Rizwanullah M. Recent advancement in chitosan-based nanoparticles for improved oral bioavailability and bioactivity of phytochemicals: Challenges and perspectives. Polymers. 2021;13(22):4036.
15. Tang CH, Chen HL, Dong JR. Solid lipid nanoparticles (SLNs) and nanostructured lipid carriers (NLCs) as food-grade nanovehicles for hydrophobic nutraceuticals or bioactives. Applied Sciences. 2023;13(3):1726.
16. Preeti, Sambhakar S, Malik R, Bhatia S, Al Harrasi A, Rani C, Saharan R, Kumar S, Geeta, Sehrawat R. Nanoemulsion: An emerging novel technology for improving the bioavailability of drugs. Scientifica. 2023;2023(1):6640103.
17. Gigliobianco MR, Casadidio C, Censi R, Di Martino P. Nanocrystals of poorly soluble Drugs: Drug bioavailability and physicochemical stability. Pharmaceutics. 2018;10(3):134.
18. Rezania N, Rahmati P, Noorbakhsh F, Farhadyar N, Lotfali E. Investigation the effects of silver nanoparticles and gold nanoparticles on expression of bap and csu genes in biofilm formation of *Acinetobacter baumannii*. Iranian Journal of Microbiology. 2022;14(4):510.
19. Ghaffari-Moghaddam M, Hadi-Dabanlou R, Khajeh M, Rakhshanipour M, Shameli K. Green synthesis of silver nanoparticles using plant extracts. Korean Journal of Chemical Engineering. 2014;31(4):548–57.
20. Liu M, Wang R, Hoi MP, Wang Y, Wang S, Li G, Vong CT, Chong CM. Nano-based drug delivery systems for managing diabetes: Recent advances and future prospects. International Journal of Nanomedicine. 2025:6221–52.

21. Ashfaq R, Rasul A, Asghar S, Kovács A, Berkó S, Budai-Szűcs M. Lipid nanoparticles: An effective tool to improve the bioavailability of nutraceuticals. International Journal of Molecular Sciences. 2023;24(21):15764.
22. Hoang NH, Le Thanh T, Sangpueak R, Treekoon J, Saengchan C, Thepbandit W, Papathoti NK, Kamkaew A, Buensanteai N. Chitosan nanoparticles-based ionic gelation method: A promising candidate for plant disease management. Polymers. 2022;14(4):662.
23. Attri N, Kaur S, Aggarwal P Spray Drying: A Promising Technique in Food Processing–Concept, Applications, and Latest Advancements. 2025.
24. Priya S, Desai VM, Singhvi G. Surface modification of lipid-based nanocarriers: A potential approach to enhance targeted drug delivery. ACS Omega. 2022;8(1):74–86.
25. Danaei MR, Dehghankhold M, Ataei S, Hasanzadeh Davarani F, Javanmard R, Dokhani A, Khorasani S, Mozafari YM. Impact of particle size and polydispersity index on the clinical applications of lipidic nanocarrier systems. Pharmaceutics. 2018;10(2):57.
26. Elshazly EM, Arafa MG, Nour SA. Development and optimization of moxifloxacin solid lipid nanoparticles via double emulsion organic solvent free technique applying Box–Behnken experimental design. Scientific Reports. 2025;15:01–25.. https://doi.org/10.1038/s41598-025-26860-x.
27. Karataş A, Bekmezci S. Evaluation and enhancement of physical stability of semi-solid dispersions containing piroxicam into hard gelatin capsules. Acta Poloniae Pharmaceutica. 2013;70(5):883–97.
28. Gómez-Lázaro L, Martín-Sabroso C, Aparicio-Blanco J, Torres-Suárez AI. Assessment of in vitro release testing methods for colloidal drug carriers: The lack of standardized protocols. Pharmaceutics. 2024;16(1):103.
29. Albertini B, Bertoni S, Perissutti B, Passerini N. An investigation into the release behavior of solid lipid microparticles in different simulated gastrointestinal fluids. Colloids and Surfaces B: Biointerfaces. 2019;173:276–85.
30. Mistry PS, Singh S, Chorawala MR, Prajapati BG, Kapoor DU. Unlocking the potential of carrier mediated nano-biomedicine in management of diabetes mellitus: A review. Chemistry & Biodiversity. 2025;22(5):e202402258.
31. Shahidi F, Samarasinghe A. How to assess antioxidant activity? Advances, limitations, and applications of in vitro, in vivo, and ex vivo approaches. Food Production, Processing and Nutrition. 2025;7(1):1–107.
32. Stoleru OA, Burlec AF, Mircea C, Felea MG, Macovei I, Hăncianu M, Corciovă A. Multiple nanotechnological approaches using natural compounds for diabetes management. Journal of Diabetes & Metabolic Disorders. 2024;23(1):267–87.
33. Almuraee AA. Nano-formulated herbal bioactives in animal-based functional foods: A nutritional approach to enhancing bioavailability and health benefits. Applied Food Research. 2025;6:101587.
34. Xue M, Yang MX, Zhang W, Li XM, Gao DH, Ou ZM, Li ZP, Liu SH, Li XJ, Yang SY. Characterization, pharmacokinetics, and hypoglycemic effect of berberine loaded solid lipid nanoparticles. International Journal of Nanomedicine. 2013:4677–87.
35. Nowak-Jary J, Machnicka B. In vivo biodistribution and clearance of magnetic iron oxide nanoparticles for medical applications. International Journal of Nanomedicine. 2023;18:4067–100.
36. Goktas Z, Zu Y, Abbasi M, Galyean S, Wu D, Fan Z, Wang S. Recent advances in nanoencapsulation of phytochemicals to combat obesity and its comorbidities. Journal of Agricultural and Food Chemistry. 2020;68(31):8119–31.
37. Redha AA, Kodikara C, Cozzolino D. Does encapsulation improve the bioavailability of polyphenols in humans? A concise review based on in vivo human studies. Nutrients. 2024;16(21):3625.
38. Kakkar S, Jha RK, Hattila D, Singh AK, Shukla PK, Yadav SP, Meena AS. Plant-derived natural product-based nanoformulations for healthcare application. Nanotheranostics. 2025;9(3):262.
39. Vaou N, Stavropoulou E, Voidarou C, Tsakris Z, Rozos G, Tsigalou C, Bezirtzoglou E. Interactions between medical plant-derived bioactive compounds: Focus on antimicrobial combination effects. Antibiotics. 2022;11(8):1014.
40. Zolkepli H, Widodo RT, Mahmood S, Salim N, Awang K, Ahmad N, Othman R. A review on the delivery of plant-based antidiabetic agents using nanocarriers: Current status and their role in combatting hyperglycaemia. Polymers. 2022;14(15):2991.
41. Barik P, Mondal S. Immunomodulatory effects of metal nanoparticles: Current trends and future prospects. Nanoscale. 2025;17(17):10433–61.
42. Behar L, Siddique H. Antioxidant delivery revisited: The promise of nanostructured lipid carriers. Medicines. 2026;13(1):2.
43. Herdiana Y. Bridging The gap: The role of advanced formulation strategies in The clinical translation of nanoparticle-based drug delivery systems. International Journal of Nanomedicine. 2025;31:13039–53.

44. Mehta J, Pathania K, Pawar SV. Recent overview of nanotechnology based approaches for targeted delivery of nutraceuticals. Sustainable Food Technology. 2025;3(4):947–78.
45. Ewii UE, Attama AA, Olorunsola EO, Onugwu AL, Nwakpa FU, Anyiam C, Chijioke C, Ogbulie T. Nanoparticles for drug delivery: Insight into in vitro and in vivo drug release from nanomedicines. Nano TransMed. 2025;4:100083.
46. Frühwein H, Paul NW. Lost in translation?" Animal research in the era of precision medicine. Journal of Translational Medicine. 2025;23(1):152.
47. Li X, Peng X, Zoulikha M, Boafo GF, Magar KT, Ju Y, He W. Multifunctional nanoparticle-mediated combining therapy for human diseases. Signal Transduction and Targeted Therapy. 2024;9(1):1.
48. Petrovic S, Bita B, Barbinta-Patrascu ME. Nanoformulations in pharmaceutical and biomedical applications: Green perspectives. International Journal of Molecular Sciences. 2024;25(11):5842.

8 Regenerative Medicine and Nanotechnology

Vaishali Shirsat, Anagha Raut, and Archana Naik
Bombay College of Pharmacy (Autonomous), Mumbai, India

8.1 INTRODUCTION

Regenerative medicine seeks to restore form and function by mobilizing cells, scaffolds, and signals rather than merely replacing damaged tissues. Three complementary paradigms guide the field: (1) cell-based therapies that deliver or recruit living cells (stem/progenitor cells) to rebuild tissue; (2) biomaterial cues to regenerate organized tissue; and (3) in situ modulation of endogenous repair using gene therapy, growth factors. or immune reprogramming to awaken the body's own regenerative capacity. These paradigms increasingly intersect with nanotechnology, for example, through the use of nanoparticles, nano topographies that direct stem cell fate, and the controlled, localized delivery of morphogens – leading to hybrid strategies that enhance regenerative outcomes [1].

The clinical need is immediate and global. Degenerative and trauma-related conditions (myocardial infarction, osteoarthritis, chronic skin wounds, spinal cord injury) continue to account for massive morbidity and health-economic burden because current replacements (prostheses, grafts, organ transplants) cannot fully restore native tissue architecture or long-term function. Translational successes are emerging: 3D-bioprinted cardiac patches and nano-reinforced scaffolds have produced contractile tissue in preclinical and early human studies, illustrating how nano-enabled design improves mechanical matching and cell integration [2].

However, limitations slow its wider impact. Biological complexity (multicellular architectures, vascularization, innervation), immunogenicity, long-term safety of nanomaterials, manufacturability, and regulatory uncertainty remain key barriers. Nanotoxicology and variable biodegradation profiles demand rigorous, standardized testing before clinical deployment. Moreover, reproducible clinical endpoints and cost-effective production are essential for global adoption beyond high-income centers. Recent reviews emphasize that convergent advances – advances combining precise nanoformulations, high throughput biomanufacturing, and rigorous clinical trial design – are needed to translate promising laboratory paradigms into durable, equitable therapies worldwide [3].

8.2 FUNDAMENTALS OF REGENERATIVE MEDICINE

Regenerative medicine is built on the integration of cellular biology, material science, and molecular signaling to restore damaged tissues toward their original structure and function. Unlike conventional therapies that often aim to replace tissue, regenerative therapies focus on functional regeneration, emphasizing biological integration, long-term durability, and physiological remodeling. Three fundamental pillars characterize this field: stem cell sources, the tissue engineering triad, and endogenous repair mechanisms.

8.2.1 Stem Cell Sources

Stem cells are the biological drivers of regeneration due to their capacity of self-renewal and differentiation. Embryonic stem cells (ESCs) offer broad pluripotency but suffer from ethical issues

DOI: 10.1201/9781003598657-8

and immunological risks. Adult stem cells, such as mesenchymal stem/stromal cells (MSCs) from bone marrow, adipose tissue, and umbilical cord are widely investigated because of their immunomodulatory properties and established safety profiles. Notably, umbilical-cord-based MSCs are increasingly favored in global clinical trials due to non-invasive sourcing and higher proliferation potential. Induced pluripotent stem cells (iPSCs) represent a major advance, enabling patient-specific regenerative therapies while reducing immune rejection. Recent studies have demonstrated that nano-patterned substrates and defined xeno-free culture systems improve the genomic stability and differentiation efficiency of iPSCs, thereby enhancing their translational potential [4].

8.2.2 Tissue Engineering Triad

The tissue engineering triad – cells, scaffolds, and bioactive signals – provides a systematic framework for designing regenerative constructs. Cells supply regenerative capacity, scaffolds provide three-dimensional structural support, and signaling molecules (growth factors, cytokines, and mechanical cues) guide tissue maturation. Advances in nanotechnology have refined this triad by enabling nanoscale control over scaffold architecture, stiffness, and ligand presentation, which directly influences adhesion and lineage commitment. For instance, nanofibrous polymeric scaffolds have shown improved osteogenic and chondrogenic differentiation compared to conventional microstructured matrices, highlighting the importance of biomimetic design [5].

8.2.3 Endogenous Repair Mechanism

Endogenous repair focuses on stimulating the body's intrinsic healing capacity without extensive cell transplantation. This approach leverages resident stem and progenitor cells, as well as immune modulation and angiogenesis, to promote regeneration in situ. There has been recent evidence that nano-enabled delivery systems have the potential to locally modulate inflammatory and growth factor gradients, which can greatly improve tissue repair in chronic wounds and ischemic tissues. Such strategies reduce manufacturing complexity and regulatory burden, positioning endogenous regeneration as scalable and globally relevant solution. Together, these fundamentals define the scientific foundation for regenerative medicine, and lay the foundation for nano-enabled and clinically translatable therapies [6].

8.3 ROLE OF NANOTECHNOLOGY IN REGENERATION

Nanotechnology has become a revolutionary enabler in regenerative medicine by allowing precise control over biological processes at length scales that very closely match natural architecture. Since most cellular interactions involve nanometers, nano-engineered systems can directly interact with the behavior of the cell, organization of tissues, and recovery of function in a way unachievable in conventional micro or macro systems.

8.3.1 Nanoscale Biointeractions

At the nanoscale, materials interact with proteins, cell membranes, and extracellular matrix (ECM) components in a highly selective manner. Nanostructured surfaces control protein adsorption, orientation, and conformation, which in turn dictate downstream cellular response such as adhesion and signaling. Recent research demonstrates that nanoparticles and nanofibrous matrices can modulate integrin binding and focal adhesion assembly, leading to enhanced osteogenesis, neurogenesis, and angiogenesis. For example, calcium-phosphate and silica-based nanoparticles have been shown to promote bone mineralization by mimicking native bone nano-apatite, while causing minimal inflammatory responses [7].

8.3.2 Nano-Cell Interface

The nano-cell interface represents a critical control where physical, chemical, and biological cues converge. Nanotopographical features – such as grooves, pits, and fibers – can direct stem cell fate without exogenous growth factors by influencing cytoskeletal tension and mechanotransduction pathways. In recent regenerative models, nano-patterned substrates have been shown to promote cardiomyocyte alignment and synchronized contraction, improving function in engineered cardiac tissues. Additionally, nano-enabled carriers facilitate intracellular delivery of genes, RNA, and proteins with higher efficiency and lower toxicity, enabling precise reprogramming and differentiation of stem cells. These advances are especially important for neural and cardiac regeneration, where spatial and temporal control is essential [8].

8.3.3 Advantage over Conventional Systems

Compared to conventional bulk biomaterials and drug delivery systems, nanotechnology offers distinct advantages. Nanoscale systems provide a high surface area, improved bioavailability, and targeted, localized delivery with controlled release of therapeutic agents, thereby minimizing systemic exposure and reducing side effects. They also enable biomimicry of native tissues environments, leading to improved cell survival, integration, and long-term function. Importantly, nano-engineered platforms can be designed as multifunctional systems – simultaneously supporting cells, delivering signals, and modulating immune responses, something rarely achievable with conventional methods. As a result, nanotechnology significantly enhances the precision, efficiency, and translational potential of regenerative therapies, establishing nanotechnology as a cornerstone of next-generation tissue repair strategies [9]. At the core of nano-enabled regeneration lies the nano–bio-interface, where nanoscale material properties directly regulate protein adsorption, cell signaling, immune response, and tissue remodeling (Figure 8.1).

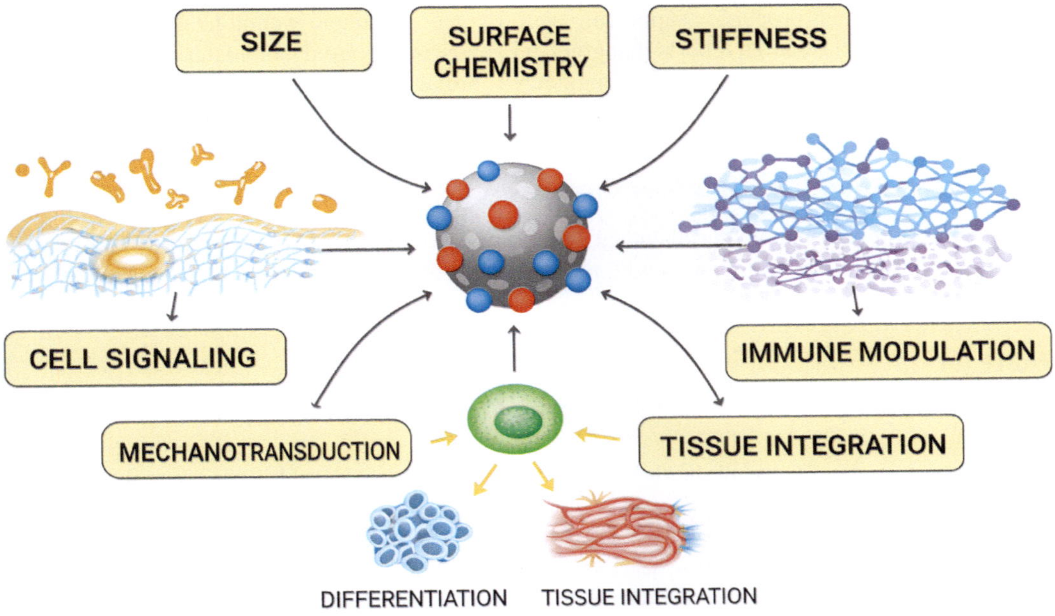

FIGURE 8.1 Nano–bio interface governing of regenerative fate.

8.4 NANOMATERIALS FOR REGENERATIVE APPLICATIONS

Nanomaterials form the structural and functional foundation of many regenerative strategies, as their physicochemical properties can be engineered to closely emulate native extracellular matrices and biological signaling environments. Advances over the past decade have expanded the repertoire of nanomaterials that support cell survival, differentiation, and tissue integration, with growing emphasis on safety, scalability, and clinical relevance. Nanotechnology has overcome several long-standing limitations in regenerative medicine by improving stem cell delivery, scaffold bioactivity, growth factor stability, immune regulation, and tissue integration. These comparative advantages of nano-enabled strategies over the conventional approaches are summarized in Table 8.1.

8.4.1 Polymeric Nanostructures

Polymeric nanostructures are widely used due to their tunable degradation, mechanical flexibility, and known biocompatibility. Natural polymers such as collagen, chitosan, gelatin, and alginate have intrinsic bioactivity and cell-recognition motifs, making them suitable for soft tissue regeneration. Synthetic polymers, such as poly(lactic-co-glycolic acid) (PLGA), polycaprolactone (PCL), or polyethylene glycol (PEG), allow precise control over nanoscale architecture and drug release kinetics. Recent research (2023–2025) demonstrates that electrospun polymeric nanofibers enhance stem cell adhesion and lineage-specific differentiation, particularly in bone, cartilage, and skin regeneration. Clinically, PLGA-based nanoparticles are increasingly used as carriers for growth factors and nucleic acids, owing to their history and predictable biodegradation [10].

8.4.2 Inorganic Nanomaterials

Inorganic nanomaterials have special mechanical, electrical, and bioactive properties essential for regenerating hard and excitable tissues. Calcium phosphate and hydroxyapatite nanoparticles closely resemble the bone mineral phase and have exhibited superior osteointegration in both preclinical and clinical orthopedics. Metallic nanoparticles, such as gold and silver, offer conductive and antimicrobial properties supporting neural regeneration and wound healing, respectively. Recent international research reports that graphene- and carbon-based nanomaterials enhance electrical coupling and signal propagation in engineered cardiac and neural tissues. However, long-term parameters of biocompatibility and clearance remain important considerations [11].

8.4.3 Hybrid and Composite Nanomaterials

Hybrid and composite nanomaterials integrate polymeric and inorganic components to combine the biological compatibility of polymers with the functional properties of inorganic materials, thereby

TABLE 8.1
Key Contributions of Nanotechnology to Regenerative Medicine

Regenerative Component	Conventional Limitation	Nano-Enabled Advancement
Stem cell delivery	Low survival; poor retention	Nanocarrier enhanced cell viability, targeting, and engraftment
Biomaterial scaffolds	Limited bioactivity; weak integration	Nano-architectures mimic ECM and improve cell signaling
Growth factor therapy	Rapid degradation; systemic toxicity	Controlled, localized, and sustained nano-delivery
Immune response	Chronic inflammation; fibrosis	Nano-immunomodulation promotes proregenerative healing
Tissue integration	Poor vascularization	Nano-engineered cues accelerate angiogenesis and remodeling

achieving enhanced therapeutic performance. These systems combine the degradability of polymers with the mechanical strength, conductivity, or bioactivity of inorganic phases. For example, polymer–ceramic nanocomposites have shown to promote bone regeneration by simultaneously supporting cell infiltration and mineral deposition. Recent advances also include smart composites capable of responding to mechanical stress or biochemical stimuli, enabling adaptive tissue regeneration. Such multifunctional platforms represent a critical step toward clinically translatable, next generation, regenerative therapies [12].

8.5 NANOENGINEERED SCAFFOLDS

Nanoengineered scaffolds are central to regenerative medicine because they recreate important aspects of the native ECM while enabling precise control over cellular behavior. By integrating nanoscale architecture with tailored mechanical and biochemical factors, these scaffolds support cells adhesion, proliferation, differentiation, and long-term tissue integration. Recent advances have emphasized scalability, reproducibility, and functional maturation critical for global clinical translation.

8.5.1 Architecture and Porosity

Scaffold architecture and porosity determine mass transport, cell infiltration, and tissue organization. At nanoscale, fibrous and porous structures mimic collagen fibrils and ECM, promising physiologically relevant cell-matrix interactions. Studies show that electrospun nanofibrous scaffolds with interconnected pores (50–300 μm) significantly enhanced vascularization and nutrient diffusion in skin and bone regeneration model. Hierarchical scaffolds that combine nanoscale and microscale porosity have demonstrated superior performance compared with uniform structures by enabling simultaneous surface-mediated cell signaling and tissue ingrowth. Such architectural optimization is particularly important for the regeneration of thick tissues, where diffusion limitations often impair effective tissue repair [13].

8.5.2 Mechanical and Biochemical Cues

Cells sense and respond to mechanical stiffness, topography, and biochemical signals through mechanotransduction pathways. Nanoengineered scaffolds allow fine-tuning of elastic modulus to match native tissues ranging from soft neural tissue to load-bearing bone, thereby guiding the lineage-specific differentiation. Recent data indicate that stem cells cultured on nanoscale substrates with tissue-matched stiffness show up to twofold improvement in differentiation efficiency, compared with rigid and non-biomimetic materials. In parallel, biochemical stimuli such as immobilized growth factors, adhesion peptides, and glycosaminoglycans can be presented at controlled densities, reducing the need for high systemic doses and minimizing adverse effects [14].

8.5.3 Smart and Responsive Scaffolds

Smart scaffolds represent the next generation of regenerative platforms. These systems respond dynamically to environmental stimuli, including pH, enzymes, mechanical stress, or by electrical signals, to modulate the degradation, drug release, or mechanical properties. Recent international studies report nanoengineered scaffolds that release angiogenic or anti-inflammatory factors in response to local tissue cues, accelerating healing in chronic wounds and ischemic tissues. Electrically conductive nanocomposite scaffolds have also shown promise in cardiac and neural regeneration by enhancing signal transmission and functional integration. Collectively, smart and responsive nanoengineered scaffolds move regenerative medicine toward adaptive, patient-specific therapies with improved clinical results [15].

8.6 NANOTECHNOLOGY IN STEM CELL ENGINEERING

Nanotechnology has become indispensable for engineering, monitoring, and manipulating stem cells, enabling higher precision, safety, and functional integration than traditional methods.

8.6.1 Stem Cell Tracking and Imaging

Magnetic and magnetic-sensitive nanomaterials (notably superparamagnetic iron oxide nanoparticles, SPIONs) remain the workhorses for non-invasive in vivo cell tracking, because they create strong MRI contrast and can persist intracellularly for long enough to map cell biodistribution and engraftment. Recent methodological advances have improved labeling efficiency and signal stability, supporting longitudinal tracking of administered cells in preclinical models and translational studies. Ferumoxytol and related iron formulations are now being repurposed as clinically acceptable cell labels and MRI enhancers, improving safety and clinical interpretability in early humans' work. In parallel, magnetic particle imaging (MPI) and optimized nanoparticle formulations are entering first-in-human evaluations of real-time, quantitative stem-cell tracking, a key step toward safer, image-guided cell therapies [16].

8.6.2 Nanocarrier-Mediated Differentiation

Nanocarriers (lipid, polymeric, inorganic) enable targeted delivery of small molecules, peptides, mRNA, and proteins to stem cells, creating programmable differentiation cues without high systemic exposure. Controlled-release nanoparticles embedded within scaffolds or used for transient ex vivo preconditioning enhance lineage specification (osteogenic, neuronal, cardiomyocyte) and improve survival after implantation. Recent advances in engineered non-viral nanocarriers have demonstrated transfection efficiencies approaching those of viral vectors for genes and mRNA delivery, while markedly reducing immunogenicity. These developments accelerate the translational feasibility of nanotechnology-based approaches for the repair of myocardial, cartilage, and nervous tissues [17].

8.6.3 Epigenetics and Gene Regulation

Nanotechnology also provides tools to reprogram cell identity through accurate epigenetic modulation and nucleic-acid delivery. Nanoparticle-mediated delivery of siRNA, miRNA mimics, and CRISPR (clustered regulatory interspaced short palindromic repeats) reagents permits transient or durable modulation of epigenetic regulators and transcriptional programs that regulate self-renewal and differentiation. However, nanoparticles themselves can influence the epigenome altering DNA methylation and histone marks in some contexts; so design must balance efficacy with genomic safety. Growing mechanistic studies emphasize standardized assays for epigenetic effects as an essential component of preclinical validation [18].

Together, these nano-enabled capabilities – reliable imaging, programmable cargo delivery, and epigenetic control – are converging to make stem-cell therapies more predictable and controllable. Ongoing clinical-grade nanoparticle refinements and rigorous safety testing will determine how rapidly these approaches scale into routine regenerative medicine [19].

8.7 NANO-ENABLED DRUG AND GROWTH-FACTOR DELIVERY

Nanotechnology has re-shaped regenerative medicine by transforming how therapeutic agents and growth factors are delivered to injured tissues. Unlike conventional formulations that have problems with fast elimination, poor targeting, and systemic toxicity, nano-enabled systems are capable of precise, controlled, and highly localized delivery, which is necessary for efficient tissue repair and regeneration.

8.7.1 Controlled Release Systems

Controlled release is an outstanding characteristic of nano-delivery. Nanocarriers such as polymeric nanoparticles, liposomes, dendrimers, solid lipid nanoparticles (SLNs), and other engineered carriers can encapsulate drugs and growth factors, protecting them from degradation and releasing them over sustained periods at the injury site, thereby maintaining therapeutic without repeating dose. This improves efficacy and reduces side effects associated with high systemic exposure. For example, nanofiber-based delivery systems with high surface area-to-volume ratios show promising controlled release profiles that support long-term regeneration in chronic wound models and orthopedic healing scenarios [20].

8.7.2 Spatiotemporal Signaling

Effective regeneration requires not just delivery, but precise timing and location of bioactive cues to mimic natural healing. Advances in stimulus-responsive nanomaterials now allow factors to be released in a spatially and temporally controlled manner. Near-by infra-red controlled release systems, for example, have been shown to release multiple growth factors like PDGF-BB (platelet-derived growth factor subunit B), VEGF (vascular endothelial growth factor), and EGF (epidermal growth factor) in a defined time sequence, to orchestrate tissue regeneration; the possibility to control patterns of delivery that are dependent on the gradients simulating developmental signals of the organism. These abilities are of paramount importance in complex tissues such as bone and vasculature, where sequential signaling is crucial for quality of repair [21, 22].

8.7.3 Microenvironment Modulation

Nanotechnology also enables direct modulation of the tissue microenvironment, a critical determinant of regeneration. Nanocarriers deliver not just drugs but also growth factors like BMP-2, VGEF, and TGF-β to enhance osteogenesis and angiogenesis in bone repair frameworks, improving stem cells engraftment and function. Beyond growth factors, smart nanomaterials can respond to pH, enzymes, or other local cues to adjust therapeutic release, reduce inflammation, and support scaffold integration, thus creating a more favorable niche for tissue regeneration [23].

Together, controlled release, spatiotemporal control, and microenvironment modulation illustrate how nanotechnology is enabling a new generation of regenerative therapies that are more effective, safer, and tailored to complex biology than ever before.

8.8 IMMUNOMODULATION AND TISSUE INTEGRATION

Successful regeneration depends not only on replacing damaged cells and tissues but also on orchestrating a supportive immune response and integrating regenerated structures with the host-environment. Nanotechnology provides powerful tools for controlling the immune milieu, reducing deleterious inflammation, and driving vascularization to enhance functional integration of engineered tissues.

8.8.1 Nano-Immunoengineering

Nanotechnology is redefining how biomaterials interact with the immune system. Instead of merely evading immune recognition, modern designs leverage nano-immunoengineering – the deliberate modulation of the immune system using nanomaterials to promote healing rather than chronic inflammation. Nanoparticles can deliver immunomodulatory agents such as cytokines or small molecules directly to target cells, minimizing systemic exposure while enhancing local efficacy. This precision enables controlled recruitment and activation of macrophages and T cells that support tissue repair rather than fibrosis. Recent reports emphasize nanomedicine-based immunotherapies that deliver immune regulators with high spatial precision, opening new avenues for designing pro-regenerative environments in complex tissues [24].

8.8.2 Inflammation Control

Inflammation is a double-edged sword in regeneration: it is essential for initial clearance of damaged tissue, but harmful if persistent. Nanotechnology supports inflammation control by modulating immune responses at injury sites, preventing prolonged inflammatory cascades that lead to scarring and impaired healing. Smart nanocarriers can release anti-inflammatory drugs or bioactive peptides in response to microenvironmental cues – for example, enzyme or pH changes – ensuring release only when and where it is needed. Such approaches have proven ineffective in preclinical chronic wounds and musculoskeletal tissues models by shifting macrophage populations toward pro-repair phenotypes and decreasing cytokines-driven fibrosis [25].

8.8.3 Vascularization Strategies

Rapid and robust vascularization is fundamental for long-term graft survival and functional integration. Without effective blood vessels formation, engineered tissues suffer ischemia and fail. Nanotechnology enhances vascularization through several approaches: the incorporation of pro-angiogenic ions or nanoscale growth factor carrier in scaffold, the sustained and localized delivery of VEGF and other angiogenic cues, and the design of nanopatterned architectures that promote endothelial cell migration and capillary networks assembly. Recent studies emphasize nanocomposite scaffolds designed to optimize immune-regulated angiogenesis, enhancing both vessel formation and tissue regeneration [26].

Collectively, nano-immunoengineering, inflammation control, and vascularization strategies comprise a next-generation toolkit to direct host response and neutralize the challenge of integrating newly formed tissues – a critical step toward obtaining durable and clinically-resolutional results in regenerative medicine [27].

8.9 APPLICATION IN REGENERATIVE MEDICINES

Nanotechnology is having transformational impact across regenerative medicine by enabling materials and devices that mimic the natural tissue environment, precisely deliver therapeutic cues, and actually regenerate a condition which is otherwise intractable. Recent research demonstrates significant advances in bone and cartilage repair, neural regeneration, cardiac and vascular repair, and skin wound healing, illustrating both basic science progress and translational potential.

8.9.1 Bone and Cartilage Repair

Bone and cartilage regeneration remains a major clinical problem due to complex structure, poor self-healing ability, and load-bearing requirements. Nanomaterials, including nano-hydroxyapatite, graphene-reinforced scaffolds, and nanocomposite hydrogels, now provide hierarchical materials that replicate native ECM while inducing osteogenic and chondrogenic differentiation of stem cells. For example, in 2025 researchers developed graphene-oxide-reinforced nanoscaffolds that achieved mature mineralization and functional bone tissue in vivo, overcoming mechanical and biological limitations of earlier biomaterials [28].

8.9.2 Neural Regeneration

Neural tissues are very sensitive and traditionally very difficult to regenerate. Nanoscale platforms such as carbon-based nanofibers, conductive hydrogels, and DNA-based nanostructures have improved axonal guidance and functional recovery in preclinical models by providing topographical and electrical cues that support neuron outgrowth and synaptic integration. Additionally, nanofiber electrodes for brain-machine interfaces are advancing regenerative approaches for spinal cord and peripheral nerve injuries. These electrodes combine structural support with bioactive signaling [29].

8.9.3 Cardiac and Vascular Repair

After myocardial infarction or chronic ischemia, promoting vasculature and functional cardiomyocyte integration is critical. Nanoengineered scaffolds containing pro-angiogenic factor (e.g., VEGF) and electroconductive nanomaterials support both vascular network formation and synchronized contraction, improving outcomes in animal models. These materials are also being combined with stem cells and controlled-release growth factors for maximum integration and minimum arrhythmogenic risk – advancements critical for future clinical translation [30].

8.9.4 Skin and Wound Healing

Chronic wounds and burns are serious causes of illness worldwide. Nanotechnology has led to antimicrobial nanofiber dressings, growth factor-rich hydrogels, and nanoparticle augmented topical formulations that together have the potential to increase the speed of re-epithelialization processes, manage infection, and modulate inflammations. Multifunctional nanoparticles (e.g., ZnO, silver and cerium oxide) are being explored for increased healing and antimicrobial activity under stressed skin conditions with encouraging early results for the aged model [31].

8.10 EMERGING TECHNOLOGIES AND CONVERGENCE

The future of regenerative medicine lies at the intersection of nanotechnology, robotics, additive manufacturing, and artificial intelligence (AI). These convergent technologies are overcoming long-standing barriers, enabling precise fabrication real-time control, adaptive design, and highly personalized therapies that were previously out of reach. Recent research and technological developments point to a transformative era, where regenerative constructs are not just biologically functional but also intelligent and adaptive. The confluence of nanotechnology with the field of stem cell engineering and/or smart scaffolds, combined with advanced fabrication strategies, allows a regenerative workflow from material design to clinical translation, which is summarized in Figure 8.2.

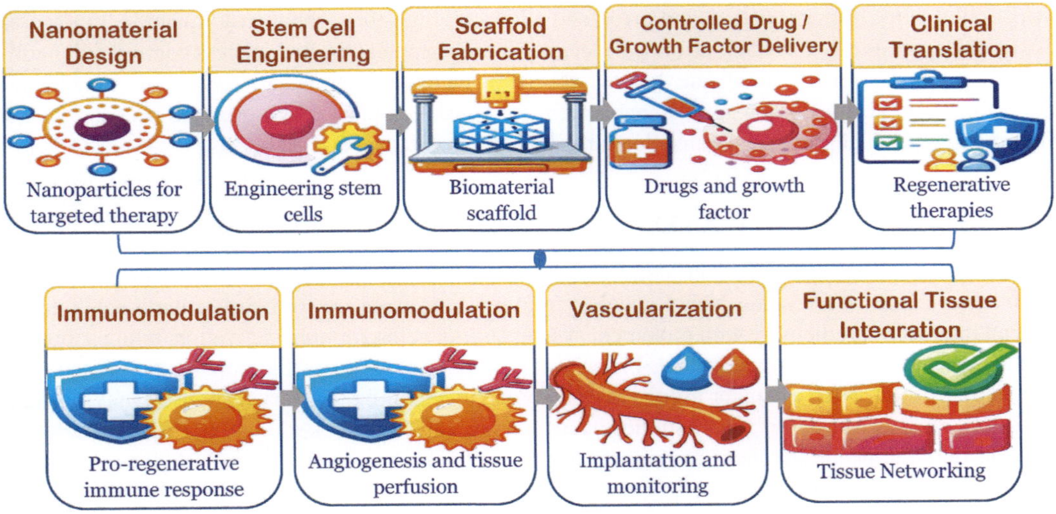

FIGURE 8.2 Nano-enabled regenerative medicine workflow from design to clinical translation.

8.10.1 Nanorobotics and Biofabrication

Nanorobotics – microscopic machines constructed on the nanoscale – is a nascent but frontier field in regenerative medicine. These systems are designed to perform extremely specific functions such as targeted drug delivery, microsurgery, and cell manipulation with unprecedented precision. For example, magnetically facilitated nanobots have been shown in preclinical models to navigate through complex tissue environments to deliver therapeutics directly to wound sites or tumors, minimizing systemic exposure and enhancing therapeutic efficacy. In addition to complementing biofabrication processes, these nano-actuated systems provide opportunities to modulate the regenerative microenvironments in situ, promoting better integration and functional maturation of engineered tissues [32].

Biofabrication, via the driving force of nanotechnology, allows the formation of multiscale architectures with embedded cells, growth factors, and supporting matrices that emulate the native tissue complexity with high fidelity. Nanomaterials, such as functionalized nanofibers and nanoparticle-reinforced inks, are beneficial for improving the print resolution, mechanical performance and biological behavior of biofabricated constructs [33].

8.10.2 3D Bioprinting and Nanocomposites

3D bioprinting has emerged as a cornerstone of regenerative biofabrication by precisely layering cells and biomaterials to construct organ-mimetic structures that were previously unattainable. Recent research shows how nanocomposite bioinks, materials infused with nanoparticles like graphene, hydroxyapatite, or nano-ceramics, enhance the biological performance of printed tissues by improving mechanical strength, electrical conductivity, or cell signaling. This enables more robust vascularization and functional integration in engineered tissues such as bone, cartilage, and myocardium [34].

Combined nano-additives also allow innovative strategies such as 4D printing, where printed constructs can adapt over time in response to physiological stimuli to better mimic dynamic biological processes.

8.10.3 AI-Guided Regenerative Design

AI is dramatically changing the way regenerative constructs will be designed, optimized, and scaled toward clinical applications. AI models woven into 3D bioprinting processes allow for data-driven bioink formulation, printed architecture, and multi-cellular configuration optimization. This improves structural fidelity, minimizes trial-and-error, and allows for high-throughput customization. Innovative AI-driven systems can also track printing processes as they happen ("in-line process control"), dynamically adapt the design, and anticipate the best fabrication paths compatible with patient-specific biological parameters. This approach greatly enables clinical translation of more complex tissue constructs by improving reproducibility, personalization, and quality control during scale-up [34].

8.11 SAFETY, TOXICITY, AND REGULATORY CONSIDERATIONS

Safety, toxicity, and regulatory considerations are critical factors for the clinical translation of nano-enabled regenerative therapies. Nanotoxicology remains a central concern because nanoscale materials can interact unpredictably with biological systems, influencing immune activation, biodistribution, persistence, and long-term clearance. Properties like particle size, surface chemistry, shape, and breakdown products have a major influence on cytotoxicity and inflammatory responses, making standardized, mechanism-based safety studies necessary instead of the traditional bulk material testing. Despite the significant advances in nano-enabled regenerative products, several challenges remain in their clinical translation, including manufacturing variability, scalability under good manufacturing practice (GMP) conditions, batch-to-batch consistency, and reproducibility. Additional concerns include potential toxicity, cellular clonality and replicability issues, pathophysiological differences between preclinical models and humans, pharmacokinetic and pharmacodynamic variations, and differences in resistance mechanisms. In parallel, the regulatory landscape continues to evolve but remains fragmented, as nano-enabled regenerative products often lie at the intersection of existing regulatory frameworks for drugs, biologics, and medical devices. Regulatory authorities are increasingly adopting risk-based classification approaches, with greater emphasis on long-term follow-up, safety evaluation, and post-market surveillance. Therefore, early engagement with regulatory agencies and the development of international consensus frameworks are essential to ensure scientific validity, clinical relevance, and timely adoption of these innovative therapies [35].

8.12 FUTURE PERSPECTIVES

Future perspectives in regenerative medicine increasingly emphasize clinical translation and personalization driven by advances in nanotechnology, bioengineering, and data-driven design. For clinical translation, the focus is shifting from proof-of-concept studies toward scalable, reproducible, and regulatory-compliant platforms that demonstrate durable functional outcomes in humans. The progress on synthesis of common nanomaterials, GMP-compatible bioprocessing, and advanced in vivo imaging is improving predictability and safety, and accelerating movement from laboratory to clinic. At the same time, personalized regenerative treatments are emerging as a paradigm change, enabled by patient-specific stem cells, tunable nanomaterials, and AI-guided design of scaffolds and delivery systems tailored to individual biological profiles. These approaches aim to optimize efficacy while minimizing immune rejection and adverse responses. Together, clinically-focused development and personalization signal a shift toward precision regeneration, where therapies are biologically effective but also customized, scalable, and globally accessible [36].

8.13 CONCLUSIONS

Regenerative medicine, empowered by nanotechnology, represents a paradigm shift from tissue replacement toward true biological restoration. By enabling precise control over cellular behavior, molecular signaling, and microenvironmental cues, nano-engineered systems have greatly improved the efficacy of stem-cell therapies, scaffolds, and targeted delivery systems. Advances in nano-enabled immunomodulation, smart biomaterials, and biofabrication are gradually overcoming old problems such as poor integration, poor vascularization, and inconsistent clinical results. While safety, scalability, and regulatory alignment remain critical hurdles, ongoing convergence with AI, advanced manufacturing, and personalized medicine is accelerating translational progress. Collectively, these developments have positioned nanotechnology as a cornerstone of the next-generation regenerative therapies with the potential to deliver durable, patient-specific, and globally relevant solutions for complex degenerative illnesses and tissue injuries.

ACKNOWLEDGMENTS

I would like to extend my heartfelt gratitude to the Department of Pharmaceutical Analysis, Bombay College of Pharmacy (Autonomous), Mumbai, India for providing an inspiring academic environment and the state-of-the-art facilities that were instrumental in the successful completion of this chapter.

REFERENCES

1. Mao AS, Mooney DJ. Regenerative medicine: Current therapies and future directions. Proceedings of the National Academy of Sciences. 2015;112(47):14452–9.
2. Coppola C, Greco M, Munir A, Musarò D, Quarta S, Massaro M, Lionetto MG, Maffia M. Osteoarthritis: Insights into diagnosis, pathophysiology, therapeutic avenues, and the potential of natural extracts. Current Issues in Molecular Biology. 2024;46(5):4063–105.

3. Shukla AK. Nanotechnology for Dentistry Applications. IOP Publishing; 2021.
4. Li F, Fu C. Stem cell revolution: Bridging the gap between research and clinical application. Stem Cell Research & Therapy. 2025;16(1):661.
5. Narayanan KB. Nanotopographical features of polymeric nanocomposite scaffolds for tissue engineering and regenerative medicine: A review. Biomimetics. 2025;10(5):317.
6. Khodve G, Banerjee S, Kumari M, Ravichandiran V, Banerjee S, Roy S. Exploration of biomaterial and stem cell-based strategies for promoting neuronal regeneration and creating engineered 3D in-vitro disease models. Journal of Translational Medicine. 2025;23(1):1–37.
7. Verma PK, Preety P, Sharma PR, Sharma P, Sharma AK. Multi-scale computational frameworks for predicting biomaterial-host interactions. Sciences des Structures et de la Matière. 2026;9(2):112–31.
8. Kumar R, Gulia K. The convergence of nanotechnology-stem cell, nanotopography-mechanobiology, and biotic-abiotic interfaces: Nanoscale tools for tackling the top killer, arteriosclerosis, strokes, and heart attacks. Nano Select. 2021;2(4):655–87.
9. Petrovic S, Bita B, Barbinta-Patrascu ME. Nanoformulations in pharmaceutical and biomedical applications: Green perspectives. International Journal of Molecular Sciences. 2024 May 27;25(11):5842.
10. Qureshi MA, Aziz R, Azim Y, Ahmad M. Polymeric hydrogels for bioprinting: A comprehensive review. Annals of 3D Printed Medicine. 2025;18:100198.
11. Burduşel AC, Gherasim O, Andronescu E, Grumezescu AM, Ficai A. Inorganic nanoparticles in bone healing applications. Pharmaceutics. 2022;14(4):770.
12. Tabrizi E, Li B. Silver integrated hybrids and nanocomposites for next-generation biomedicine: Beyond antimicrobial coatings toward smart sense–response–heal platforms. Materials Today Bio. 2025:102609.
13. Chan SS, Black JR, Franks GV, Heath DE. Hierarchically porous 3D-printed ceramic scaffolds for bone tissue engineering. Biomaterials Advances. 2025;169:214149.
14. Selig M, Lauer JC, Hart ML, Rolauffs B. Mechanotransduction and stiffness-sensing: Mechanisms and opportunities to control multiple molecular aspects of cell phenotype as a design cornerstone of cell-instructive biomaterials for articular cartilage repair. International Journal of Molecular Sciences. 2020; 21(15):5399.
15. Liang D, Wang H, Jiang Y, Zhang Z, Zhou T, Ge S, Tan S, Qin K, Wang Y, Lin X, Xie Y. Smart biomaterials for skeletal aging repair and regeneration. Bone Research. 2026;14(1):24.
16. Andreas K, Georgieva R, Ladwig M, Mueller S, Notter M, Sittinger M, Ringe J. Highly efficient magnetic stem cell labeling with citrate-coated superparamagnetic iron oxide nanoparticles for MRI tracking. Biomaterials. 2012;33(18):4515–25.
17. Yadav N, Debnath N, Das S. Stimuli-responsive nanocarriers for targeted mRNA therapeutics: A paradigm shift in mRNA delivery for biomedical applications. Drug Delivery and Translational Research. 2026:1–27.
18. Mujtaba M, Wang D, Carvalho LB, Oliveira JL, Espirito Santo Pereira AD, Sharif R, Jogaiah S, Paidi MK, Wang L, Ali Q, Fraceto LF. Nanocarrier-mediated delivery of miRNA, RNAi, and CRISPR-Cas for plant protection: Current trends and future directions. ACS Agricultural Science & Technology. 2021;1(5):417–35.
19. Gupta V, Kumar D, Gupta S, Tanwar R, Jaiswal NK, Islam MM, Singh S, Choudhary N, Gowri S, Webster TJ, Faiyazuddin M. Nanotechnology-driven cancer therapies for precision oncology: Advances and clinical outlook. International Journal of Nanomedicine. 2026;31:1–33.
20. Mall J, Naseem N, Haider MF, Rahman MA, Khan S, Siddiqui SN. Nanostructured lipid carriers as a drug delivery system: A comprehensive review with therapeutic applications. Intelligent Pharmacy. 2025;3(4):243–255.
21. Parvin N, Joo SW, Mandal TK. Biodegradable and stimuli-responsive nanomaterials for targeted drug delivery in autoimmune diseases. Journal of Functional Biomaterials. 2025;16(1):24.
22. Zhang X, Gong B, Rao F, Hu H, Tian F, Lu Y, Zhang L, Xia Y, Xue J. Spatiotemporally controlled delivery of biological effectors from nanofiber scaffolds accelerates skin wound healing in porcine models. Science Advances. 2025;11(42):eadz5302.
23. Liang W, Zhou C, Liu X, Xie Q, Xia L, Liu L, Bao W, Lin H, Xiong X, Zhang H, Zheng Z. Current status of nano-embedded growth factors and stem cells delivery to bone for targeted repair and regeneration. Journal of Orthopaedic Translation. 2025;50:257–73.
24. Aljabali AA, Obeid MA, Gammoh O, El-Tanani M, Mishra V, Mishra Y, Kapre S, Srivatsa Palakurthi S, Hassan SS, Nawn D, Lundstrom K. Nanomaterial-driven precision immunomodulation: A new paradigm in therapeutic interventions. Cancers. 2024;16(11):2030.

25. Zhuang ZM, Guo K, Wu ZR, Wang Y, Zhong XC, Chen CY, Feng ZX, Yu YZ, Zhang HQ, Tan MH, Zhang T. Skin regeneration axis under metal-based nanozymes: From chronic wound healing to structural and functional restoration. Journal of Advanced Research. 2026 (Article in Press. Available online).
26. Wang H, Lin F, Zhang Y, Lin Y, Gao B, Kang D. Biomaterial-based vascularization strategies for enhanced treatment of peripheral arterial disease. Journal of Nanobiotechnology. 2025;23(1):103.
27. Li S, Lu L, Xiong Y, Xiao J. Nanomedicine-based immunotherapy for tissue regeneration. Burns & Trauma. 2025;13:tkaf015.
28. Mondal S, Bal T. Composite systems based on hyaluronic acid and natural, polysaccharides for cartilage and bone tissue regeneration: An updated, review. Tissue and Cell. 2026; 100 :103358.
29. Zhang H, Sha J, Cao S, Feng J, Pang X, Xu D, Hu Y, Li M, Zhang C, Wang Y, Wang H. Engineering neural recovery: Micro/nano-structured materials for nerve regeneration. Materials Today Bio. 2025;10: 102538.
30. Lv Q, Zhou D, He Y, Xu T, Qiu X, Zeng J. Engineering functional electroconductive hydrogels for targeted therapy in myocardial infarction repair. Bioactive Materials. 2025;49:172–92.
31. Jiang T, Li Q, Qiu J, Chen J, Du S, Xu X, Wu Z, Yang X, Chen Z, Chen T. Nanobiotechnology: Applications in chronic wound healing. International Journal of Nanomedicine. 2022:3125–45.
32. Henly H. Nanomedicine-Advances in Medical Technology. On The Risk. 2022;38(3):74–76.
33. Chen J, Huang D, Wang L, Hou J, Zhang H, Li Y, Zhong S, Wang Y, Wu Y, Huang W. 3D bioprinted multiscale composite scaffolds based on gelatin methacryloyl (GelMA)/chitosan microspheres as a modular bioink for enhancing 3D neurite outgrowth and elongation. Journal of Colloid and Interface Science. 2020;574:162–73.
34. Ramadan Q, Zourob M. 3D bioprinting at the frontier of regenerative medicine, pharmaceutical, and food industries. Frontiers in Medical Technology. 2021;2:607648.
35. Maria MF, Thangam T, Prakashini RS, Hemamalani AU, Parthasarathy K, Phoebe M. Evaluating nanoparticle-induced cytotoxicity: Mechanisms and methods. Nano Biomedicine & Engineering. 2025; 17(4). 481–504.
36. Hoang VT, Nguyen QT, Phan TT, Pham TH, Dinh NT, Anh LP, Dao LT, Bui VD, Dao HN, Le DS, Ngo AT. Tissue engineering and regenerative medicine: Perspectives and challenges. MedComm. 2025; 17(4):481–504.

9 Wearable and Injectable Nanotechnologies for Personalized Diabetes Management

Allenki Venkatesham
SVS Group of Institutions, Hanamakonda, India

Errepalli Kavya Sri
Sri Venkateswara College of Pharmacy (Autonomous), Chittoor, India

Ruchi Tiwari
PSIT-Pranveer Singh Institute of Technology (Pharmacy), Kanpur, India

Vaibhav Dagaji Aher
Maharashtra University of Health Sciences, Nashik, India

Nadeem Hasan
Mam College of Pharmacy, Kalaburagi, India

Vaishali Shirsat
Bombay College of Pharmacy (Autonomous), Mumbai, India

Sirajuddin Khan
Aurosri Institute of Pharmaceutical Education & Research, Cuttack, India

9.1 INTRODUCTION

Diabetes mellitus remains one of the most significant global health burdens in the 21st century. According to the most recent estimates, more than 422 million adults worldwide are living with diabetes, and recent projection suggests that this number could rise to nearly 783 million by 2045 if current trends continue. Around 10.5% of adult population of 20–79 years are currently affected, and almost half are unaware they have the disease, leading to delayed management and higher rates of complications such as cardiovascular disease, nephropathy, retinopathy, and neuropathy [1, 2].

Despite increased access to conventional therapies – including insulin analogs and oral hypoglycemics – optimal glycemic control remains elusive for most patients. Recent data show that although a high percentage of diagnosed cases receive treatment, only about 40% achieve effective glucose control, with even fewer maintaining stable blood glucose over time. This failure stems from several factors: the inherent variability in glucose metabolism in various individuals, fixed dosing regimens, lifestyle factors, and the absence of tools to record real-time physiological changes [3].

DOI: 10.1201/9781003598657-9

These gaps highlight a "personalization gap" in diabetes care: monitoring devices and drug delivery systems are currently reactive rather than adaptive; relying on periodic finger prick monitoring or fixed insulin dosing that cannot dynamically adjust to rapid metabolic changes. Moreover, many monitoring technologies are invasive, uncomfortable, or require high compliance – barriers that reduce adherence and worsen long-term outcomes [4].

Nanotechnology has emerged as a promising approach to bridge this personalization gap by providing highly sensitive, minimally-invasive tools that can continuously monitor glucose and deliver therapeutics in a more physiological fashion. Nanomaterials like carbon-based nanostructures and quantum dots are being incorporated into wearable sensors capable of real-time glucose tracking from sweat or interstitial fluid. Early research shows that wearable plasmonic nanowire sensors can accurately detect glucose within physiological ranges. These sensors can be integrated into personal health dashboards to stream real-time, continuous data [5].

On the therapeutic side, nanocarriers and stimuli-responsive delivery systems are enabling precise insulin release, potentially reducing hypoglycemia events, and glycemic stability. These innovations are a good sign for the future applicability of tailored adaptive diabetes management, and they may even become a matter of routine [6].

9.2 NANOTECH FUNDAMENTALS

At the nanoscale (1–100 nm), materials have unique characteristics that greatly differ from their bulk analogs due to two fundamental facts: an extreme high surface-to-volume ratio and size-dependent electronic/optical behavior. These features produce improved chemical reactivity, quantum effects, mechanical strength, and novel optical responses such as size-tunable fluorescence – characteristics that are pivotal in biosensing and drug delivery. Such characteristics allow the physicochemical interaction of nanoparticles with biological systems at resolutions approaching the molecular level for improved sensitivity, specificity, and response times in diagnostic devices and delivery systems [7].

Carbon-based nanomaterials form one of the most exploited classes. Carbon nanotubes (CNTs) and graphene derivatives provide good electrical conductivity and large surface areas, facilitating rapid electron transfer in electrochemical biosensors. Graphene quantum dots (GQDs) combine these electrical properties with photoluminescence, making them suitable for optical sensing and imaging, with minimal cytotoxicity compared to traditional semiconductor quantum dots [8].

Metal and metal-oxide nanoparticles, including gold, silver, and platinum, are also extensively leveraged. Their plasmonic properties (collective oscillations of conduction electrons) enable highly sensitive optical detection modalities, while their catalytic surfaces enhance reaction rates in electrochemical sensors. Novel synthesis methods that are recently developed, including confined dewetting methods, allow scalable production of uniform metal nanoparticles, expanding their practical applicability in disease sensors [9].

Polymeric nanomaterials – from biodegradable polymers like poly(lactic-co-glycolic) acid (PLGA) to conductive polymers such as polyaniline – serve as versatile scaffolds for drug encapsulation or flexible sensors matrices. Their tunable mechanical and chemical properties allow for controlled drug release and integration with soft wearable devices. Polymer nanocomposites can be engineered to blend mechanical robustness with biological activity [10].

Emerging classes of peptide-based nanostructures leverage biological building blocks for inherent biocompatibility and biofunctionality, enabling targeted delivery and decreased immune clearance.

For any biomedical application, biocompatibility is a central design criterion. Nanomaterials interact at the cellular level through surface chemistry, size, shape, and charge – factors that govern protein adsorption, cellular uptake, and potential immune response. Surface functionalization (e.g., PEGylation or peptidation) is regularly used to reduce nonspecific immune activation and increase circulation time. Comprehensive testing – from in vitro cytotoxicity testing to in vivo immunological profiling – is crucial for ensuring safety alongside performance [11].

9.3 WEARABLE NANOTECH: SENSING

9.3.1 Electrochemical Sensors (Enzymatic, Mediator-Based)

Electrochemical sensing remains the workhorse for wearable glucose detection due to high sensitivity, low power, and compatibility with miniaturized electronics. Traditional enzymatic sensors use glucose oxidase (GOx) or glucose dehydrogenase immobilized on nanostructured electrodes surfaces to catalyze glucose oxidation while nanomaterials (CNTs, graphene, and metal nanoparticles) increase active surface area and enable direct or mediated electron transfer. The most recent reviews stress on the progress in enzymatic and non-enzymatic wearable electrochemical platforms in terms of stability, response time, and integration into textile and patch form factors. For instance, non-enzymatic flexible electrodes fabricated from vertically aligned gold nanowires on flexible substrates showed good electrocatalysis and mechanical strength that can be applied to continuous monitoring [12].

9.3.2 Optical and Fluorescence Sensors (Quantum Dots, CQDs)

Optical approaches – fluorescence, Raman, and plasmonical detection – exploit the size-tunable optical properties of quantum dots and carbon quantum dots (CQDs). CQDs offer low toxicity and excellent tunable photoluminescence and their nanocomposites have been used in ex vivo and wearable fluorescence-based glucose assays. Such optical sensors are attractive because they can be interrogated with compact LEDs/photodiodes and lend themselves to multiplexing (simultaneous detection of several analytes). Recent attempts demonstrate CQD-polymer composites with sensitive glucose response in biologically relevant ranges, making them promising building blocks for wearable optical patches [13].

9.3.3 Photonic Nanostructures and Nanochains

Photonic nanostructures (nanopillars, metasurfaces, plasmonic nanochains) enable “hot spots” for enhanced light-matter interaction and label-free detection via refractive index change or SERS (surface enhancement of Raman-scattering). Wearable photonic sensors have progressed from proof-of-concept substrates to prototypes integrated with wrist-worn optics or contact lenses for tear sensing. These platforms provide high analytical sensitivity and the potential for non-invasive, label-free readouts, although they currently face challenges in motion tolerance and optical coupling in skin-adjacent environment [14].

9.3.4 Skin-Interface Materials and Flexible Electrodes

Reliable skin contact is as important as the sensing chemistry. Advances in stretchable conductors, conductive hydrogels, and microneedle (MN) electrodes reduce motion artifacts and eliminate skin preparation. MN and dry-electrode arrays that bypass the stratum corneum offer stable access to interstitial fluid or low impedance electrophysiological signals with enhanced comfort for multi-day wear. These interface materials enable tighter coupling between nanosensors and the biological environment, increasing signal fidelity in a real-world application [15].

9.4 WEARABLE PLATFORMS: INTEGRATION

9.4.1 Patch and Textile Form Factors

Wearable glucose platforms have evolved beyond rigid device into soft, skin-conformal systems for long-term use. Two dominating architectures are emerging: adhesive skin patches and smart textiles. Patch-based systems typically combine thin-film electrochemical or optical nanosensors with microelectronic on flexible substrates such as polyimide or thermoplastic polyurethane. Many incorporate MN arrays to access interstitial fluid painlessly, improving signal stability compared with sweat-only sensing. Advances in stretchable conductors and nanocomposite inks have enabled multi-day wear with minimal motion artifact [16].

Textile-based systems embed conductive fibers, graphene-coated yarns, or printed nanomaterial electrodes directly into garments. These platforms aim for unobtrusive, continuous monitoring during daily activities. Recent research demonstrates stretch-tolerant, washable, e-textiles that can be used to acquire stable biosignals, representing a step toward the trend of incorporating metabolic monitoring into clothing. While still largely investigational for glucose monitoring, textile wearables are making significant progress in durability, wash stability, and signal consistency [17].

9.4.2 Data Fusion and Low-Power Electronics

Integration is not only mechanical but also computational. Modern wearable platforms increasingly employ sensor fusion and combine glucose signals with temperature, pH, motion, and sweat rate data to correct artifacts and improve analytical reliability. Motion artifacts and physiological variability remain major barriers in ambulatory sensing; multi-parameter calibration improves robustness under real-world conditions [18].

Low-power microcontrollers and edge-AI architectures are central to wearable integration. By performing signal preprocessing and anomaly detection directly on the device, power consumption and latency can be reduced. Advances in ultra-low-power Bluetooth Low Energy (BLE) communications and energy-efficient analog front-end circuits allow continuous operation for several days without frequent recharging. Edge computing also improves privacy, as sensitive metabolic data can be partially processed locally before cloud transmission [19].

9.4.3 Interfacing with CGMs and Apps

For clinical translation, wearable nanosensors must interface seamlessly with established continuous glucose monitoring (CGM) ecosystems and digital health platforms. Contemporary CGMs offer minute-level glucose readings transmitted to smartphone applications and cloud dashboards, enabling remote monitoring and data sharing with clinicians. Increasingly, manufacturers are enabling interoperability through application programming interfaces (APIs) and electronic health record (EHR) integration pilots [20].

Integration with mobile applications allows visualization of trends, alerts for hypo- or hyperglycemia, and AI-driven insights for dose adjustment. The convergence of nanosensors, wireless communication, and app-based analytics is slowly changing wearables from passive monitor into active components of individual diabetes management system, bridging real-time sensing with decision support and remote care infrastructure [21].

9.5 INJECTABLE NANOMEDICINES

Injectable nanomedicines aim to improve the pharmacokinetics, stability, and precision of insulin and adjunct antidiabetic therapies. Conventional subcutaneous insulin injections usually result in non-physiological absorption profiles resulting in glycemic variability and risk of hypoglycemia. Nanotechnology provides ways to control release kinetics, protect labile biomolecules, and add glucose-responsive behavior that more closely mimics the functions of pancreatic β-cells [22].

9.5.1 Nanoparticle-Based Insulin Carriers (Lipid, Polymeric, Peptide NPs)

Lipid nanoparticle (LNPs) and liposomal systems have been investigated to encapsulate insulin and improve its stability while enabling controlled release. Lipid-based carriers offer biocompatibility and ability to fuse with biological membranes for better absorption subcutaneously. Advances in solid lipid nanoparticles and nanostructured lipid carriers have exemplified better encapsulation efficacy, as well as a longer duration of release of insulin in preclinical models [23].

Polymeric nanoparticles, especially those based on biodegradable polymers such as PLGA, chitosan, and polyethylene glycol (PEG) derivatives have been widely studied for insulin delivery. These systems can protect insulin from enzymatic degradation and allow tunable release profiles through polymer composition and molecular weight control. In experimental diabetic models, PLGA nanoparticles have demonstrated sustain insulin release over 24–72 hours, reducing injection frequency compared with rapid-acting insulin formulations. Surface modification (e.g., PEGylation) can improve circulation time and reduce aggregation [24].

Peptide-based and self-assembling nanostructures represent a newer class of carriers. Amphiphilic peptides can form nanofibers or nanospheres capable of encapsulating insulin while offering intrinsic biocompatibility and reduced immunogenicity. Such biomimetic systems are particularly attractive for personalized therapy because they can be engineered for targeted tissues interaction or environmental-responsive release [25].

9.5.2 Bioresponsive (Glucose-Sensing) Nanoparticles

A great development in injectable nanomedicine is the development of glucose-responsive nanoparticles designed to release insulin in correlation with ambient glucose concentration. These systems usually use one of three sensing mechanisms, which include glucose oxidase (GOx)-mediated enzymatic reactions, phenylboronic acid (PBA)-glucose binding interactions, or glucose binding proteins such as concanavalin A [26].

In GOx-based systems, glucose oxidation generates local pH or hypoxic that destabilizes the nanoparticle matrix, which in turn triggers insulin release. PBA-containing polymer nanoparticles exploit reversible covalent binding between boronic acid groups and glucose, enabling concentration-dependent swelling and drug release. Preclinical studies have demonstrated that glucose-responsive nanoparticles can maintain normoglycemia in diabetic rodents for prolonged periods following a single injection, causing fewer hypoglycemic episodes than conventional insulin [27].

Although most systems remain in preclinical or early translational stages, the concept of "smart insulin" continues to attract significant research attention because of its potential to create a closed-loop, self-regulated therapy without external electronics.

9.5.3 Depot Systems and Sustained Release Formulations

Injectable nanotechnology also facilitates depot formulations that provide prolonged insulin action from a single administration. Nano-in-microparticle composites, hydrogel-aided nanoparticles, and thermoresponsive polymers depots are being explored to achieve multi-day or even weekly release. Such systems rely on diffusion-controlled release, polymer degradation, and environmental triggers to maintain therapeutic levels [28].

Sustained-release depots can reduce injection burden, enhance adherence, and balance pharmacodynamic fluctuations. Long-acting insulin analogs already improve basal coverage; nanostructured depots aim to further control kinetics and maintain biological activity. However, translational challenges remain, including reproducible large-scale manufacturing, long-term biocompatibility, and regulatory classification as combination products. Collectively, injectable nanomedicines represent a promising avenue toward more physiological, personalized diabetes management by combining drug protection, responsiveness, and prolonged delivery of the drug into one nanoscale platform [29].

9.6 MICRONEEDLE AND MINIMALLY INVASIVE DELIVERY

MN technology represents one of the most promising minimally invasive strategies for insulin and biologic delivery in diabetes treatment (Table 9.1). Unlike conventional hypodermic needles, MNs are microscopic projections (usually 100–900 µm in height) that penetrate the stratum corneum without reaching deep pain receptors, enabling painless or minimally painful transdermal delivery.

TABLE 9.1
Comparative Performance Metrics of Current and Emerging Diabetes Technologies [33, 36–39]

Technology Category	Example System Type	Mean Absolute Relative Difference (MARD, %)	Time in Range (70–180 mg/dL, %)	Hypoglycemia Reduction	Clinical Status	Key Limitation
Real-time CGM	Factory calibrated enzymatic CGM	~8–10%	60–70% (Standalone use)	Moderate	FDA/CE approved	Requires sensor replacement (7–14 days)
Hybrid closed-loop	CGM + Insulin pump (automated basal adjustment)	8–10% (sensor dependent)	70–75%	Significant nocturnal reduction	FDA/EMA approved	Mela bolus still user-dependent
Advanced hybrid closed-loop	Adaptive algorithm + automated correction boluses	7–9% (sensor dependent)	75–80%	Reduced severe hypoglycemia	FDA approved (recent generation)	Cost and training burden
Injectable long-acting insulin analogs	Basal analog formulations	Not sensor-based	Improves fasting glucose; HbA1c ↓ ~0.5–1.0%	Moderate	Approve	Fixed pharmacokinetics
Glucose-responsive nanoparticles (preclinical)	GOx- or PBA-based smart NPs	Experimental	Normoglycemia maintained in rodent models up to 24 h	Reduced hypoglycemia in animals	Preclinical	Human data lacking
Glucose-responsive MN patches (preclinical)	Smart MN + nanoparticle reservoir	Experimental	Sustained euglycemia in diabetic	Reduced hypoglycemia (animal studies)	Preclinical	Scale-up and regulatory pathway

By targeting the dermal interstitial fluid compartment, rich in capillary networks, MNs offer effective systemic absorption while improving patient comfort and compliance [30].

9.6.1 Dissolving and Hydrogels Microneedles (Insulin and Biologics)

Dissolving MNs are made from biodegradable polymers that include hyaluronic acid, polyvinylpyrrolidone (PVP), or carboxymethyl cellulose. Insulin or other biologics are loaded into the needle matrix and are released as the MNs dissolve after insertion. Preclinical studies have demonstrated rapid insulin absorption with pharmacodynamic profiles comparable to subcutaneous injection, while eliminating sharps waste and reducing needle-dependent anxiety. Importantly, polymer choice impacts the mechanical strength and the dissolution kinetics, both crucial for reliable dose delivery [31].

Hydrogel forming MNs operate differently. These systems swell upon insertion into the skin, creating a diffusion-controlled process between a drug reservoir and the systemic circulation. Crosslinked polymers such as methacrylated hyaluronic acid or polyethylene glycol diacrylate allow tunable swelling behavior and sustained release. In diabetic animal models, hydrogel MN systems have achieved controlled insulin delivery over several hours with reduced peak-trough fluctuations compared to bolus injection. As MNs are structurally intact during use and are removed after swelling, they reduce polymer deposition in tissue [32].

9.6.2 Smart/Glucose-Responsive (GR) MN Patches

Recent studies integrate glucose-responsive nanoparticles within MN matrix to create self-controlled delivery platforms. These smart MN patches contain glucose oxidase, phenylboronic acid-modified polymers, or hypoxia-sensitive vesicles that trigger insulin release when glucose levels rise. In rodent models of diabetes, a single application of glucose-responsive MN patches has maintained normoglycemia longer (up to 24 hours) with lower rates of hypoglycemia compared to standard insulin injections. Such systems conceptually go close enough to a "closed-loop" therapy without the need for external electronics, but human clinical translation is still underway [33, 34].

9.6.3 User Acceptability and Comparative Benefits

User acceptability is a major driver of MN development. Surveys consistently indicate strong patient preference for MN patches over conventional injections due to reduced pain, ease of self-administration, and improved convenience. Compared to insulin pumps or traditional injections, MN systems decrease the risk, eliminate needle disposal issue, and potentially enable more discrete therapy [35].

While challenges – including large-scale production, dosing precision, and regulatory categorization – remain, MN technologies offer a compelling link between wearable sensing and injectable nanomedicine, advancing minimally invasive, patient-centered diabetes care.

9.7 CLOSED-LOOP AND DIGITAL CONVERGENCE

Closed-loop diabetes management systems – often referred to as "artificial pancreas" platforms – integrate continuous sensing, automated control algorithms, and insulin delivery into a feedback-regulated loop. These systems represent the convergence of wearable nanotechnology, digital health, and smart drug delivery. Modern CGMs show mean absolute relative difference (MARD) values of about 8–10%, reflecting high analytical accuracy [36]. Hybrid closed-loop systems enhance time in range to ~70–75% as compared with ~60–65% using standard sensor augmented therapy [37]. Advanced systems are able to get 75–80% time in range with major reductions in hypoglycemia [38]. Glucose-responsive nanoparticle and MN systems have been able to achieve normoglycemia for up to 24 hours [33, 39] in rodent models.

9.7.1 Sensor → Controller → Actuator Loops

A closed-loop system consists of three main components: a continuous glucose sensor, control algorithm, and an insulin delivery actuator (usually an insulin pump). The CGM measures interstitial glucose at intervals of around 1–5 minutes and sends data onto a controller (integrated into a pump or smartphone). The algorithm computes insulin dosing adjustment in real time, which is then executed by the pump [40].

Recent hybrid closed-loop systems have demonstrated clinically beneficial improvements in glycemic outcomes. Time in range (70–180 mg/dL) improvements have been reported in large multicenter trials of automated insulin delivery systems as being approximately 70–75% compared with approximately 60–65% under conventional sensor-augmented pump therapy. Reductions in HbA1c of 0.3–0.5% and substantial reductions in nocturnal hypoglycemia have also been recorded. These results demonstrate the clinical value of integrating continuous sensing with automated actuation [37, 41].

9.7.2 Role of AI/ML and Personalization Algorithms

While early closed-loop systems used proportional-integral-derivative (PID) or model predictive controls (MPC) algorithms, newer platforms increasingly incorporate ML to improve personalization. ML models can analyze historical glucose trends, meals pattern, physical activity, and insulin sensitivity variability to adapt dosing parameters dynamically. Personalization is important because insulin requirements vary widely among individuals and fluctuate due to stress, illness, circadian rhythms, and hormonal changes. Data-driven adaptive algorithms can refine insulin-to-carbohydrate ratios and basal rates over time, reducing glycemic variability. Emerging work examines reinforcement learning frameworks that continuously update control policies based on real-world outcomes, potentially enhancing long-term glycemic stability beyond rule-based systems [42].

9.7.3 Security, Privacy, and Interoperability

As closed-loop systems depend on wireless data transmission and cloud connectivity, cybersecurity and data privacy are essential considerations. The design requirements also involve encrypted Bluetooth communication, secure firmware updates, and meeting data protection standards of a healthcare application (e.g., HIPAA-equivalent standards). Interoperability is also equally important. Modern CGMs and pumps increasingly support standardized communication protocols and APIs, enabling integration with smartphones, telemedicine platforms, and electronic health records. Such digital convergence supports remote monitoring, data sharing with clinicians, and integration into broader personalized care ecosystems ensuring that technological innovation translates into scalable, real-life diabetes management solution. Closed-loop platforms (Figure 9.1) integrating continuous glucose sensing with automated insulin delivery have demonstrated significant improvements in time in range compared to regular therapy [43].

9.8 SAFETY AND TOXICOLOGY/IMMUNOLOGY

The clinical translation of wearable and injectable nanotechnologies for diabetes management depends not only on performance but also on rigorous safety evaluation. Nanomaterials interact with biological systems at the molecular and cellular scale, and their small size, high surface reactivity, and tunable surface chemistry can influence biodistribution, clearance, and immune recognition. Both acute and long-term effects must therefore be systematically assessed before regulatory approval.

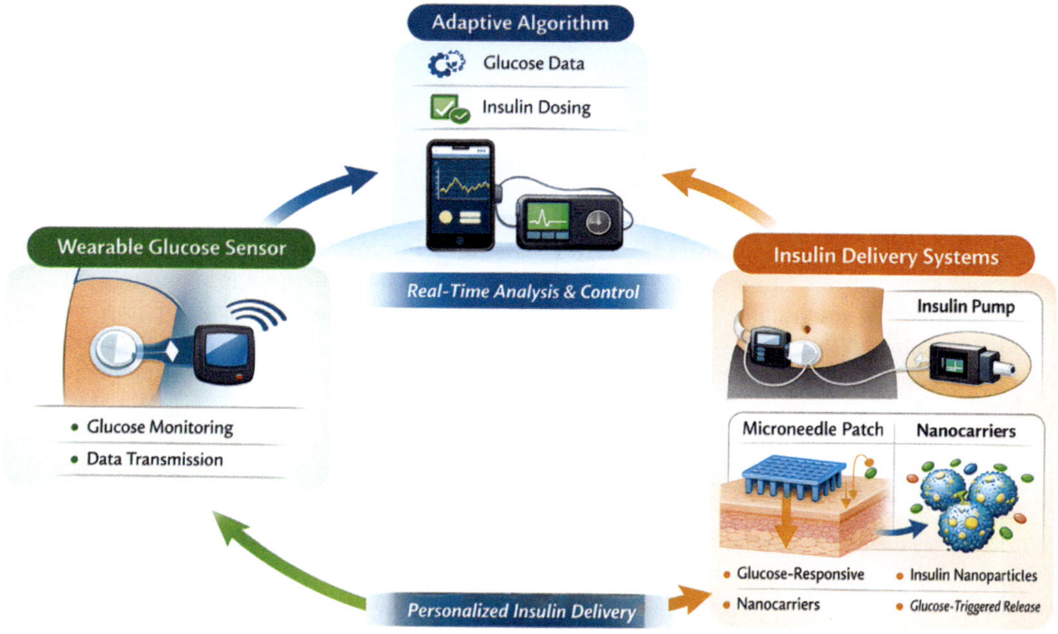

FIGURE 9.1 Integrated nano-enabled closed-loop diabetes management system.

9.8.1 Acute and Chronic Safety Concerns

Acute safety issues involve local irritation, inflammation, oxidative damage, and cytotoxicity after exposure of nanomaterials. For injectable nanoparticles, risks could include vascular embolism (if aggregation occurs), rapid immune activation, or unexpected biodistribution to organs such as liver and spleen. Wearable nanosensors can cause skin irritation, contact dermatitis, or microbiome disruption with prolonged use, especially when adhesives or metallic nanomaterials are involved [44].

Chronic safety considerations are particularly important for long-term diabetes management. Persistent exposure may lead to bioaccumulation, especially for non-biodegradable materials such as some metallic nanoparticles. Studies show that nanoparticle size, shape, and the surface charge significantly influence tissue retention and clearance pathways. For example, particles ~10 nm are generally cleared renally, whereas larger particles may undergo hepatic uptake. Chronic low-grade inflammations and oxidative stress are potential risks if materials are not totally biodegradable or well surface-modified [45].

9.8.2 Nanotoxicology Testing Approaches

Nanotoxicology assessment follows a stepwise strategy integrating in vitro, in vivo, and increasingly in silico approaches. Standard in vitro assays evaluate cytotoxicity (e.g., MTT/XTT assay), oxidative stress markers, membrane integrity, and inflammatory cytokine production in relevant cell lines. Advanced 3D skin and vascular models are increasingly used to stimulate realistic exposure conditions for wearing system [46].

In vivo studies measure biodistribution, pharmacokinetics, immunological response, and organ toxicity. Imaging modalities such as fluorescence or radiolabeling help track nanoparticle fate. Regulatory agencies emphasize comprehensive physicochemical characterization including size distribution, aggregation behavior, zeta potential, and surface chemistry because these parameters directly affect biological response [47].

Emerging computational toxicology models and high-throughput screening platforms are being developed to predict hazard profiles and reduce animals testing, aligning with modern regulatory demands for nanomedicine safety assessment.

9.8.3 Immunogenicity and Foreign Body Reactions

Nanomaterials can trigger immune responses through protein adsorption and recognition by innate immune cells. A protein corona forms when nanoparticles contact biological fluids, which changes the particle's identity and affects its uptake by macrophages. If materials are not properly engineered, they can trigger complement activation, release cytokines, and form a foreign-body granuloma. Surface functionalization strategies such as PEGylation, zwitterionics coatings, or biomimetic peptide layers are commonly employed to reduce immune recognition and prolong circulation time. For implantable or long-term MN systems, minimizing chronic inflammation and fibrosis is vital for maintaining device function [48].

A comprehensive safety framework integrating material design, rigorous preclinical testing, and post-market surveillance is therefore essential to ensure that nanotechnology-enabled diabetes therapies deliver clinical outcomes without unintended immunological or toxicological consequences.

9.9 REGULATORY AND TRANSLATIONAL PATHWAYS

9.9.1 Device vs Drug vs Combination Product Pathways

The regulatory classification of wearables and nanotechnology-based injectables depends on their primary mode of action. Continuous glucose monitoring (CGM), wearable sensing patches, and smart insulin pumps are generally regulated as medical devices (Class II or III devices under the US FDA rules), requiring analytical validation, electrical safety testing, biocompatibility evaluation, and clinical proof of accuracy [49].

Nanoparticle-based insulin formulations or long-acting injectable depots are regulated as drugs or biologics, which require comprehensive preclinical toxicology, pharmacokinetics, pharmacodynamics, and phased clinical trials approval. Emerging systems such as glucose-responsive MN patches – combining insulin delivery with device-based sensing – are classified as combination products. In the United States, these products are managed by the FDA's Office of Combination Products. The review is led by the FDA center that regulates the product's primary mode of action. Such platforms must comply with device and pharmaceutical manufacturing standards (including Good Manufacturing Practice [GMP] compliance) [50].

9.9.2 Key Regulatory Cautions (Non-Approved Consumer Devices)

Regulatory agencies have made warnings of non-approved consumer wearables that claim non-invasive glucose monitoring without validated clinical data. Inaccurate readings by unapproved smartwatches or mobile applications may lead to inappropriate insulin dosing and serious harm. Authorities emphasize that only devices with demonstrated clinical accuracy, often evaluated using metrics such as MARD, should guide therapeutic decisions. Robust analytical validation and post-market surveillance are thus mandatory for market authorization [51].

9.9.3 Clinical Trial End Points and Real-World Evidence

Clinical trials for advanced diabetes technologies usually measure HbA1c reduction, time in range (70–180 mg/dL), frequency of hypoglycemia, and device-related adverse events. Regulators are increasingly incorporating real-world evidence (RWE) from digital platforms and remote

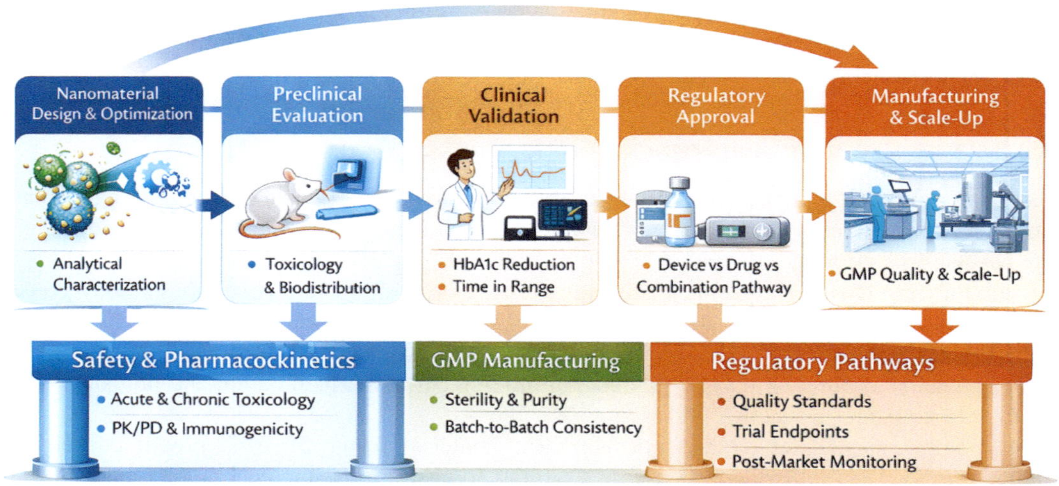

FIGURE 9.2 Translational pathway of injectable and wearable nanotechnologies.

monitoring systems to complement randomized controlled trials. This integration of traditional clinical endpoints with large-scale real-world datasets is accelerating translation while maintaining rigorous standards of safety and performance[52]. Combination nano-enabled systems must satisfy both pharmaceutical and device regulatory requirement, including GMP and clinical requirements for performance validation (Figure 9.2).

9.10 MANUFACTURING AND SCALE-UP

9.10.1 GMP for Nanomaterials

Manufacturing nanotechnology-based diabetes therapeutics and wearable components requires strict adherence to GMP standards to ensure quality, safety, and consistency. For injectable nanoparticle systems, GMP compliance involves validated synthesis protocols, sterile processing, endotoxins control, and batch-to-batch physicochemical characterization (particle size distribution, polydispersity index, zeta potential, drug loading, and release kinetics). Regulatory agencies require full documentation of raw material sourcing, in-process controls, and stability testing under the International Council for Harmonisation (ICH) guidelines [53].

For device-integrated nanomaterials (e.g., nanosensor-coated electrodes or MN arrays), manufacturing must conform to medical device quality systems (such as ISO 13485). This includes validation of coating uniformity, mechanical integrity, electrical performance, and biocompatibility testing under ISO 10993 standards. Scalable methods like roll-to-roll printing, micro-molding, and automated nanoparticle synthesis reactors are increasingly used to transition laboratory fabrication industrial production [54].

9.10.2 Reproducibility and Cost Considerations

Reproducibility is a central challenge in nanomanufacturing because small differences in synthesis conditions can significantly alter biological behavior. Tight control over precursor purity, reaction temperature, and mixing dynamics is essential for consistent particle size and surface chemistry. Cost considerations are equally critical for diabetes technologies intended for chronic use. Materials such as gold nanoparticles or complex peptide nanostructures can increase production costs, whereas biodegradable polymers and scalable printing methods offer more economically sustainable options. Achieving large-scale reproducibility while maintaining affordability remains a key determinant of successful clinical translation [55].

9.11 FUTURE DIRECTIONS

Future diabetes management is moving toward totally personalized biosystems that integrate nanosensors, adaptive algorithms, and responsive drug delivery into seamless smart closed-loop platforms. Advances in multi-analyte sensing, combining glucose with lactate, ketones, cortisol, and activity metrics, will enable context-aware insulin modulation rather than glucose-only control. Next-generation closed-loop systems are expected to incorporate adaptive machine learning models that constantly recalibrate insulin-sensitivity parameters based on circadian rhythms, hormonal fluctuations, illness, and lifestyle patterns. In parallel, hybrid-biological and nanotechnology methods are emerging, including nanoengineered encapsulation systems for pancreatic islet transplantation, biomimetic nanoparticles that emulate β-cells glucose responsiveness, and immunomodulatory nanocoatings to reduce graft rejection. Integration of synthetic biology with nanomaterials may further enable programmable, self-regulating therapeutic platforms. Together, these innovations aim to shift diabetes care from reactive management to predictive, autonomous metabolic regulation with improved safety, precision, and quality of life [56].

9.12 CONCLUSIONS

Wearable and injectable nanotechnologies are redefining the landscape of personalized diabetes management by integrating high-sensitivity sensing, adaptive drug delivery, and digital intelligence into cohesive therapeutic ecosystem. Nanoscale materials enhance analytical precision, enable minimally invasive monitoring, and support glucose-responsive insulin release strategies that more closely replicate physiological regulation. When coupled with closed-loop algorithms and interoperable digital platforms, these innovations move diabetes care from episodic intervention toward continuous, data-driven control. However, for successful translation, there are demanding safety, long-term compatibility, reproducibility of manufacturing, compliance considerations, as well as a robust cost structure. As the convergence of material science, artificial intelligence and biomedical engineering goes on, the next generation of nano-enabled systems has the potential to offer safer, more autonomous, and truly individual metabolic management.

REFERENCES

1. Saeedi P, Petersohn I, Salpea P, Malanda B, Karuranga S, Unwin N, Colagiuri S, Guariguata L, Motala AA, Ogurtsova K, Shaw JE. Global and regional diabetes prevalence estimates for 2019 and projections for 2030 and 2045: Results from the International Diabetes Federation Diabetes Atlas. Diabetes Research and Clinical Practice. 2019;157:107843.
2. Hossain MJ, Al-Mamun M, Islam MR. Diabetes mellitus, the fastest growing global public health concern: Early detection should be focused. Health Science Reports. 2024;7(3):e2004.
3. Naeem MH, Raza M, Aziz MB, Ullah N, Wahab A, Khan ZA, Farooq H. Effectiveness of insulin versus Oral agents in patients with uncontrolled type 2 diabetes mellitus: A retrospective comparative study. Cureus. 2025;17(8):01–07.
4. Rao LT, Mandal CK, Patolsky F. Body biofluids for minimally-invasive diagnostics: Insights, challenges, emerging technologies, and clinical potential. Advanced Healthcare Materials. 2025;10:e03096.
5. Haider R, Das ZA, Zameer GK. S. Revolutionizing patient care: Multidimensional approaches to 21st-century diabetes management. Journal of Heart and Vasculature. 2025;4(6):01–05.
6. Yao Y, Ji K, Wang Y, Gu Z, Wang J. Materials and carriers development for glucose-responsive insulin. Accounts of Materials Research. 2022;3(9):960–70.

7. Hoque MA, Yao CW. Nanoscale characterization of nanomaterial-based systems: Mechanisms, experimental methods, and challenges in probing corrosion, mechanical, and tribological properties. Nanomaterials. 2025;15(23):1824.
8. Batool I, Anwar A, Imran M, Alvi ZI. Prospecting carbon-based nanomaterials for harnessing multienzyme-like activities. Topics in Catalysis. 2025;68(9):823–55.
9. Rejeeth C, Chaudhary S. Plasmonic metal nanoparticles in spectroscopic biosensing: Innovation in label free detection. Analytical Letters. 2026:1–24.
10. Biglari N, Zare EN. Conjugated polymer-based composite scaffolds for tissue engineering and regenerative medicine. Alexandria Engineering Journal. 2024;87:277–99.
11. Bilardo R, Traldi F, Vdovchenko A, Resmini M. Influence of surface chemistry and morphology of nanoparticles on protein corona formation. Wiley Interdisciplinary Reviews: Nanomedicine and Nanobiotechnology. 2022;14(4):e1788.
12. Soranzo T, Ben Tahar A, Chmayssem A, Zelsmann M, Vadgama P, Lenormand JL, Cinquin P, Martin DK, Zebda A. Electrochemical biosensing of glucose based on the enzymatic reduction of glucose. Sensors. 2022;22(19):7105.
13. Giordano MG, Seganti G, Bartoli M, Tagliaferro A. An overview on carbon quantum dots optical and chemical features. Molecules. 2023;28(6):2772.
14. Gu P, Zhang W, Zhang G. Plasmonic nanogaps: From fabrications to optical applications. Advanced Materials Interfaces. 2018;5(19):1800648.
15. Kim H, Lee J, Heo U, Jayashankar DK, Agno KC, Kim Y, Kim CY, Oh Y, Byun SH, Choi B, Jeong H. Skin preparation–free, stretchable microneedle adhesive patches for reliable electrophysiological sensing and exoskeleton robot control. Science Advances. 2024;10(3):eadk5260.
16. Banitaba SN, Khademolqorani S, Jadhav VV, Chamanehpour E, Mishra YK, Mostafavi E, Kaushik A. Recent progress of bio-based smart wearable sensors for healthcare applications. Materials Today Electronics. 2023;5:100055.
17. Meena JS, Choi SB, Jung SB, Kim JW. Electronic textiles: New age of wearable technology for healthcare and fitness solutions. Materials Today Bio. 2023;19:100565.
18. Cheng J, Xue N, Zhou W, Qin B, Qiu B, Fang G, Sun X. Recent progress in flexible wearable sensors for real-time health monitoring: Materials, devices, and system integration. Micromachines. 2025; 16(10):1124.
19. Zhang D, Wei B. Smart sensors and devices in artificial intelligence. Sensors. 2020;20(20):5945.
20. Chen J, Jastrzebska-Perfect P, Chai P, Say MG, Tu J, Gao W, Halperin F, Korzenik J, Huang HW, Katabi D, Traverso G. Barriers to translating continuous monitoring technologies for preventative medicine. Nature Biomedical Engineering. 2025;14:1–9.
21. Fraser RA, Walker RJ, Campbell JA, Ekwunife O, Egede LE. Integration of artificial intelligence and wearable technology in the management of diabetes and prediabetes. npj Digital Medicine. 2025; 8(1):687.
22. Kamankesh M, Yadegar A, Llopis-Lorente A, Liu C, Haririan I, Aghdaei HA, Shokrgozar MA, Zali MR, Miri AH, Rad-Malekshahi M, Hamblin MR. Future nanotechnology-based strategies for improved management of *Helicobacter pylori* infection. Small. 2024;20(3):2302532.
23. Ashfaq R, Rasul A, Asghar S, Kovács A, Berkó S, Budai-Szűcs M. Lipid nanoparticles: An effective tool to improve the bioavailability of nutraceuticals. International Journal of Molecular Sciences. 2023; 24(21):15764.
24. Mansoor S, Kondiah PP, Choonara YE, Pillay V. Polymer-based nanoparticle strategies for insulin delivery. Polymers. 2019;11(9):1380.
25. Yu D, Han N, Son H, Kim SJ, Kweon S. Functional peptide-based biomaterials for pharmaceutical application: Sequences, mechanisms, and optimization strategies. Journal of Functional Biomaterials. 2026;17(1):37.
26. Liu J, Yi X, Zhang J, Yao Y, Panichayupakaranant P, Chen H. Recent advances in the drugs and glucose-responsive drug delivery systems for the treatment of diabetes: A systematic review. Pharmaceutics. 2024; 16(10):1343.
27. VandenBerg MA, Webber MJ. Biologically inspired and chemically derived methods for glucose-responsive insulin therapy. Advanced Healthcare Materials. 2019;8(12):1801466.
28. Zeng J, Tang X, Qin D, Yu L, Zhou X, Feng C, Mi J, Pan H, Wu J, Huang B, Wu A. Engineered GLP-1R-targeting nanoplatforms: Multimodal therapeutics in human diseases. Journal of Nanobiotechnology. 2025;23(1):682.
29. Chen W, Yung BC, Qian Z, Chen X. Improving long-term subcutaneous drug delivery by regulating material-bioenvironment interaction. Advanced Drug Delivery Reviews. 2018;127:20–34.

30. Zhao J, Xu G, Yao X, Zhou H, Lyu B, Pei S, Wen P. Microneedle-based insulin transdermal delivery system: Current status and translation challenges. Drug Delivery and Translational Research. 2022; 12(10):2403–27.
31. Meng F, Qiao X, Xin C, Ju X, He M. Recent progress of polymeric microneedle-assisted long-acting transdermal drug delivery. Journal of Pharmacy & Pharmaceutical Sciences. 2024;27:12434.
32. Aroche AF, Nissan HE, Daniele MA. Hydrogel-forming microneedles and applications in interstitial fluid diagnostic devices. Advanced Healthcare Materials. 2025;14(1):2401782.
33. Yu J, Zhang Y, Ye Y, DiSanto R, Sun W, Ranson D, Ligler FS, Buse JB, Gu Z. Microneedle-array patches loaded with hypoxia-sensitive vesicles provide fast glucose-responsive insulin delivery. Proceedings of the National Academy of Sciences. 2015;112(27):8260–65.
34. Martínez-Navarrete M, Pérez-López A, Guillot AJ, Cordeiro AS, Melero A, Aparicio-Blanco J. Latest advances in glucose-responsive microneedle-based systems for transdermal insulin delivery. International Journal of Biological Macromolecules. 2024;263:130301.
35. Nagarkar R, Singh M, Nguyen HX, Jonnalagadda S. A review of recent advances in microneedle technology for transdermal drug delivery. Journal of Drug Delivery Science and Technology. 2020; 59:101923.
36. Heinemann L, Deiss D, Siegmund T, Schlüter S, Naudorf M, von Sengbusch S, Lange K, Freckmann G. Glucose measurement and control in patients with type 1 or type 2 diabetes. Experimental and Clinical Endocrinology & Diabetes. 2019;127(S 01):S8–26.
37. Brown SA, Kovatchev BP, Raghinaru D, Lum JW, Buckingham BA, Kudva YC, Laffel LM, Levy CJ, Pinsker JE, Wadwa RP, Dassau E. Six-month randomized, multicenter trial of closed-loop control in type 1 diabetes. New England Journal of Medicine. 2019;381(18):1707–17.
38. Rapini N, Martino M, Arnaldi C, Deodati A, Anagnostopoulou L, Amodeo ME, Ciampalini P, Pampanini V, Lorubbio A, Tosini D, Cianfarani S. Efficacy and safety of advanced hybrid closed loop systems in children with type 1 diabetes younger than 6 years. Frontiers in Endocrinology. 2024;15: 1382920.
39. Yu J, Qian C, Zhang Y, Cui Z, Zhu Y, Shen Q, Ligler FS, Buse JB, Gu Z. Hypoxia and H2O2 dual-sensitive vesicles for enhanced glucose-responsive insulin delivery. Nano Letters. 2017;17(2):733–9.
40. Ware J, Hovorka R. Closed-loop insulin delivery: Update on the state of the field and emerging technologies. Expert Review of Medical Devices. 2022;19(11):859–75.
41. Boughton CK, Hartnell S, Lakshman R, Nwokolo M, Wilinska ME, Ware J, Allen JM, Evans ML, Hovorka R. Fully closed-loop glucose control compared with insulin pump therapy with continuous glucose monitoring in adults with type 1 diabetes and suboptimal glycemic control: A single-center, randomized, crossover study. Diabetes Care. 2023;46(11):1916–22.
42. Fabris C, Kovatchev B. The closed-loop artificial pancreas in 2020. Artificial Organs. 2020;44(7):01–10.
43. Ahamad SS, Khan Pathan AS. A formally verified authentication protocol in secure framework for mobile healthcare during COVID-19-like pandemic. Connection Science. 2021;33(3):532–54.
44. He Y, Li X, Zhang T. Nanoparticles-induced potential toxicity on human health. 2023.
45. Murali S, Thomas J, Abraham J, Kanna V, Ramachandiran S, SS Suruthi. Nanodiagnostics and nanotoxicology: A systematic review and meta-analysis on nanoparticle applications and safety in metabolic organs. OpenNano. 2025:100266.
46. Galanki V, Rangala M, Tejolahari I, Niharika G, Likhita A. Evaluating nanotoxicity: Integrating invitro and invivo models for risk assessment. Biosciences Biotechnology Research Asia. 2025;22(2):435.
47. Tamarov K, Wang JT, Kari J, Happonen E, Vesavaara I, Niemela M, Peramaki P, Al-Jamal KT, Xu W, Lehto VP. Comparison between fluorescence imaging and elemental analysis to determine biodistribution of inorganic nanoparticles with strong light absorption. ACS Applied Materials & Interfaces. 2021; 13(34):40392–400.
48. Panico S, Capolla S, Bozzer S, Toffoli G, Dal Bo M, Macor P. Biological features of nanoparticles: Protein corona formation and interaction with the immune system. Pharmaceutics. 2022;14(12):2605.
49. Abhinav V, Basu P, Verma SS, Verma J, Das A, Kumari S, Yadav PR, Kumar V. Advancements in wearable and implantable BioMEMS devices: Transforming healthcare through technology. Micromachines. 2025;16(5):522.
50. Nasira AS (2025). Nanoparticle-enabled insulin delivery systems for optimizing glycemic control in diabetes mellitus. IDOSR JOURNAL OF EXPERIMENTAL SCIENCES 11(2):5–11.
51. US Food and Drug Administration. Do not use smartwatches or smart rings to measure blood glucose levels: FDA safety communication. FDA; 2024.
52. Goshrani A, Lin R, O'Neal D, Ekinci EI. Time in range—A new gold standard in type 2 diabetes research? Diabetes, Obesity and Metabolism. 2025;27(5):2342–62.

53. Singh P, Joshi AS, Singh H, Mijakovic I. Medical importance and pharmacokinetics of gold nanoparticles in the human body. Molecular Cancer. 2025;24(1):252.
54. Gurav SR, Waikar MR, Rasal AS, Sonker RK, Sonkawade RG. Current Development and Challenges in textile-Based Flexible Supercapacitors. In Smart and Flexible Energy Devices (pp. 539–550). CRC Press; 2022.
55. Kumari S, Raturi S, Kulshrestha S, Chauhan K, Dhingra S, András K, Thu K, Khargotra R, Singh T. A comprehensive review on various techniques used for synthesizing nanoparticles. Journal of Materials Research and Technology. 2023;27:1739–63.
56. Zhang K, Qi Y, Wang W, Tian X, Wang J, Xu L, Zhai X. Future horizons in diabetes: Integrating AI and personalized care. Frontiers in Endocrinology. 2025;16:1583227.

10 Ethical Considerations in Nanomedicine

Mahesh Kumar Posa
School of Health and Medical Sciences, Adamas University Barasat, Kolkata, India

Guarav Tiwari
PSIT-Pranveer Singh Institute of Technology (Pharmacy), Kanpur, India

Nidhi Singh
Teerthanker Mahaveer College of Pharmacy (TMCOP), Teerthanker Mahaveer University, Muradabad, India

Shipra Omar
School of Pharmaceutical Sciences, Shri Guru Ram Rai University, Dehradun, India

Shahzad Chohan
College of Clinical Pharmacy, King Faisal University, Al-Ahsa, Saudi Arabia

10.1 INTRODUCTION

Nanomedicine – therapeutics, diagnostics, and devices that exploit structures at the 1–100 nm scale – has transitioned from proof-of-concept to clinical reality, with a growing pipeline of human trials and a growing number of regulatory/safety guidelines. As of late 2024, systematic surveys found numerous ongoing and planned clinical trials using nanoparticle platforms across oncology, gene therapy, and diagnostics, underlining rapid clinical translations [1].

For this chapter, "nanomedicine" will include: (1) engineered nanoparticle drug carriers (lipid, polymeric, inorganic); (2) nanoscale implantable or surface-modified medical devices (e.g., graphene-based neural interfaces); and (3) nano-enabled diagnostic platforms and biosensors. Regulatory bodies often treat these as "complex" or "non-biological complex drugs" requiring case-by-case evaluation because nanoscale properties can change pharmacokinetics, toxicity, and environmental fate. Recent EU and US regulatory reviews explicitly highlight the need for specific quality, safety, and characterization approaches for nanomedicines [2, 3].

Three converging factors make ethical analysis timely. First, faster clinical translation: reviews in 2024 show many first-in-human and later-phase trials for nanoparticle therapeutics, increasing the urgency of informed-consent and long-term follow-up considerations. Second, novel device examples highlight unique societal stakes. For example, a graphene brain-chip, currently emerging in UK clinical testing for tumor surgery, demonstrates both therapeutic promise and profound questions about identity, data capture, and dual-use potential. Third, regulatory and occupational frameworks are evolving but incomplete: recent European Medicines Agency (EMA) horizon-scanning and the U.S. Food and Drug Administration (FDA) nanomaterials guidance emphasize adaptive governance, while the World Health Organization (WHO) and national occupational guidance underline gaps in

DOI: 10.1201/9781003598657-10

worker protection and life cycle stewardship. These developments mean ethicists, regulators, clinicians, and industry must collaborate now to address consent, equity, environmental stewardship, and governance before technologies scale widely [4].

10.2 KEY ETHICAL PRINCIPLES

The foundational ethical framework used in medicine – autonomy, beneficence, non-maleficence, and justice – also underpins ethical evaluation in nanomedicine, though its application here presents unique challenges. These principles, formalized in clinical ethics literature and widely endorsed by bioethics bodies, guide morally responsible action in situations of risk and uncertainty. At its core, autonomy prioritizes respect for people's rights to make informed decision about their care, grounded in transparent communication and voluntary consent [5]. In the United States, the FDA's Office of Combination Products manages these items, while the specific FDA center responsible for the product's primary therapeutic action handles the actual review (Table 10.1).

10.2.1 Autonomy, Beneficence, Non-Maleficence, Justice

Beneficence requires clinicians and researchers to act in the best interests of patients, promoting benefits, such as improved targeting, reduced side effects, and improved diagnostics – advantages vividly present in nano-enabled oncology and regenerative medicine applications. Non-maleficence, encapsulated in the Hippocratic "do no harm" maxim, obliges minimization of potential harms. Nanomedicines often involve novel materials whose short- and long-term toxicological profiles (e.g.,

TABLE 10.1
Major Ethical Domains in Nanomedicine: Risks, Evidence Gaps, and Governance Responses

Ethical Domain	Key Risk/Concern	Example	Governance Response
Risk and toxicology	Reactive oxygen species (ROS) generation, immune activation, organ accumulation	Metallic nanoparticle shown to induce oxidative stress and inflammatory responses in preclinical [6, 7]	Nano-specific safety testing; enhanced post-marketing surveillance
Clinical trials and consent	Long-term uncertainty in nanoparticle biodistribution	Ethical concerns about informed consent in early-phase nanomedicine trials [8]	Transparent uncertainty disclosure; adaptive trial monitoring
Benefit-risk assessment	Complex immunogenicity and pharmacokinetics	FDA guidance on nanomaterial-containing drug product [9]	Iterative regulatory review; real-world evidence integration
Privacy and data governance	Continuous biomonitoring and data ownership ambiguity	Expansion of nano-enabled sensors and digital health governance debates [10]	Dynamic consent; strengthened data protection regulation
Equity and access	High development cost; global disparities	Disproportionate early access to nano-enabled vaccines in high-income countries [11]	Tiered pricing; global procurement coordination
Environmental impact	Release of engineered nanoparticles into ecosystems	Ecotoxicity of Ag and TiO_2 nanoparticles in aquatic systems [12]	Life cycle assessment; nanowaste management standards
Dual-use risks	Potential misuse in military or surveillance applications	Dual-use concerns in nano-neurotechnology [13]	International risk governance; cross-sector oversight
Responsible innovation	Lack of binding nano-specific ethical codes	EU Code of Conduct for Responsible Nanosciences [14]	Ethics-by-design; accountability frameworks

biodistribution, bioaccumulation) are actively researched, highlighting the ethical necessity of rigorous safety assessment before clinical deployment. Distributive justice requires the fair allocation of healthcare resources. In nanomedicine, this means ensuring equal access to expensive, advanced therapies. Without affordable and widespread distribution, these innovations risk widening existing health inequalities. Together, these principles form a prima facie ethical structure where no single principle always overrides another, and balancing them depends on context [15].

10.2.2 Precautionary Approach

Given pervasive scientific uncertainty of specific risks related to nanoscale interactions with biological systems, applying the precautionary approach is ethically salient. Originating in environmental and public health ethics, this approach asserts that lack of full scientific certainty should not delay protective action when there are plausible risks of serious harm. In nanomedicine, where long-term effects and environmental fate of nanomaterials are not fully known, a precautionary approach encourages increased safety testing, adaptive regulation, and ongoing risk assessment before wide clinical or environmental release. This aligns with broader ethical imperatives to protect patients and the ecosystems in the face of uncertain but potentially significant harm [16].

10.3 RISK, SAFETY, AND TOXICOLOGY

10.3.1 Unique Nanoscale Hazards

Nanomedicine utilizes materials designed at the 1–100 nm scale, where physicochemical properties vary greatly from bulk counterparts. Increased surface-area-to-volume ratio, increased surface reactivity, quantum effects, and changes in electrical charge allow for increased drug solubility, targeted delivery, and barrier crossing (e.g., blood-brain barrier crossing). However, these same properties may also create special toxicological threats [17].

One major concern is the generation of ROS, which can induce oxidative stress, DNA damage, mitochondrial dysfunction, and inflammatory responses. Experimental studies have shown that certain metallic nanoparticles (e.g., silver, titanium dioxide, zinc oxide) can accumulate in liver, lung, and renal tissues following systemic exposure. Size, shape, surface coating, and aggregation state significantly influence biodistribution and toxicity. Unlike conventional drugs, nanoparticles may evade rapid renal clearance, resulting in prolonged tissue retention [18].

Another nanoscale-specific issue is the formation of a protein corona upon contact with biological fluids. This dynamic adsorption of proteins alerts particle identity, cellular uptake, immune recognition, and toxicity profiles, making safety prediction complex and context-dependent. Additionally, some nanoparticles can cross placental or neural barriers, raising the intergenerational and neurotoxicity concerns that require long-term evaluation [19]. Ethical risks in nanomedicine emerge progressively along the translational pathway from material design to post-market exposure (see Figure 10.1).

10.3.2 Preclinical Testing Gaps

Despite advances in nanotoxicology, important preclinical safety gaps remain. Traditional toxicological assays were developed for small-molecule drugs, but they may not adequately capture nanoparticle behavior. Standard 2D cell cultures often fail to replicate tissue architecture, immune interactions, or long-term exposure dynamics. Consequently, in vitro results may not correlate reliably with in vivo results [20].

Animal models also present translational limitations. Differences in immune response, metabolism, and clearance mechanisms complicate extrapolation to humans. Furthermore, chronic exposure studies and long-term biodistribution tracking remain limited for many emerging nanotherapeutics [21].

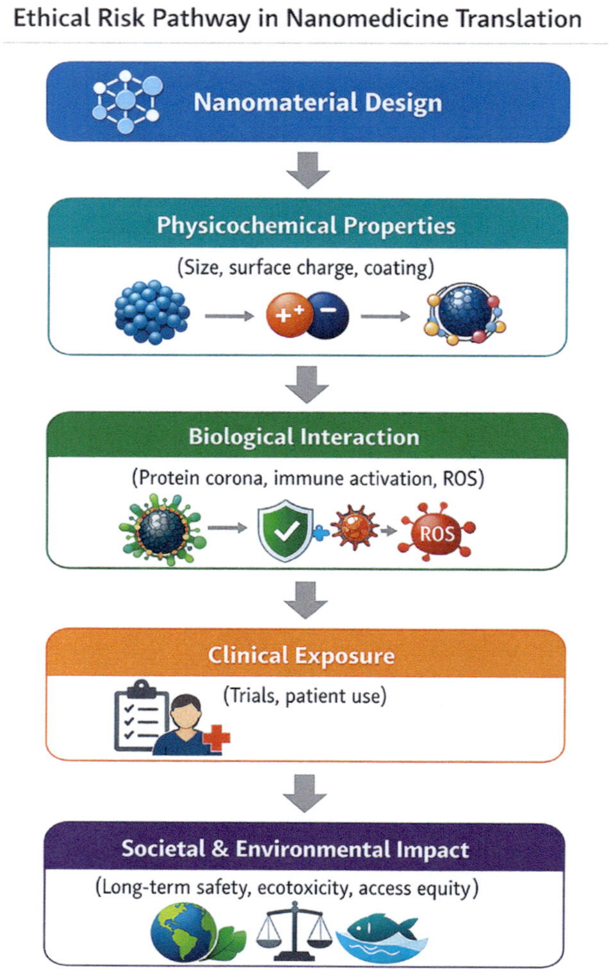

FIGURE 10.1 Ethical risk pathway in translation of nanomedicine.

There is currently no universally harmonized global testing framework specific to nanomedicine. Variability in particle characterization methods (size distribution, zeta potential, surface chemistry) further affects reproducibility across laboratories. Regulatory agencies increasingly recommend comprehensive physicochemical profiling, immunotoxicity testing, and life cycle analysis, yet standardized endpoints are still evolving. Strengthening predictive models such as organ-on-chip systems, 3D organoids, and advanced computational toxicology will be critical to improving risk assessment and ensuring responsible clinical translation [22].

10.4 CLINICAL TRIALS AND CONSENT

Clinical research involving nanomedicine has expanded rapidly. Today, you can find thousands of nanomedical clinical trials registered globally. Recent growth is driven by oncology and emerging infectious-disease applications linked to lipid nanoparticle technologies, which were first widely used in mRNA vaccines for COVID-19. This diversification highlights the need for robust trial design and ethical oversight [23].

10.4.1 Informed Consent Challenges

Nanomedicine trials pose specific informed-consent challenges because novel risks and scientific uncertainty about long-term effects and mechanisms persist even at later phases. Many formulations entering human trails, including targeted lipid and polymeric carriers, have complex biodistribution and immune interactions that are not fully predictable from preclinical data, making it difficult for participants to understand all potential harms and benefits before enrollment. Regulators and ethicists stress that consent materials must transparently communicate such uncertainties, particularly for first-in-human studies involving nanoparticles with limited human exposure history. Additionally, the legal and ethical requirement that subjects understand risk-benefit profiles becomes harder to satisfy where long-term safety data are limited, raising concerns about truly "informed" consent in early-phase nanomedicine trials [24].

10.4.2 Trial Design and Monitoring

Nanomedicine trial design must take into account an increased safety monitoring because of unpredictable biodistribution and immune response. Many nanoparticle trials are still in Phase I/II where close monitoring for acute & delayed adverse events is critical. Adaptive trial designs and independent data-monitoring committees are increasingly recommended to identify safety signals early and adjust protocols in real time [25].

10.5 BENEFIT-RISK ASSESSMENT

Assessing the balance between benefits and risks is central to ethical evaluation and regulatory decision-making in nanomedicine. Nanotechnology-based medical products must demonstrate evidence of therapeutic efficacy while ensuring that potential harms are identified, quantified, and minimized. Regulatory authorities such as the FDA and the EMA require that nanomedicines should meet the same standards of safety, efficacy, and quality as other medicinal products, even where unique nanoscale properties complicate evaluation. This includes comprehensive characterization of nanomaterials, functional performance data, and clinically relevant outcomes. Recent guidance from the FDA emphasizes issues of nominating and controlling risks relating to nanomaterials and advocating detailed physicochemical characterization related to the clinical impact [26].

Many on-going and completed clinical trials – especially in oncology and immunotherapy – that show meaningful improvements in treatment outcomes must be weighed against safety-profile. For example, lipid nanoparticle formulations used in RNA delivery have shown improved targeted delivery and therapeutic efficacy over conventional formulations, but regulators and ethics committees continue to emphasize the need for robust data on adverse effects, immune reactions, and long-term outcomes to inform benefit-risk ratio assessments [27].

10.5.1 Evidence Standards of Efficacy and Harm

Nanomedicines are evaluated through standard clinical endpoints such as survival, disease progression, and symptoms improvement, supplemented by mechanistic biomarkers specific to nano-delivery systems. Regulators also require detailed safety data, including immunotoxicity, biodistribution, and metabolism. Because nanomaterials may behave differently in vivo compared with traditional drugs, enhanced analytical techniques and tailored testing strategies are increasingly needed to reliably characterize both efficacy and harm [28].

10.5.2 Uncertainty Handling

Uncertainty is inherent in nanomedicine benefit-risk assessments due to limited long-term human data and complex biological interactions. Regulatory risk frameworks endorse adaptive risk assessment approaches – i.e., acceptability of ongoing data review throughout clinical development and after-market use surveillance. Approaches such as integrated testing strategies, modeling, and simulation or real-world evidence collection support dealing with uncertainty and inform decision-making [29].

10.6 PRIVACY AND DATA GOVERNANCE

10.6.1 Biomonitoring, Sensors, Long-Term Tracking

Nanomedicine is increasingly intertwined with advanced sensing and biomonitoring technologies, including implantable or wearable nanosensors capable of continuous health tracking. These devices can generate high-resolution physiological data over extended periods, offering unprecedented insight into individual health trajectories as well as raising significant privacy concerns. Continuous tracking produces extensive personal data – often including biomarkers, movement patterns, and other sensitive health indicators – thus creating a rich digital profile that could be misused if inadequately protected. Ethical literature on nanomedical tech highlights that extensive data collection must be accompanied by robust privacy safeguards and transparent governance frameworks to retain patient trust [30].

Long-term monitoring also poses data governance challenges released to data retention, transfer, and de-identification, especially as data may persist beyond the period of direct clinical use. Healthcare systems increasingly store health information in large datasets for ongoing analysis and research, but without careful data life cycle governance, this creates risks of unauthorized access or re-identification of individuals even from anonymized datasets. Recent broader healthcare data privacy research underscores those traditional protections (e.g., HIPAA in the U.S.) may offer incomplete coverage when wearables and third-party services are involved; leaving gaps in long-term privacy protections [31].

10.6.2 Data Ownership and Secondary Use

A central ethical concern in nanomedicine data governance is the ownership of biometric and clinical data, especially as analytic capabilities grow. Patients increasingly question who "owns" health data generated by nanotechnologies and how they may be used beyond the original clinical purpose – so-called secondary use. Worries about data being shared for commercial analytics, AI model training, or insurance profiling without explicit on-going consent are well documented. Ethical frameworks and recent proposals advocate for models where patients retain control over their data and are managed dynamically, preventing unauthorized secondary use and reinforcing trust in nanomedical innovation [32].

10.7 EQUITY, ACCESS, AND JUSTICE

10.7.1 Global Distribution, Cost, Health Disparities

Nanomedicine holds promise for transforming healthcare with targeted therapies and improved diagnostics, but equitable distribution of benefits remains a core ethical concern. Research shows that medical innovation, including nanomedicine, is often concentrated in high-income countries where research funding, industry capacity, and regulatory infrastructure are strongest. Consequently, conditions that mainly affect low-and-middle-income regions may receive disproportionally less attention, and reinforce existing health inequities. Analyses of clinical trial distribution and disease burden data indicate that nanomedicine research does not currently bridge the gap between wealthier and poorer nations, reflecting broader patterns of global health research inequality [33].

The COVID-19 pandemic offered a concrete example: although several approved vaccines relied on nanoparticle delivery platforms, high-income countries secured the majority of early doses – around 75% of nano-vaccine procurement, while middle and low-income countries received far fewer. This disparity illustrates how cost, production capacity, and intellectual property constraints can limit access to nanomedicine technologies where these are most needed [34].

Affordability is also a challenge within countries; early nanotherapeutics and diagnostics often come with higher price tags than conventional alternatives, risking unequal access based on ability to pay. Such disparities can exacerbate health outcomes across socio-economic groups, unless policy measures address affordability and coverage [35].

10.7.2 Prioritization and Fairness

Ethical principles of justice and non-discrimination require that priority setting nanomedicine development and distribution be transparent and equitable. This includes ensuring that research agendas reflect the global disease burden and that allocation frameworks prioritize the most vulnerable populations, rather than focusing solely on affluent markets [36].

Fair prioritization mechanisms can include public-private partnerships to subsidize access in resource-limited settings, cross-subsidization pricing strategies, and global governance coordination to avoid "first-come, first served" advantages for wealthy nations. Without such measures, nanomedicine risks deepening rather than alleviating existing health disparities [37].

10.8 ENHANCEMENT AND HUMAN IDENTITY

The ethical line between therapy and enhancement in nanomedicine is increasingly debated as technologies designed to treat disease could be repurposed to augment human capacities. Traditional medical interventions aim to restore function or minimize illness, but new nano-enabled devices and biological interfaces blur the difference. For example, advanced implantable systems, such as brain-computer interfaces (BCIs) are being developed not only to restore motor function in paralysis but also to potentially improve cognitive or sensory performance beyond typical human norm. Debates surrounding companies like Neuralink highlight a growing ethical tension: while current brain–computer interface (BCI) trials aim to restore communication and mobility for paralyzed individuals, critics worry about the future of elective cognitive enhancement and potential alterations to human identity [38].

10.8.1 Therapeutic vs Enhancement Lines

This blurring raises questions about human identity, autonomy, and authenticity. If technologies change cognition, memory, or emotional response, individuals and societies must grapple with what constitutes the "authentic self," a theme explored in research on neurotechnology ethics. Scholars argue that enhancement technologies may change conventional concepts of personal identity and agency, particularly if external implants increasingly shape thought or behavior [39].

10.8.2 Social/Psychological Impacts

Ethicists also highlight potential social and psychological impacts: pressure to adopt enhancement technologies could create new inequalities, stigmatization of those who choose not to augment, and shifts in societal norms about ability and performance. These concerns underscore the need for broad ethical and social dialogue as nanomedicine evolves beyond therapeutic use and into the realm of human enhancement [40].

10.9 DUAL-USE AND MISUSE RISKS

Nanotechnology's capability to precisely manipulate matter at the molecular scale carries dual-use risk – technologies intended for health benefits could also be misused for harmful purposes. For example, research in nano-neurotechnology highlights concerns that targeted delivery systems capable of crossing the blood-brain barrier might one day be repurposed to interfere with neural functions if misappropriated, raising biothreat considerations alongside therapeutic applications [41].

10.9.1 Biothreats, Surveillance; Military Applications

Nanomaterials also present surveillance and military application risk. Ethical analyses suggest that nano-enabled devices could be used for covert monitoring or battlefield sensing, and hypothetical "nano-weapons" concerns have been raised in security discussion, though practical deployment is limited and theoretical [42].

10.9.2 Governance Responses

In terms of governance, international regulation of nanotechnology's military or misuse potential is currently limited or absent, with no comprehensive framework to monitor R&D or restrict harmful applications. Experts argue that this governance gap allows innovation to outpace policy, underscoring the need for integrated risk governance strategies that coordinate national policies, international norms, and multidisciplinary oversight to manage dual-use risks with nanotech [43].

10.10 ENVIRONMENTAL IMPACT AND STEWARDSHIP

10.10.1 Ecotoxicology and Life Cycle Impacts

Nanomedicines and other nanotechnology-enabled products inevitably contribute nanoparticles to the environment at various points in their life cycle – from manufacturing and use to disposal. Engineered nanoparticles (ENPs) can enter aquatic ecosystems through waste-water streams, where they undergo physical and chemical transformations and affect their fate and toxicity. For instance, nanoparticles released during washing fabrics or disposal of personal care products can leach into water systems and affect microbial communities and fish, raising concerns about biomagnification up the food chain. ENPs may aggregate, dissolve, or adsorb complex environmental media affecting their lifespan and ecotoxicological properties [44].

Laboratory studies and environmental assessments point to potential problems caused by certain nanoparticles. For example, silver and titanium dioxide can disrupt soil invertebrate populations and inhibit nutrient cycling, thereby indirectly affecting ecosystem health. Smaller particles (≤10 nm) more easily penetrate soil and biological membranes, thus increasing risk to organisms and altering ecological equilibrium. The life cycle analysis approach advocated by environmental scientists examines emissions, transformation, and ecological effects from production to disposal, in order to predict and reduce impacts [45].

10.10.2 Waste Management

Current waste management systems are generally not suited to capture and neutralize nanomaterials. Wastewater treatment plants may remove only a fraction of ENPs, leading to their accumulation in sludge or release into water bodies. Without specific recycling and disposal standards for nanowaste, nanoparticles can persist in landfills or natural environments, with potential long-term ecological consequences. Stakeholders urges policy-making from incorporating life-cycle stewardship, safe disposal protocols, and more funding for environmental nanotoxicology research to ensure sustainable use of nanotechnologies [46].

10.11 REGULATION AND GOVERNANCE

10.11.1 Regulatory Gaps and Adaptive Governance

The rapid emergence of nanomedicine has outpaced traditional regulatory frameworks in many jurisdictions, creating significant regulatory gaps. Conventional drug and device regulatory pathways were developed for small molecules and biologics, and although they are being applied to nanomedicines, they often lack tailored provisions for nano-specific issues, such as unique biodistribution, immune interactions, and particle behavior at the nanoscale. As a result, regulators frequently rely on guidance documents rather than statutes to govern nanomedicine evaluation, leading to uncertainty for developers and potential safety oversight gaps. Notably, the FDA and the EMA have issued guidance documents to help sponsors characterize nanomaterial-based therapeutics, but these remain evolving and sometimes lack harmonized global standards. Adaptive governance approaches, such as iterative assessment, post-market surveillance enhancements, and nanomedicine-specific testing protocols, are increasingly advocated to manage uncertainty and rapidly incorporate scientific advances into the regulatory decision-making [47].

10.11.2 International Coordination

Effective oversight of nanomedicine also requires international coordination, as regulatory fragmentation can hinder cross-border research and product approval. Bodies like the International Coalition of Medicines Regulatory Authorities (ICMRA) bring national regulators together to discuss the emerging issues and harmonies evaluation methodologies. Similarly, international fora and observatories (e.g., the European Union Observatory for Nanomaterials) promote transparency and shared data on nanomaterial uses and safety, and facilitate coordinated regulatory responses. However, global alignment remains incomplete: many countries still lack nanomedicine, and harmonization of definitions, testing standards, and risk-benefit frameworks is an ongoing effort. Strengthening international governance mechanisms, including collaborative guideline development and mutual recognition agreements, will be critical for ensuring that nanomedicines are regulated effectively and equitably worldwide [48]. An adaptive, multi-level governance structure is required to manage uncertainty and ensure responsible innovation (see Figure 10.2).

10.12 PUBLIC ENGAGEMENT AND TRUST

Effective risk communication is necessary for establishing and maintaining public confidence in nanomedicine and broader nanotechnology. Experiences across emerging tech fields show that public attitudes are strongly shaped by how information about benefits and risks are framed and shared. Studies on public perception of nanotechnology find that knowledge levels correlate with attitudes, and that clear, balanced communication, especially early in technology development, can reduce misperceptions and build trust. Citizens often express desire for more transparent information and clearer explanations of safety and regulatory processes, not just promotional messages about innovation [49].

Risk communication strategies now increasingly focus on a two-way communication approach instead of one-way dissemination. Engagement methods vary from stakeholder deliberations to interactive online engagement platforms collecting varying perceptions about nanotechnology applications, including health-related applications. These approaches make it easier for the public to input by enabling innovation that reflects societal values [50].

Deliberative processes, such as structured public forums and co-creation workshops involving scientists, patients, policymakers, and community members, are recommended because they allow participants to discuss uncertainties, ethical concerns, and priorities openly. Such participatory involvement can improve legitimacy and trust in governance decisions and enhance transparency in nanomedicine development [51].

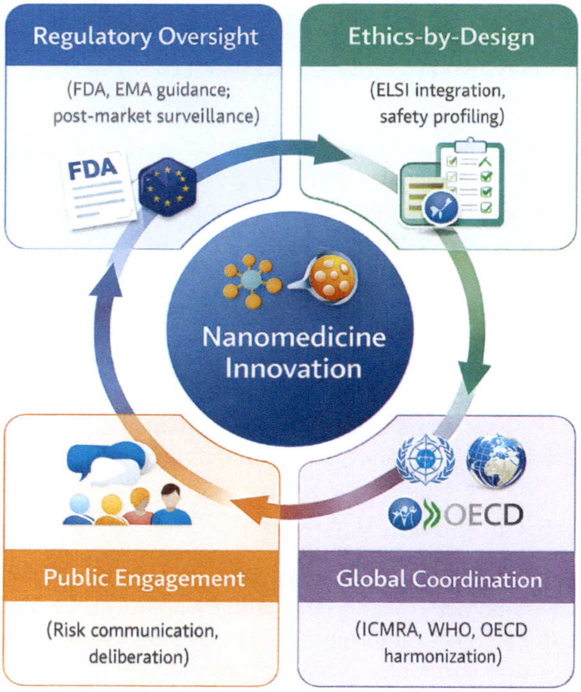

FIGURE 10.2 Adaptive governance framework of ethical nanomedicine.

10.13 RESPONSIBLE INNOVATION AND INDUSTRY PRACTICE

Ethics-by-design, transparency, and responsible R&D are increasingly considered critical for trustworthy nanomedicine development. Responsible Research and Innovation (RRI) frameworks emphasize integrating ethical reflection, anticipatory assessments of impacts, stakeholder inclusion, and responsiveness to societal needs throughout research life cycle, rather than only when products reach the market. This approach promotes the researchers and companies address downstream risks and societal implications early in design and testing, thereby promoting sustainability and public trust. Such principles – anticipation, inclusion, reflexivity, and responsiveness – are widely discussed in nanotechnology ethics scholarship and applied in emerging innovation governance models [52].

Industry transparency – safety data, mechanism, and rationale of design choices – is open. For instance, certain consortia of nanomedical researchers now publish safety guidelines and participate in multi-stakeholder conversations with clinicians, regulators, and ethicists about making technological trends align with people's values [53].

Industry codes and accountability also play a role. Although formal, binding ethical codes specific to nanomedicine are still developing, voluntary frameworks – such as the European Commission's code of Conduct for Responsible Nanosciences and Nanotechnologies Research – support guiding principles for ethical practices and accountability. These emphasize transparency in reporting, stakeholder engagement, and monitoring of social and environmental impacts. Continued adoption of industry-specific codes and ethical standards help strengthen accountability and social legitimacy as nanomedicine technologies mature [54].

10.14 RECOMMENDATIONS (POLICY INDICATORS AND PRACTICE)

Policymakers, researchers, industry, and funders should adopt clear ethics-by-design practices that integrate ethical, safety, and social impact assessments throughout nanomedicine R&D to anticipate risks and guide responsible innovation. Enhanced transparency in data, methodologies, and decision processes improves trust and governance. Regulators should develop adaptive oversight frameworks with tailored criteria for nanoparticle characterization, risk-benefit evaluation, and post-market surveillance, closing gaps in governance. Cross-sectorial collaboration and international coordination can harmonize standards and ensure fair access. Funders should prioritize projects that include ethical, legal, and social implication (ELSI) component alongside scientific aims. Emphasizing public engagement and accountability mechanisms ensures that nanomedicine development aligns with societal values and equity goals.

10.15 CONCLUSION

Nanomedicine represents one of the most transformative frontiers in contemporary healthcare, offering unprecedented precision in diagnosis, drug delivery, and regenerative therapies. Yet its nanoscale nature – though scientifically advantageous – introduces ethical complexities that extend beyond traditional biomedical concerns. Issues of long-term safety, informed consent under uncertainty, equitable access, and privacy in continuous biomonitoring, dual-use risks, and environmental stewardship demand proactive and coordinated.

As innovation accelerates, ethical reflection must evolve in parallel. Strengthening of adaptive regulatory systems, ethics-by-design in research and industry practice, and promoting global collaboration are essential to ensure responsible translation. Equally important is sustained public engagement to maintain trust and legitimacy. Ultimately, the ethical governance of nanomedicine is not a barrier to progress, but a foundation for it, ensuring that technological advancement advances human well-being, while safeguarding individual rights, social justice, and environmental sustainability.

REFERENCES

1. Kazi RN, Hasani IW, Khafaga DS, Kabba S, Farhan M, Aatif M, Muteeb G, Fahim YA. Nanomedicine: The effective role of nanomaterials in healthcare from diagnosis to therapy. Pharmaceutics. 2025;17(8):987.
2. Wang B, Hu S, Teng Y, Chen J, Wang H, Xu Y, Wang K, Xu J, Cheng Y, Gao X. Current advance of nanotechnology in diagnosis and treatment for malignant tumors. Signal Transduction and Targeted Therapy. 2024;9(1):200.
3. Joseph TM, Kar Mahapatra D, Esmaeili A, Piszczyk, Hasanin MS, Kattali M, Haponiuk J, Thomas S. Nanoparticles: Taking a unique position in medicine. Nanomaterials. 2023;13(3):574.
4. Desai N, Rana D, Patel M, Bajwa N, Prasad R, Vora LK. Nanoparticle therapeutics in clinical perspective: Classification, marketed products, and regulatory landscape. Small. 2025;21(29):2502315.
5. Plöckinger U, Auga U. The "Four principles" of Western medical bioethics and the bioethics of Shīʿī Islam in Iran—Is the claim of universality by both justified? Religions. 2022;13(11):1118.
6. Nel AE, Mädler L, Velegol D, Xia T, Hoek EM, Somasundaran P, Klaessig F, Castranova V, Thompson M. Understanding biophysicochemical interactions at the nano–bio interface. Nature Materials. 2009; 8(7):543–57.
7. Fadeel B, Farcal L, Hardy B, Vázquez-Campos S, Hristozov D, Marcomini A, Lynch I, Valsami-Jones E, Alenius H, Savolainen K. Advanced tools for the safety assessment of nanomaterials. Nature Nanotechnology. 2018;13(7):537–43.
8. Resnik DB, Tinkle SS. Ethical issues in clinical trials involving nanomedicine. Contemporary Clinical Trials. 2007;28(4):433–41.
9. de Vlieger JS, Crommelin DJ, Tyner K, Drummond DC, Jiang W, McNeil SE, Neervannan S, Crist RM, Shah VP. Report of the AAPS guidance forum on the FDA draft guidance for industry: Drug products, including biological products, that contain nanomaterials. The AAPS Journal. 2019;21(4):56.
10. Mittelstadt B. The ethics of biomedical 'big data' analytics. Philosophy & Technology. 2019;32(1):17–21.
11. Privor-Dumm L, Excler JL, Gilbert S, Karim SS, Hotez PJ, Thompson D, Kim JH. Vaccine access, equity and justice: COVID-19 vaccines and vaccination. BMJ Global Health. 2023;8(6):e011881.
12. Leppanen MT, Sourisseau S, Burgess RM, Simpson SL, Sibley P, Jonker MT. Sediment toxicity tests: A critical review of their use in environmental regulations. Environmental Toxicology and Chemistry. 2024;43(8):1697–716.
13. Nixdorff K, Borisova T, Komisarenko S, Dando M. Dual-use nano-neurotechnology: An assessment of the implications of trends in science and technology. Politics and the Life Sciences. 2018;37(2):180–202.

14. Dorbeck-Jung B, Shelley-Egan C. Meta-regulation and nanotechnologies: The challenge of responsibilisation within the European Commission's code of conduct for responsible nanosciences and nanotechnologies research. Nanoethics. 2013;7(1):55–68.
15. Bester JC. Beneficence, interests, and wellbeing in medicine: What it means to provide benefit to patients. The American Journal of Bioethics. 2020;20(3):53–62.
16. Van Herten J, Bovenkerk B. The precautionary principle in zoonotic disease control. Public Health Ethics. 2021;14(2):180–90.
17. Kurul F, Turkmen H, Cetin AE, Topkaya SN. Nanomedicine: How nanomaterials are transforming drug delivery, bio-imaging, and diagnosis. Next Nanotechnology. 2025;7:100129.
18. Fu PP, Xia Q, Hwang HM, Ray PC, Yu H. Mechanisms of nanotoxicity: Generation of reactive oxygen species. Journal of Food and Drug Analysis. 2014;22(1):64–75.
19. Huang W, Xiao G, Zhang Y, Min W. Research progress and application opportunities of nanoparticle–protein corona complexes. Biomedicine & Pharmacotherapy. 2021;139:111541.
20. Silvani G, Stenzel MH, Kilian KA. Precision nanomedicine: A necessary convergence of nanodrug development, organotypic models and microphysiological systems. ACS Nano Medicine. 2025;1(1): 54–73.
21. Peplow PV. Animal models in medical translation: The grand challenge of developing new treatments for human diseases. Frontiers in Medical Technology. 2024;6:1367521.
22. Havelikar U, Ghorpade KB, Kumar A, Patel A, Singh M, Banjare N, Gupta PN. Comprehensive insights into mechanism of nanotoxicity, assessment methods and regulatory challenges of nanomedicines. Discover Nano. 2024;19(1):165.
23. Nirmala MJ, Kizhuveetil U, Johnson A, Nagarajan R, Muthuvijayan V. Cancer nanomedicine: A review of nano-therapeutics and challenges ahead. RSC Advances. 2023;13(13):8606–29.
24. Chehelgerdi M, Chehelgerdi M, Allela OQ, Pecho RD, Jayasankar N, Rao DP, Thamaraikani T, Vasanthan M, Viktor P, Lakshmaiya N, Saadh MJ. Progressing nanotechnology to improve targeted cancer treatment: Overcoming hurdles in its clinical implementation. Molecular Cancer. 2023;22(1):169.
25. Gupta PK. Nanotoxicology in Nanobiomedicine. Springer International Publishing; 2023.
26. Malik S, Muhammad K, Waheed Y. Emerging applications of nanotechnology in healthcare and medicine. Molecules. 2023;28(18):6624.
27. Han J, Lim J, Wang CP, Han JH, Shin HE, Kim SN, Jeong D, Lee SH, Chun BH, Park CG, Park W. Lipid nanoparticle-based mRNA delivery systems for cancer immunotherapy. Nano Convergence. 2023;10(1):36.
28. Pandey H, Pandey RK. Ensuring Safe Nanotechnology: A Biosafety and Regulatory Perspective. In Green Nanomaterials: An Agriculture and Circular Economy Alternative (pp. 257–272). Springer Nature Switzerland; 2025.
29. Giubilato E, Cazzagon V, Amorim MJ, Blosi M, Bouillard J, Bouwmeester H, Costa AL, Fadeel B, Fernandes TF, Fito C, Hauser M. Risk management framework for nano-biomaterials used in medical devices and advanced therapy medicinal products. Materials. 2020;13(20):4532.
30. Gulati S, Yadav R, Kumari V, Nair S, Gupta C, Aishwari M. Nanosensors in healthcare: Transforming real-time monitoring and disease management with cutting-edge nanotechnology. RSC Pharmaceutics. 2025;2(5):1003–18.
31. Shinta Oktaviana R, Handayani PW, Hidayanto AN. Health organization challenges in health data governance implementation: A systematic review. Journal of Infrastructure, Policy and Development. 2024;8(6):3892.
32. Wylde V, Prakash E, Hewage C, Platts J. Ethical Challenges in the Use of Digital Technologies: AI and Big Data. In Digital Transformation in Policing: The Promise, Perils and Solutions (pp. 33–58). Springer International Publishing; 2023.
33. Fortune A, Aime A, Raymond D, Kumar S. Nanotechnology in medicine: A double-edged sword for health outcomes. Health Nanotechnology. 2025;1(1):9.
34. Das JK, Chee HY, Lakhani S, Khan MH, Islam M, Muhammad S, Bhutta ZA. COVID-19 vaccines: How efficient and equitable was the initial vaccination process? Vaccines. 2022;11(1):11.
35. Tsatsakis AM, Vliora M, Paraskevi K, Kalkach-Aparicio M. Emerging Social Issues on Targeted Drug Delivery. Scientific Research Publishing; 2024.
36. Moroşteş A, Stoicu NM. Principle of non-discrimination and equal treatment. Journal of Legal Studies. 2021;28(42):202–12.
37. Abdul S, Adeghe EP, Adegoke BO, Adegoke AA, Udedeh EH. Public-private partnerships in health sector innovation: Lessons from around the world. Magna Scientia Advanced Biology and Pharmacy. 2024;12(1):045–59.

38. Ma X, Tian Y, Yang R, Wang H, Allahou LW, Chang J, Williams G, Knowles JC, Poma A. Nanotechnology in healthcare, and its safety and environmental risks. Journal of Nanobiotechnology. 2024;22(1):715.
39. Horne J. Does AI represent authentic intelligence, or an artificial identity? Journal of Systemics, Cybernetics and Informatics. 2025;23(7):49–68.
40. Siala H, Wang Y. SHIFTing artificial intelligence to be responsible in healthcare: A systematic review. Social Science & Medicine. 2022;296:114782.
41. Prasanth MI, Mallya AR, Cho WC, Mundekkad D. Nano-structured strategies in combatting neurodegeneration. Frontiers in Bioengineering and Biotechnology. 2025;13:1638668.
42. Kosal ME. Military Applications of Nanotechnology: Implications for Strategic Security I. Georgia Institute of Technology; 2014.
43. Amutha C, Gopan A, Pushbalatatha I, Ragavi M, Reneese JA. Nanotechnology and Governance: Regulatory Framework for Responsible Innovation. In Nanotechnology in Societal Development (pp. 481–503). Springer Nature Singapore; 2024.
44. Abbas Q, Yousaf B, Ali MU, Munir MA, El-Naggar A, Rinklebe J, Naushad M. Transformation pathways and fate of engineered nanoparticles (ENPs) in distinct interactive environmental compartments: A review. Environment International. 2020;138:105646.
45. Abd EL-Aziz MA, Saeed AM, Ibrahim MK, El-Sayed WS. Impact of TiO_2, ZnO, and Ag nanoparticles on anammox activity in enriched river Nile sediment cultures: Unveiling differential effects and environmental implications. BMC Microbiology. 2024;24(1):468.
46. Bolan S, Sharma S, Mukherjee S, Zhou P, Mandal J, Srivastava P, Hou D, Edussuriya R, Vithanage M, Truong VK, Chapman J. The distribution, fate, and environmental impacts of food additive nanomaterials in soil and aquatic ecosystems. Science of the Total Environment. 2024;916:170013.
47. Parvin N, Aslam M, Alam MN, Mandal TK. Nanotechnology driven innovations in modern pharmaceutics: Therapeutics, imaging, and regeneration. Nanomaterials. 2025;15(22):1733.
48. Mudyiwenyama LG, Khoza S, Dube A. Situation analysis on the regulation of nanomedicines in Southern Africa. Frontiers in Medicine. 2023;10:1098830.
49. Capon A, Gillespie J, Rolfe M, Smith W. Perceptions of risk from nanotechnologies and trust in stakeholders: A cross sectional study of public, academic, government and business attitudes. BMC Public Health. 2015;15(1):424.
50. Maxim L, Mazzocchi M, Van den Broucke S, Zollo F, Robinson T, Rogers C, Vrbos D, Zamariola G, Smith, European Food Safety Authority (EFSA). Technical assistance in the field of risk communication. EFSA Journal. 2021;19(4):e06574.
51. Douglas H, Halpern MK, Louson E. Engaging publics in science: A practical typology. Journal of Responsible Innovation. 2024;11(1):2419238.
52. Lukkien DR, Nap HH, ter Stal M, Boon WP, Peine A, Minkman MM, Moors EH. Embedding responsible innovation into R&D practices: A case study of socially assistive robot development. Journal of Responsible Technology. 2024;19:100091.
53. Safarlou CW, Jongsma KR, Vermeulen R, Bredenoord AL. The ethical aspects of exposome research: A systematic review. Exposome. 2023;3(1):osad004.
54. Bowman DM, Hodge GA. Counting on Codes: An Examination of Transnational Codes as a Regulatory Governance Mechanism for Nanotechnologies. In Emerging Technologies (pp. 467–486). Routledge; 2020.
55. Brey PA. Ethical impact assessment: Theoretical foundations, methodology, and applications. Science and Engineering Ethics. 2026;32(1):6.

11 Regulatory Framework for Nano-Based Therapies

Deepak Maramwar
Karnataka College of Pharmacy, Bidar, India

Ajay Kumar Gupta
School of Pharmaceutical Sciences (formerly University Institute of Pharmacy), C.S.J.M. University Campus (formerly Kanpur University), Kanpur, India

Piyali Dey
Assam Down Town University, Guwahati, India

Vaibhav Dagaji Aher
Maharashtra University of Health Sciences, Nashik, India

Shaveta Ahalwat
University Institute of Pharma Sciences and Research Chandigarh University, Mohali, India

Vaishali Shirsat
Bombay College of Pharmacy (Autonomous), Mumbai, India

Ashish Singhai
Teerthanker Mahaveer College of Pharmacy, Teerthanker Mahaveer University, Moradabad, India

11.1 INTRODUCTION

Nanotechnology has reshaped drug development by enabling materials engineered at the 1–1000 nm scale to alter pharmacokinetics, biodistribution, and target engagement compared with traditional formulations. Regulatory attention has intensified because these size-dependent properties can have clinically relevant implications in safety, efficacy, and manufacturing control – issues not covered by the traditional categorization of "small-molecule" drugs and devices. Recent regulatory activity – for example, the U.S. Food and Drug Administration (FDA)'s focused guidance documents and outreach – broadly flags the necessity of product-specific risk assessment and enhanced characterization for products containing nanomaterials [1].

Practically, "nanomaterial" and "nanomedicine" are used with variable definitions across stakeholders. Regulators increasingly define nanomaterials' operationally (i.e., engineered materials with intentional nanoscale features that impart new properties) and evaluate them case-by-case rather than by single blanket rule. This approach is reflected in established FDA guidance and more recent clarifications, which advise sponsors to describe how nanoscale attributes influence critical quality attributes, in vitro/in vivo performance, and comparability [2].

DOI: 10.1201/9781003598657-11

Real-world examples illustrate regulatory stakes. Lipid-nanoparticle (LNP) delivery systems enabled the rapid use of mRNA COVID-19 vaccines, demonstrating how nanoscale carriers can transform public-health responses while raising complex questions about stability, cold-chain logistics, and immunogenicity. Similarly, systemically administered LNP therapeutics such as patisiran (Onpattro; approved in 2018) required detailed chemistry, manufacturing, and control (CMC), biodistribution, and immunotoxicity data to satisfy regulators, underscoring the depth of evidence expected for approval [3].

European regulators have paralleled these developments: recent EMA horizon-scanning and reflection reports reiterate that nanomedicines merit tailored data packages addressing physicochemical characterization, absorption, distribution, metabolism, and excretion (ADME), and post-market monitoring to manage both patient and environmental risks. These evolving expectations frame the regulatory pathway and justify the structured, multidisciplinary approach this chapter outlines [4].

11.2 GLOBAL REGULATORY LANDSCAPE

The global regulatory landscape for nano-based therapies is shaped by science-based, case-by-case evaluation within existing drug, biologic, and device frameworks. Major authorities such as the FDA, the EMA, and Asia-Pacific regulators emphasize rigorous characterization, safety assessment, and life cycle oversight of nano-characteristics. Greater international cooperation through harmonization initiatives supports consistency in standards while accommodating regional regulatory requirements [5]. The regulatory life cycle for nano-based therapies is summarized in Figure 11.1.

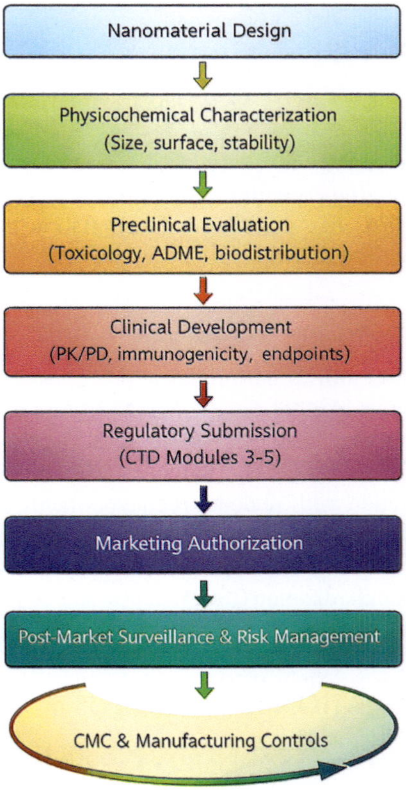

FIGURE 11.1 Life cycle regulatory framework for nano-based therapies.

11.2.1 United States: FDA Approach

In the United States, the FDA regulates nano-based therapies under existing human drug, biologic, or device statutes rather than via standalone "nanomedicine" category. This product-focused, science-based approach means nano-enabled products are evaluated on how their nanoscale attributes influence quality, safety, and efficacy within the applicable regulatory framework. The FDA guidance such as "Drug Products, Including Biological Products, that Contain Nanomaterials" (2022) emphasizes rigorous characterization and risks consideration for engineered nanomaterial components [6].

Unlike legacy small molecules, tiny differences in particle size, surface charge, or morphology can alter recognition or biodistribution, prompting the FDA to want improved data packets for these characteristics. The agency also participates in nanotechnology research collaborations and international standards efforts to inform regulatory science [7].

11.2.2 Europe: EMA and National Authorities

In the European Union, the European Medicines Agency (EMA) manages nano-based medicinal products within established medicinal product regulations, providing scientific guidelines and reflection papers to assist applicants. EMA's horizon-scanning reports and specific guidance on products such as liposomal or colloidal iron preparations indicate the need for detailed characterization and clinical justification related to nanoscale design [8].

Many EU member states also enforce complementary frameworks; for example, the European Chemicals Agency (ECHA) regulates nanoforms of chemicals under REACH (Registration, Evaluation, Authorisation and Restriction of Chemicals), demanding comprehensive safety dossiers for manufactured nanomaterials used in medical and non-medical products [9].

11.2.3 Asia Pacific and Other Regions

Across the Asia Pacific, regulatory styles vary. Japan's Pharmaceuticals and Medical Devices Agency (PMDA) issues guideline on liposomal drugs and nanoformulations, emphasizing robust CMC data, while Health Canada and the Therapeutic Goods Administration (TGA) in Australia apply product-based assessment aligned with the FDA/EMA principles. China's National Medical Products Administration (NMPA) has drafted nanoformulation guidance reflecting its growing domestic pipeline and global ambitions [10].

11.2.4 International Coordination (ICMRA, WHO)

International coordination efforts aim to harmonies approaches across regions. The International Coalition of Medicines Regulatory Authorities (ICMRA) fosters dialogue on emerging regulatory science challenges, including nanotechnology's role in advanced therapies [11].

While the World Health Organization (WHO) activities focus broadly on health product regulation and capacity building, collaboration with regional regulators helps align evidence expectations and safety monitoring, especially for products with global distribution. Regular workshops and contributions to standards bodies (e.g., Organisation for Economic Co-operation and Development [OECD], International Organization for Standardization [ISO]) support shared frameworks for nano-based health products [12]. Table 11.1 summarizes life cycle regulatory requirements for nano-based therapies.

11.3 PRODUCT CLASSIFICATION LEGAL STATUS

11.3.1 Nano-Drug, Devices, and Combination Products

Nano-based therapies do not fall under a unique legal category; rather, they are classified by regulators based on how they achieve their primary intended effect – as drugs, devices, or biologics – under

TABLE 11.1
Regulatory Life Cycle Requirements for Nano-Based Therapies

Development Stage	Key Regulatory Focus	Nano-Specific Considerations	Typical Regulatory Output
Product classification	Legal category (drug/device/biologic/combination)	Primary mode of action; nanoscale functional contribution	Regulatory pathway determination
Quality and CMC	Manufacturing controls, specifications, stability	Particle size distribution, surface chemistry, morphology, aggregation, drug loading	Defined critical quality attributes (CQAs); validated analytical methods
Preclinical safety	Toxicology, pharmacology, ADME	Biodistribution, persistence, immunotoxicity, protein corona effects	Good laboratory practice (GLP) toxicology reports; investigational new drug (IND) / clinical trial application (CTA) readiness
Clinical development	Safety, efficacy, PK/PD	Altered pharmacokinetics, immune activation, nanoparticle clearance	Phase I–III clinical data
Regulatory submission	Common Technical Document (CTD) modules (quality, safety, efficacy)	Justification of nano-specific assays and comparability data	Marketing authorization review
Post-market surveillance	Pharmacovigilance and risk management	Long-term safety, batch variability impact, environmental exposure	Risk management plan (RMP; safety updates)
Follow-on products	Comparability and interchangeability	Manufacturing sensitivity; non-biological complex drug considerations	Bridging data; hybrid or 505 (b)(2) pathways

existing regulatory frameworks. In the United States, the FDA categorizes a product as a drug, device, biologic, or a combination product depending on its mode of action. If a nano-enabled product achieves its principal therapeutic effect via chemical or pharmacological action, it is regulated as a drug or biologic. If the effect is predominantly physical or mechanical, it is regulated as a medical device. When multiple mechanisms overlap (e.g., a drug encapsulated within a nanocarrier delivering therapy interacting with tissue interfaces), the product may be designated as a combination product and reviewed accordingly. Sponsors can formally request a designation through the FDA's Office of Combination Products to confirm the regulatory pathway [13].

In the European Union, nanomedicines are treated as medicinal products when they meet the legal definition under the EU pharmaceutical law, even if nanomaterials are present to enhance delivery or targeting. EMA reflection papers acknowledge that nanoscale components can impart unique properties such as controlled release or preferential distribution, but classification remains grounded in the existing legal frameworks rather than a separate nano-category [14].

11.3.2 Regulatory Implications of Classification

Accurate classification has profound implications for regulatory expectations, evidentiary standards, and timelines. For example, a nano-drug will be subject to the same stringent safety, efficacy, and benefit-risk considerations as other pharmaceuticals, with additional emphasis on nanoscale characterization and biodistribution data. A device incorporating nanomaterials may be subject to a higher risk class (e.g., Class III under Rule 19 of the EU MDR); this requires robust clinical evidence and a conformity assessment by a notified body. A misclassification can lead to inappropriate regulatory pathways, delayed review cycles, or additional data requests, emphasizing the need for early engagement with regulators and a clear justification of the product's primary mode of action [15].

11.4 QUALITY AND CHARACTERIZATION REQUIREMENTS

11.4.1 Physicochemical Characterization

Robust physicochemical characterization is fundamental to ensuring the quality, performance, and safety of nano-based therapies because nanoscale properties critically influence biological behavior. Regulatory guidance, including the FDA's "Drug Products, Including Biological Products, that Contain Nanomaterials," stresses that engineered nanomaterial attributes such as particle size and distribution, morphology, surface charge, composition, and stability must be systematically defined and controlled during development and manufacturing. These attributes directly affect ADME, immunogenicity, and therapeutic efficacy. For example, the size and uniformity of LNPs used in mRNA vaccines like Comirnaty and Spikevax were essential quality parameters required by regulators, as small changes can alter cellular uptake and immune responses [16].

Analytical techniques such as dynamic light scattering (DLS), electron microscopy, and zeta-potential measurements are routinely used to quantify these critical quality attributes. Regulators also scrutinize batch-to-batch consistency to ensure reproducible performance and minimize safety risk. Recent literature highlights that physicochemical characterization remains a regulatory priority globally, including for nanomaterial-enabled medical devices where surface and structural properties can affect biocompatibility [17].

11.4.2 Analytical Standard and Reference Material

Despite advances, a key regulatory challenge is the lack of harmonized, consensus, reference materials and standardized methods tailored specifically for nanomedicines. International standards like ISO/TR 13014 (guidance on physicochemical characterization of engineered nanoscale materials) and ISO/TR 10993-22 (biological evaluation of nanomaterials) provide framework for evaluating properties relevant to safety and toxicology, although uptake varies across jurisdiction to another. Collaborative efforts - including the Nanotechnology Characterization Laboratory (NCL) in the United States, jointly supported by the FDA, the National Institute of Standards and Technology (NIST), and the National Cancer Institute, develop and disseminate reference materials and protocols to harmonize preclinical characterization, thereby aiming to streamline regulatory review and facilitate global comparability. The current landscape thus balances a science-based push for rigorous characterization with the need for continued development of widely accepted analytical standards for nano-based therapies [18].

11.5 PRECLINICAL SAFETY ASSESSMENT

11.5.1 In Vitro Toxicology Nano-Specific Assays

Preclinical safety assessment for nano-based therapies begins with in vitro toxicity and nano-specific assays designed to evaluate cellular responses that may be influenced by nanoscale properties. Unlike traditional drugs, nanomaterials can interact uniquely with cell membranes, proteins, and immune cells, making tailored assays critical. Advanced in vitro models employ human cell lines – such as peripheral blood leukocytes or macrophages – to measure inflammatory cytokines release, oxidative stress, and uptake potential because conventional assays may not be fully predictive of nano-specific effects. These evaluations are important in early screening to determine possible cytotoxic, immunotoxic, and genotoxic reactions before animal testing. The scientific literature highlights the importance of combined panels of assays due to varying mechanisms of nanoparticles toxicity, such as oxidative stress or immune activation [19].

For example, LNPs used in mRNA vaccines and siRNA therapies are routinely tested in vitro for effects on cell viability, membrane integrity, and cytokines induction before advancing to in vivo studies. This ensures that lipid composition, size, and surface characteristics do not trigger excessive inflammatory responses or unintended cellular uptake [20].

11.5.2 In Vivo Studies: ADME, Immonotoxicity, Biodistribution

In vivo safety studies examine ADME, immunotoxicity, and biodistribution, which are all deeply influenced by nanoscale attributes. Regulatory expectations require quantitative data on how nanoparticles distribute across organs, accumulate, and clear over time, as this impacts safety and efficacy. For example, lipid-based nanoparticles like those in patisiran (Onpattro) show preferential liver uptake, a crucial determinant of both therapeutic effect and off-target safety [21].

Immunotoxicity evaluation includes monitoring for complement activation and cytokine signaling, as some nanomaterials can elicit hypersensitivity or exaggerated immune responses. Biodistribution studies employing imaging methods or radiolabeling determine tissue kinetics, ensuring that systemic exposure does not lead to unintended toxicity. These integrated in vivo assessments build the safety foundation required by regulators before clinical trials can proceed [22].

11.6 CMC (Chemistry, Manufacturing, and Controls) Considerations

11.6.1 Manufacturing Challenges and Scale-Up

The CMC phase for nano-based therapies is more complex than for conventional pharmaceuticals because many nanoscale properties such as particle size distribution, surface chemistry, and drug loading are sensitive to manufacturing conditions and directly influence clinical performance. Even small process variations can alter these critical quality attributes (CQAs), affecting efficacy and safety, which regulators scrutinize closely. Studies highlight that translating laboratory processes to industrial scale poses particular hurdles due to the multi-parameter nature of nanoparticle formulation and the need to preserve physicochemical uniformity at larger volumes. This can include challenges in mixing, solvent removal, lipid assembly (for LNPs), or the control of aggregation tendencies, all of which can impact product consistency [1, 23].

Recent reviews demonstrate that developers increasingly use advanced manufacturing techniques such as microfluidics, iterative design-of-experiments (DoE), and real-time process analytics to achieve reproducible scale-up. These strategies help define the design space and maintain targeted CQAs during scale transition, which not only supports regulatory submissions but also improves yield and product quality [24].

11.6.2 Batch Consistency and GMP

Batch-to-batch consistency under good manufacturing practice (GMP) is critical for regulatory approval because nanomedicines are notably sensitive to production variability. Regulators expect you to document that CQAs – including size, morphology, drug encapsulation efficiency, and stability – remain within predefined limits across all batches. For example, LNP-based products like siRNA therapeutics and mRNA vaccines have stringent release criteria for particle size and encapsulation characteristics because deviations can affect biodistribution immunogenicity [16, 25].

Quality systems under GMP must integrate validated analytical methods capable of accurately characterizing nanoscale attributes, robust facility controls, and clear change-control strategies when scaling or updating process. Without such controls, sponsors may face additional regulatory queries or delayed approvals, underscoring the strategic importance of early CMC planning strategy and continuous quality assurance throughout development [26].

11.7 CLINICAL DEVELOPMENT

11.7.1 Trial Design and Endpoints for Nanotherapies

Clinical development of nano-based therapies integrates traditional drug development principles with design features tailored to nanomaterials behavior in humans. Early-phase trials usually start with Phase I studies of dose escalation to determine safety and maximum tolerated dose (MTD) with observation of pharmacokinetics (PK) and indications of initial efficacy. For instance, liposomal cisplatin (Lipoplatin) has completed Phase I–III clinical trials for non-small cell lung cancer with an extended half-life of circulation (~120 h) and improved tumor uptake over free cisplatin. These properties informed the endpoint selection, such as response rate and progression-free survival [27].

Across oncology and infectious diseases, study designs for nano-based agents often include target engagement and biomarkers-based endpoints that directly reflect nanocarrier performance, such as tumor accumulation or immune activation. Clinical investigations have deployed nanoparticle-enabled formulations like GBP511, a protein nanoparticle vaccine candidate now in Phase I/II trials aimed at eliciting broad protective immunity against coronaviruses, with some immunogenicity endpoints including antibody titers and T-cell responses [28].

11.7.2 Pharmacokinetics, Immunogenicity, and Biomarkers

Nanostructured therapies demonstrate complex PK compared with conventional small molecules because particle size, surface chemistry, and carrier composition influence absorption, distribution, metabolism, and excretion. Regulators require detailed PK profiling to understand biodistribution and clearance mechanisms. For liposomal carriers, prolonged circulation and altered tissue distribution require careful modeling to predict systemic exposure and toxicity [29].

Immunogenicity is another critical outcome, especially for carriers triggering innate immune responses or cytokine release. Biomarkers such as cytokine panels, complement activation markers, and specific tissue markers are often incorporated into trials to monitor immune reactions and guide dose selection. Adaptive trial designs leverage biomarkers alongside traditional safety and efficacy endpoints, enabling early signals of therapeutic benefit or adverse immunological events – a practice increasingly common in nanoparticle clinical research [30].

11.8 COMPARABILITY AND FOLLOW-ON PRODUCTS

11.8.1 Generics, Nanosimilars, and NBCDs

For conventional small molecule drugs, follow-on versions are usually approved as generics based on pharmaceutical equivalence and bioequivalence. However, there are many nano-enabled products with non-biological complex drugs (NBCDs) which cannot be fully characterized with standard physicochemical methodology alone because of their heterogeneous structures and nanoscale properties. Because of this the traditional generic paradigm may not be applicable to follow-ons of complex nanomedicines [31].

Examples of NBCDs include iron carbohydrate complexes and certain liposomal drugs. These products have complex compositions where small manufacturing differences can meaningfully impact biodistribution, tissue targeting, immunological responses, making simple equivalence testing unreliable. Accordingly, regulators increasingly recognize such follow-on products as nanosimilars rather than classic generic [32].

In the European Union nanomedicine follow-on approvals are trending toward the hybrid application process (Article 10(3)), which may require additional clinical or non-clinical data beyond standard generic requirements to support therapeutic equivalence. This evolution reflects acknowledgment that nanomedicine follow-ons must demonstrate similarity in performance, not just analytical sameness [33].

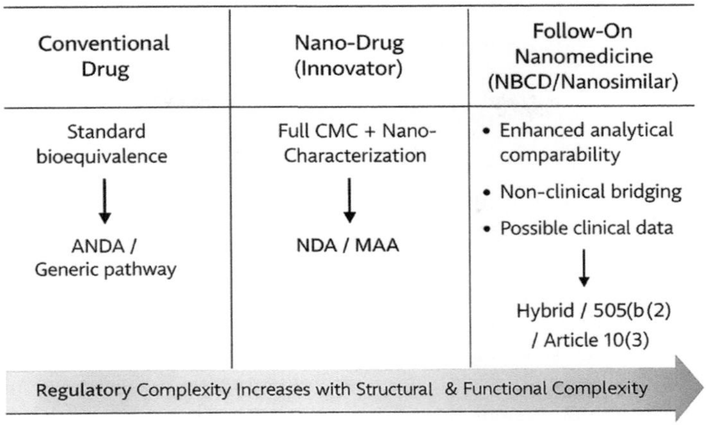

FIGURE 11.2 Comparative regulatory pathways for nano-product.

11.8.2 Regulatory Strategies and Bridging Studies

To demonstrate comparability between an originator nanomedicine and its follow-on version, regulators may require a "totality of evidence" approach involving extensive analytical characterization, non-clinical studies (e.g., biodistribution comparisons) and, where appropriate, head-to-head clinical trials in relevant patient populations. Such data help bridge gaps where in vitro assays alone cannot confirm therapeutic equivalence. [34]

Regulatory strategies emphasize early engagement with agencies to define data requirements, including bridging studies to show that any physicochemical differences do not meaningfully affect safety or efficacy. Without such evidence, automatic substitution or interchangeability common for small-molecule generics is generally discouraged for nanosimilars and NBCDs due to potential clinical and immunological differences [35]. Differences in the regulatory pathway between conventional drugs and nano-based products are shown in Figure 11.2.

11.9 REGULATORY SUBMISSIONS AND REVIEW

11.9.1 Dossier Requirements (Quality, Safety, Efficacy)

Regulatory submissions for nano-based therapies must follow the internationally accepted, CTD/eCTD format, which structures data on quality, non-clinical safety, and clinical efficacy for review by agencies such as the FDA or the EMA. The CTD offers harmonized modules covering manufacturing controls (Module 3), toxicology and pharmacology (Module 4), and clinical evidence (Module 5), facilitating regulatory review across regions [36].

For products containing nanomaterials, regulators expect the same standards for safety, efficacy, and quality as for conventional medicines, but with enhanced detail on nanomaterial characterization and controls. The FDA's recent guidance on "Drug Products, Including Biological Products, that Contain Nanomaterials" requires sponsors to describe how nanoscale attributes impact critical quality attributes, in vitro and in vivo performance, and justify testing strategies tailored to novel material behavior [2, 37].

Dossiers have to incorporate robust CMC documentation showing physicochemical characterization of the product, controls over manufacturing processes, and/or stability profiles unique to nanoscale formulations. Safety sections require thorough toxicological and biodegradation data and clinical sections must have sufficient evidence of benefit-risk based on well-designed studies.

EMA's scientific guidelines likewise give an emphasis to harmonized interpretation of clinical efficacy and safety data under existing medicinal product directives [38].

11.9.2 Common Deficiencies and Agency Expectations

Common deficiencies in nanomedicine submissions arise from incomplete characterization of nanostructures, insufficient linkage between physicochemical properties and biological behavior, and unclear controls over manufacturing variability. Regulators frequently request additional data on batch-to-batch consistency, biodistribution, immunological effects, and process validation. Early and proactive scientific advice meetings with agencies are expected to clarify data expectations and prevent review delays [39].

Agencies also watch if the analytical methods match regulatory expectations. Common problem areas include stability testing, comparability studies, and rationale for assay selection. Clear demonstration that the totality of quality and clinical data support the claimed therapeutic profile is critical for successful review and approval [40].

11.10 POST-MARKET SURVEILLANCE AND RISK MANAGEMENT

11.10.1 Pharmacovigilance and Nano-Specific Monitoring

Once nano-based therapies reach the market, regulators require robust post-market surveillance to monitor safety and real-world performance because clinical trials often include limited patient populations that may not reveal rare or long-term effects. Post-market surveillance (PMS) systems such as spontaneous reporting databases, electronic health records, and patient registries enable ongoing monitoring of adverse events and safety signals once a product is in widespread use. These systems help detect issues that pre-approval trials might miss due to smaller sample sizes and controlled condition [39, 41].

For nanomedicines, this general pharmacovigilance framework must be complemented with nano-specific monitoring strategies because nanoparticles behavior including biodistribution and clearance can vary based on subtle changes in formulation or manufacturing controls. For example, LNPs used in COVID-19 vaccines and siRNA therapies require careful tracking of adverse reactions, immune response, and batch-specific performance to identify trends that could be linked to nanocarrier properties. Regulatory authorities often ask sponsors to establish tailored risk management plans that describe how they will monitor and mitigate such risks over the life cycle of the product [42].

11.10.2 Environmental and Occupational Risk

Risk management of nano-based therapies must also extend beyond patients to workers and the environment. Nanomaterials used in manufacturing or present as by-products (e.g., wear particles) can pose occupational exposure hazards, such as inhalation or dermal contact leading to inflammation or respiratory effects, underscoring the need for exposure controls and personal protective equipment. Agencies such as Occupational Safety and Health Administration (OSHA) in the U.S. mandate hazard communication and monitoring of workplace safety where nanomaterials are handled; however, specific occupational exposure limits exist for only a few nanomaterials [43].

Environmental considerations are crucial because nanoparticles released during production use or disposal may interact differently in nature than bulk materials. Although environmental monitoring frameworks for nanotechnologies are still evolving, risk management strategies increasingly include assessment of environmental fate and toxicity, life cycle impacts, and safe disposal practices as part of sustainability planning. Integrating these elements supports comprehensive oversight of nano-based therapies from clinical to environmental realms, aligning innovation, safety, and public trust [44].

11.11 STANDARDS, HARMONIZATIONS, AND GUIDANCES

11.11.1 Current Standards Landscape

The regulatory framework for nanomedicines operates largely within existing pharmaceutical, chemical, and device standards, but several international efforts aim to shape consistent practices for nano-related evaluation. The ISO/TS 80004 series provides internationally agreed vocabulary and terminology for nanotechnology, helping to align definitions used by scientists, industry, and regulators worldwide [14, 45].

Organizations such as the ISO, the OECD, the American Society for Testing and Materials (ASTM), and the European Committee for Standardization (CEN) are active in developing guidance, tests, and test methods associated with regulatory submissions, particularly for nanoscale characterization, measurement protocols, and safety assessment models. For example, the OECD Test Guidelines Program, in collaboration with the Working Party on Manufactured Nanomaterials, has adapted and created test methods specific for nanomaterials (e.g., dispersion stability and inhalation toxicity) to promote mutual acceptance of data across jurisdictions [46].

Regulatory agencies like the U.S. FDA and the EMA issue product type guidance on nanomaterials in drugs and devices, emphasizing how nanoscale features influence key quality and safety criteria using existing frameworks [13, 47].

11.11.2 Gaps and Harmonization Needs

Despite these frameworks, significant gaps remain. There is no fully harmonized set of nano-specific regulatory standards globally, and differences in terminology, classification, and testing expectations can create uncertainty for sponsors and regulators alike. Efforts such as the International Standardisation Roadmap for Nanomedicine (2023) – involving regulators, metrology institutes, and standards bodies – are bridging these gaps by prioritizing common methods and reference materials tailored to nanomedicine characteristics [16, 25, 48].

Continued coordination and consensus on standardized test methods, data reporting formats, and risk assessment frameworks are essential for facilitating international regulatory harmonization and supporting innovation while safeguarding public health.

11.12 EMERGING CHALLENGES AND FUTURE DIRECTIONS

Advances in computational science and regulatory science are transforming how nano-based therapies are developed and regulated. Artificial intelligence (AI) and machine learning (ML) are increasingly applied to predict the nanomaterial safety profile, optimize formulation design, and accelerate toxicology assessments, promising quicker identification of viable candidates and reduced preclinical costs. However, these tools also create new regulatory complexity because models can behave as "black boxes," thereby complicating explainability, validation, and regulatory acceptance, especially when adaptive learning systems update in real time. Researchers and regulators are actively exploring standards to enhance transparency and algorithmic accountability so that AI/ML outputs can trustworthily inform decision-making, without compromising safety [49].

Emerging innovative regulatory pathways such as adaptive licensing, rolling reviews, and regulatory sandboxes for AI-assisted tools are being discussed globally to better accommodate rapidly evolving technologies, including nano-based therapies augmented by AI insights. These frameworks aim to balance the need for robust evidence with flexibility so that promising technologies can reach patients in a responsible timeframe, particularly in areas with high unmet medical need [50].

At the same time, ethical, legal, and societal issues (ELSI) are playing a key role in governing nanomedicine. Risk communication and informed consent are further complicated because patients may not fully understand the role of AI in therapeutic decisions of how nanoscale drug delivery systems work. Trust is based on transparent communication regarding potential benefits and uncertainties. This is especially true because nano-enabled treatments typically involve dense interdisciplinary ideas from materials science, biology, and data science [51].

Also, equitable and fair access to cutting-edge nano-based treatments is paramount. AI/ML has to ensure that they do not perpetuate existing health inequities. Regulations like the EU's Artificial Intelligence Act are establishing risk categories, transparency requirements, and human oversight for high-risk health applications. This framework protects fundamental rights while continuing to promote innovation [52].

11.13 CONCLUSION

Nano-based therapies are a revolutionary new frontier in modern medicine, offering targeted delivery, enhanced pharmacokinetics, and novel mechanisms of action beyond the scope of traditional pharmaceuticals. However, their nanoscale complexity requires strict control of their whole product lifespan – from characterization and preclinical evaluation to clinical development, submission, and post-market surveillance. Global regulatory agencies include the FDA, the EMA, and others in regional areas, which more regularly utilize science-based and case-by-case assessments, ensuring that nanospecific traits are adequately governed and connected to safety and efficacy outcomes.

Harmonization efforts through international standards bodies and collaborative regulatory networks are gradually addressing gaps in terminology, testing methods, and comparability frameworks. Looking ahead, integration of AI-enabled regulatory science, adaptive pathways, and strengthened ethical governance will be critical to balancing innovation with patient protection. A coordinated, transparent, and evidence-based regulatory framework remains essential to realizing the therapeutic potential of nano-based medicines.

ACKNOWLEDGMENTS

The authors express special thanks to the editors for providing necessary support and guidance.

REFERENCES

1. Patra JK, Das G, Fraceto LF, Campos EV, Rodriguez-Torres MD, Acosta-Torres LS, Diaz-Torres LA, Grillo R, Swamy MK, Sharma S, Habtemariam S. Nano based drug delivery systems: Recent developments and future prospects. Journal of Nanobiotechnology. 2018;16(1):71.
2. de Vlieger JS, Crommelin DJ, Tyner K, Drummond DC, Jiang W, McNeil SE, Neervannan S, Crist RM, Shah VP. Report of the AAPS guidance forum on the FDA draft guidance for industry: Drug products, including biological products, that contain nanomaterials. The AAPS Journal. 2019;21(4):56.
3. Xu L, Wang X, Liu Y, Yang G, Falconer RJ, Zhao CX. Lipid nanoparticles for drug delivery. Advanced NanoBiomed Research. 2022;2(2):2100109.
4. Nuevo Y, Hemmrich E, Virto R, Nuñez A, Cerrato C, Thürmer R, Dri DA, McNeil S, Boráň T. Horizon scanning to shape nanomedicines through researcher–regulator collaboration. Nature Reviews Materials. 2025;10(12):877–79.
5. Vyas H, Bhardwaj M, Das A, Agarwal J, Tiwari AK. Safety and Regulatory Considerations in Nano-Bio-Medicine. In Nano-Bio-Medicine for Gastrointestinal Diseases (pp. 311–328). Academic Press; 2026.
6. Zhang X, Chan HW, Shao Z, Wang Q, Chow S, Chow SF. Navigating translational research in nanomedicine: A strategic guide to formulation and manufacturing. International Journal of Pharmaceutics. 2025;671:125202.
7. Rauscher H, Roebben G, Amenta V, Boix SA, Calzolai L, Emons H, Gaillard C, Gibson P, Linsinger T, Mech A, Quiros PL. Towards a review of the EC Recommendation for a definition of the term "nanomaterial"; Part 1: Compilation of information concerning the experience with the definition. 2014.
8. Musazzi UM, Franzè S, Condorelli F, Minghetti P, Caliceti P. Feeding next-generation nanomedicines to Europe: Regulatory and quality challenges. Advanced Healthcare Materials. 2023;12(30):2301956.
9. Allan J, Belz S, Hoeveler A, Hugas M, Okuda H, Patri A, Rauscher H, Silva P, Slikker W, Sokull-Kluettgen B, Tong W. Regulatory landscape of nanotechnology and nanoplastics from a global perspective. Regulatory Toxicology and Pharmacology. 2021;122:104885.

10. Haschek WM, Rousseaux CG, Wallig MA, Bolon B, editors. Haschek and Rousseaux's Handbook of Toxicologic Pathology, Volume 1: Principles and Practice of Toxicologic Pathology. Academic Press; 2021.
11. Dangy-Caye A, Mousset A, Kermad A, Bouché-Bazerolle L, Bujar M, De Lucia ML, McAuslane N, Lumsden R. Harmonizing health: A global analysis of pharmaceutical regulatory activities by international regulatory organizations. Frontiers in Medicine. 2025;12:1636269.
12. Preston C, Dias MF, Peña J, Pombo ML, Porrás A. Addressing the challenges of regulatory systems strengthening in small states. BMJ Global Health. 2020;5(2): e001912.
13. Lin C, Huang X, Xue Y, Jiang S, Chen C, Liu Y, Chen K. Advances in medical devices using nanomaterials and nanotechnology: Innovation and regulatory science. Bioactive Materials. 2025;48:353–69.
14. European Medicines Agency (EMA). "Nanotechnology-Based Medicinal Products for Human Use: EU-IN Horizon Scanning Report." 2025.
15. D'Avenio G, Daniele C, Grigioni M. Nanostructured medical devices: Regulatory perspective and current applications. Materials. 2024;17(8):1787.
16. Desai N, Rana D, Patel M, Bajwa N, Prasad R, Vora LK. Nanoparticle therapeutics in clinical perspective: Classification, marketed products, and regulatory landscape. Small. 2025;21(29):2502315.
17. Hallan SS, Sguizzato M, Esposito E, Cortesi R. Challenges in the physical characterization of lipid nanoparticles. Pharmaceutics. 2021;13(4):549.
18. Rodríguez-Gómez FD, Monferrer D, Penon O, Rivera-Gil P. Regulatory pathways and guidelines for nanotechnology-enabled health products: A comparative review of EU and US frameworks. Frontiers in Medicine. 2025;12:1544393.
19. Thomas J, Kumar V, Sharma N, John N, Umesh M, Huligowda LK, Kaur K, Utreja D. Recent approaches in nanotoxicity assessment for drug delivery applications: Challenges and prospects. Medicine in Drug Discovery. 2025;25:100204.
20. Estapé Sentí M. *Expanding lipid nanoparticle platforms for effective mRNA therapeutics* (Doctoral dissertation, Utrecht University). 2024.
21. Ma X, Tian Y, Yang R, Wang H, Allahou LW, Chang J, Williams G, Knowles JC, Poma A. Nanotechnology in healthcare, and its safety and environmental risks. Journal of Nanobiotechnology. 2024;22(1):715.
22. Hofer S, Hofstätter N, Punz B, Hasenkopf I, Johnson L, Himly M. Immunotoxicity of nanomaterials in health and disease: Current challenges and emerging approaches for identifying immune modifiers in susceptible populations. Wiley Interdisciplinary Reviews: Nanomedicine and Nanobiotechnology. 2022; 14(6):e1804.
23. Singh K, Singhal S, Pahwa S, Sethi VA, Sharma S, Singh P, Kale RD, Ali SW, Sagadevan S. Nanomedicine and drug delivery: A comprehensive review of applications and challenges. Nano-Structures & Nano-Objects. 2024;40:101403.
24. Qiao D, Li H, Zhang X, Chen X, Zhang J, Zou J, Zhao D, Zhu W, Qian X, Li H. The convergence of artificial intelligence and microfluidics in drug research and development. Engineering. 2025;55:125–174.
25. Kumarasamy RV, Natarajan PM, Umapathy VR, Roy JR, Mironescu M, Palanisamy CP. Clinical applications and therapeutic potentials of advanced nanoparticles: A comprehensive review on completed human clinical trials. Frontiers in Nanotechnology. 2024;6:1479993.
26. Fabio P, Alessandro C, Stefania S, Iolanda G, Elena M, Aldo C. The requirements for manufacturing highly active or sensitising drugs comparing good manufacturing practices. Acta Bio Medica: Atenei Parmensis. 2019;90(2):288.
27. Gupta YK, Dinda AK, Pradhan AK, Dhawan A, Ninawe S Guidelines for Evaluation of Nanopharmaceuticals in India: Jointly prepared by Department of Biotechnology, GoI. 2019.
28. Chehelgerdi M, Chehelgerdi M, Allela OQ, Pecho RD, Jayasankar N, Rao DP, Thamaraikani T, Vasanthan M, Viktor P, Lakshmaiya N, Saadh MJ. Progressing nanotechnology to improve targeted cancer treatment: Overcoming hurdles in its clinical implementation. Molecular Cancer. 2023;22(1):169.
29. Patel MP, Patel KM, Vhora SZ, Gajjar AK, Patel JK, Patel AK. Model-Based pharmacokinetic approaches. Basics and Clinical Applications of Drug Disposition in Special Populations. 2025;7:11–51.
30. Yang TY, Braun M, Lembke W, McBlane F, Kamerud J, DeWall S, Tarcsa E, Fang X, Hofer L, Kavita U, Upreti VV. Immunogenicity assessment of AAV-based gene therapies: An IQ consortium industry white paper. Molecular Therapy Methods & Clinical Development. 2022;26:471–94.
31. Gaspar RS, Silva-Lima B, Magro F, Alcobia A, da Costa FL, Feio J. Non-biological Complex drugs (NBCDs): Complex pharmaceuticals in need of individual robust clinical assessment Before any therapeutic equivalence decision. Frontiers in Medicine. 2020;7:590527.
32. Rodríguez-Gómez FD, Penon O, Monferrer D, Rivera-Gil P. Classification system for nanotechnology-enabled health products with both scientific and regulatory application. Frontiers in Medicine. 2023; 10:1212949.

33. Pita R, Ehmann F, Papaluca M. Nanomedicines in the EU—Regulatory overview. The AAPS Journal. 2016;18(6):1576–82.
34. Flühmann B, Ntai I, Borchard G, Simoens S, Mühlebach S. Nanomedicines: The magic bullets reaching their target? European Journal of Pharmaceutical Sciences. 2019;128:73–80.
35. Amthaniwala BK, Rathod JA. Comparative insights into biosimilar development in the UAE and India: Opportunities, challenges, and global trends. 2025.
36. Mahaparale S, Desai B. Role and overview of drug regulatory affairs in pharmaceutical industry with implementation of CTD and ECTD. World J Pharm Res. 2018;7:201–15.
37. Shah S, Nene S, Rangaraj N, Raghuvanshi RS, Singh SB, Srivastava S. Bridging the gap: Academia, industry and FDA convergence for nanomaterials. Drug Development and Industrial Pharmacy. 2020; 46(11):1735–46.
38. Javed S, Mangla B, Almoshari Y, Sultan MH, Ahsan W. Nanostructured lipid carrier system: A compendium of their formulation development approaches, optimization strategies by quality by design, and recent applications in drug delivery. Nanotechnology Reviews. 2022;11(1):1744–77.
39. Mundekkad D, Cho WC. Nanoparticles in clinical translation for cancer therapy. International Journal of Molecular Sciences. 2022;23(3):1685.
40. Kaur S, Yadav S, Sahu V, Sharma N, Shukla VK. Biosimilar regulations: Current framework and future prospects. Current Drug Safety. 2025. https://doi.org/10.2174/0115748863360017250509063745.
41. Awasthi R, Roseblade A, Hansbro PM, Rathbone MJ, Dua K, Bebawy M. Nanoparticles in cancer treatment: Opportunities and obstacles. Current Drug Targets. 2018;19(14):1696–709.
42. Petrovic S, Bita B, Barbinta-Patrascu ME. Nanoformulations in pharmaceutical and biomedical applications: Green perspectives. International Journal of Molecular Sciences. 2024;25(11):5842.
43. Giubilato E, Cazzagon V, Amorim MJ, Blosi M, Bouillard J, Bouwmeester H, Costa AL, Fadeel B, Fernandes TF, Fito C, Hauser M. Risk management framework for nano-biomaterials used in medical devices and advanced therapy medicinal products. Materials. 2020;13(20):4532.
44. Dhall S, Nigam A, Harshavardhan M, Mukherjee A, Srivastava P. A comprehensive overview of methods involved in nanomaterial production and waste disposal from research labs and industries and existing regulatory guidelines for handling engineered nanomaterials. Environmental Chemistry and Ecotoxicology. 2024;6:269–82.
45. Grewal AS, Lather V, Sharma N, Singh S, Narang RS, Narang JK, Pandita D. Recent updates on nanomedicine based products: Current scenario and future opportunities. Applied Clinical Research, Clinical Trials and Regulatory Affairs. 2018;5(2):132–44.
46. Sachana M, Shafer TJ, Terron A. Toward a better testing paradigm for developmental neurotoxicity: OECD efforts and regulatory considerations. Biology. 2021;10(2):86.
47. Ray SS, Bandyopadhyay J. Nanotechnology-enabled biomedical engineering: Current trends, future scopes, and perspectives. Nanotechnology Reviews. 2021;10(1):728–43.
48. Mangla B, Kumar P, Javed S, Pathan T, Ahsan W, Aggarwal G. Regulating nanomedicines: Challenges, opportunities, and the path forward. Nanomedicine. 2025;20(15):1911–27.
49. Mim JJ, Al Mamun A, Nayem MH, Mahmud S, Nath A, Rahman SM, Fidal SA, Hossain N. Machine learning-driven advances in nanotechnology: From materials design to process optimization-a review. Materials Today Communications. 2025:114485.
50. Nikolai NM, Celine CK The Regulatory Future of Emerging Technologies–A Scoping Paper on Gaps and Opportunities. 2018.
51. Al-Amiery A. The ethical implications of emerging artificial intelligence technologies in healthcare. Med Mat. 2025;2(2):85–100.
52. Maleki Varnosfaderani S, Forouzanfar M. The role of AI in hospitals and clinics: Transforming healthcare in the 21st century. Bioengineering. 2024;11(4):337.

12 Challenges in the Clinical Implementation of Nanotechnology for Diabetes Management

Vishwajeet K. Chatekar
SGVSS's Adsul College of Pharmacy, Ahilyanagar, India

Jyothirmayee Devineni
KVSR Siddhartha College of Pharmaceutical Sciences, Vijayawada, India

D. Thangamani
Institute of Forest Genetics and Tree Breeding, Coimbatore, India

Nidhi Singh
Teerthanker Mahaveer College of Pharmacy (TMCOP), TMU, Muradabad, India

Tirthankar Choudhury
School of Pharmacy, ITM University, Gwalior, India

12.1 INTRODUCTION

Diabetes represents a rapidly escalating global health crisis: recent analyses estimate more than 828 million adults had diabetes in 2022, and prevalence among adults roughly doubled from 1990 to 2022, with particularly large treatment and diagnosis gaps in low-and middle-income countries [1].

Clinically, diabetes drives microvascular and macrovascular complications (retinopathy, nephropathy, neuropathy, cardiovascular disease) that require continuous metabolic control, frequent monitoring, and timely therapeutic adjustments – needs that traditional care models and periodic glucose testing struggle to meet. Improved glycemic control via continuous glucose monitoring (CGM) has been associated with reduced hypoglycemia and hospitalizations, yet access remains uneven globally [2].

Nanotechnology is positioned to address several persistent shortcomings. Nanoscale drug carriers and glucose-responsive systems aim to protect peptides, increase mucosal uptake for oral insulin, and provide on-demand release to decrease hypoglycemia risk. Recent translational examples include an oral, glucose-responsive nanoformulation reported in Nature that improved duodenal absorption in explant models, illustrating practical progress toward non-injectable insulin [3].

On the monitoring front, nanomaterial-augmented wearable sensors (graphene, metal nanoparticles [NPs], functionalized electrodes) promise improved sensitivity for minimally invasive or noninvasive CGM, and enable continuous data streams for closed-loop systems and remote care.

DOI: 10.1201/9781003598657-12

Systematic reviews from 2024 highlight rapid advances in wearable electrochemical biosensors while underscoring variability in real-world performance and signal stability [4].

However, clinical implementation faces major hurdles – safety and long-term toxicology, reproducible large-scale manufacturing, regulatory ambiguity, cost and reimbursement barriers, and equity of access – that must be resolved before these technologies can scale safely and fairly. Regulatory agencies have issued specific guidance on drug products containing nanomaterials, signaling both recognition of potential and the need for rigorous quality and nonclinical testing to support human use [5].

This chapter reviews clinical needs, technological opportunities, translation barriers, and policy considerations, grounding recommendations in recent data and tangible examples.

12.2 PRACTICAL PATHWAYS FOR ADOPTION

12.2.1 Nano-Drug Delivery (Injectable, Oral, Inhaled)

Nanocarriers – polymeric NPs, liposomes, solid lipid NPs, and inorganic quantum-dot systems – are being developed to enhance insulin stability, mucosal uptake, and pharmacokinetics. Oral strategies aim to protect insulin from gastric degradation and promote intestinal absorption using surface-modified carriers (poly(lactic-co-glycolic) acid [PLGA], PEGylated hydroxyapatite, chitosan derivatives) that show glucose-lowering in preclinical models and high uptake in human intestinal explants. One recent example described an insulin-conjugated quantum dot formulation with a pH-responsive chitosan/glucose coating that enhanced duodenal absorption in explant and in vivo models, illustrating real progress toward non-injectable insulin [6].

Inhaled formulations exploit the large alveolar surface area for rapid systemic uptake; Technosphere® (Afrezza®) is the clinically approved microparticle inhaled insulin and continues to inform design and safety expectations for aerosolized nano- and microcarriers in diabetes care. Ongoing trials continue to evaluate inhaled systems in pediatric and adult populations [7].

12.2.2 Smart Glucose-Responsive Nanocarrires

"Smart" carriers incorporate glucose-sensing chemistries (phenylboronic acids, glucose oxidase, competitive lectin systems) or acid-labile linkers that trigger insulin release when glycemia rises. Preclinical studies demonstrate pulsatile/sustained, glucose-correlated release that reduces hypoglycemia risk in rodent models. Work on acetylated-dextran and other acid- or enzyme-sensitive polymers has demonstrated tunable on-demand kinetics; recent reviews and experimental reports highlight promising in vivo performance but also note translational gaps in durability, scale-up, and human safety [8].

12.2.3 Nanomaterial-Based Sensors and CGMs (Wearable/Implantable)

Nanomaterials (graphene, carbon nanotube, metal-NP-modified electrodes) are at the core of next-generation electrochemical and optical glucose sensors. These materials enhance surface area and electron transfer rates, improving sensitivity and enabling thinner, flexible sensor platforms for minimally invasive or noninvasive continuous glucose monitoring (CGM). Recent 2024 reviews summarize rapid laboratory advances toward flexible, wearable, biosensors but emphasize signal drift, biofouling, calibration, and reproducibility as barriers to clinical deployment. Pilot wearable prototypes using graphene-platinum nanocomposites report encouraging accuracy in short-term studies but require long-term validation [9].

12.2.4 Regenerative and Tissue-Engineering Nanoplatforms

In regenerative medicine, nanoscale coatings and nanoencapsulation strategies are applied to pancreatic islets and stem-cell derived β-cells to reduce immune recognition, improve oxygenation,

TABLE 12.1
Major Nanotechnology Platforms in Diabetes and Key Translational Challenges

Nanotechnology Platform	Clinical Objectives	Representative Examples	Major Translational Barriers
Polymeric/lipid NPs	Improved insulin stability and bioavailability	PLGA NPs; lipid-based oral insulin systems [11]	Variable oral absorption; scale-up reproducibility; long-term safety
Glucose-responsive nanocarriers	On-demand insulin release	Phenylboronic acid systems; glucose oxidase microneedle patches [12]	Release predictability; immunogenicity; regulatory validation
Nanomaterial-based CGMs	CGM	Graphene-based electrodes; metal NP sensors [13]	Biofouling; signal drift; cybersecurity; interoperability
Nanoencapsulation for islet therapy	Immune protection of transplanted cells	Alginate/chitosan nano-coatings [14]	Fibrosis; oxygen diffusion limits; long-term graft survival

and promote vascularization. Conformal nanocoatings (alginate/chitosan multilayers, functionalized polymers) and immunomodulatory NPs administered peri-transplant show improved graft survival in preclinical models; however, human translation still faces immune-compatibility, scale, and durability challenges. Recent translational studies indicate that combining nano-encapsulation with local immunomodulation or hypoimmune cell engineering is the most promising path to clinically durable islet grafts [10]. The major nanotechnology platforms and their translational status are summarized in Table 12.1.

12.3 PRECLINICAL TO CLINICAL TRANSLATION: KEY HURDLES

The transition of nanotechnology-based interventions for diabetes from laboratory innovation to approved clinical products remains slow, despite promising preclinical data. Major translational bottlenecks include limited predictive validity of animal models, complex pharmacokinetics and biodistribution profiles of NPs, and uncertainties in dose scaling and therapeutic windows [15].

12.3.1 Animal Model Relevance and Predictive Validity

Most nano-enabled insulin delivery and glucose-responsive carriers are tested in streptozotocin (STZ)-induced diabetic rodents or genetically diabetic animals such as db/db mice. While these models are useful for assessing glucose-lowering efficacy, they do not fully replicate the chronic inflammatory environment, autoimmune mechanisms (in type 1 diabetes), or metabolic heterogeneity seen in humans. Differences in gastrointestinal physiology, mucus thickness, immune response, and NP uptake pathway markedly affect oral or transdermal nanoformulation [16].

Regulatory reviews continually note that nanomedicine candidates demonstrate robust glycemic control in rodents but fail to demonstrate comparable pharmacodynamic consistency in large animals or early human trials. The U.S. Food and Drug Administration (FDA) has emphasized that nonclinical programs for products containing nanomaterials must justify model selection and demonstrate relevance to human exposure and safety profiles. This is especially true for glucose respond systems where the kinetics of enzymes and immune activation may differ significantly between species [17].

Furthermore, long-term toxicity and accumulation data are frequently restricted to short-duration studies in rodents. Chronic diseases such as diabetes require lifelong therapy, yet many preclinical studies evaluate outcomes over weeks rather than months, reducing predictive validity for chronic exposure scenarios [18].

12.3.2 Pharmacokinetics and Biodistribution of Nanoparticles

Unlike conventional small molecules, NPs have size-, charge- and surface chemistry-dependent biodistribution. Minor alterations in surface functionalization such as PEGylated density or attachment of ligand can significantly change circulation time, reticuloendothelial system uptake, and tissue accumulation [19].

The FDA's recent guidance on drug products containing nanomaterials highlights the need for comprehensive characterization of particle size distribution, agglomeration behavior, surface properties, and in vivo fate. NPs may accumulate in liver, spleen, or lymphatic tissues, raising concerns about long-term biopersistence. For glucose-responsive insulin systems, premature degradation or off-target sequestration can compromise therapeutic precision and increase variability in glycemic outcomes [20].

In oral nano-insulin research, variability in intestinal permeability and first-pass hepatic extraction contributes to inconsistent systemic exposure. Even when preclinical models show enhanced absorption, human gastrointestinal differences – pH gradients, enzymatic activity, and microbiome composition – can substantially alter bioavailability. This unpredictability complicates translation to clinical pharmacokinetic (PK) profiles [21].

12.3.3 Dose Scaling and Therapeutic Windows

The dose extrapolation from rodents to humans presents another significant challenge. Traditional allometric scaling approaches are often inadequate for NP systems because their disposition is governed not only by mass but also by physicochemical attributes and biological interactions [22].

For insulin-loaded NPs, both under-dosing and overdosing pose risks: insufficient release leads to hyperglycemia, whereas uncontrolled burst release may trigger hypoglycemia. Establishing a reproducible therapeutic window is extremely important. Regulatory agencies stress the importance of integrating PK, pharmacodynamic (PD), and toxicological data to define exposure-response relationships specific to nanomaterials [23].

Additionally, batch-to-batch variability in particle size or encapsulation efficiency can alter effective dose, thereby further complicating clinical scaling. For chronic diabetes management, maintaining tight glycemic control (often defined as HbA1c <7% in many adult populations) requires predictable, sustained PK – an exacting standard for nanoformulations [24]. The multidimensional obstacles hindering translation in nano-enabled diabetes technology are outweighed in Figure 12.1.

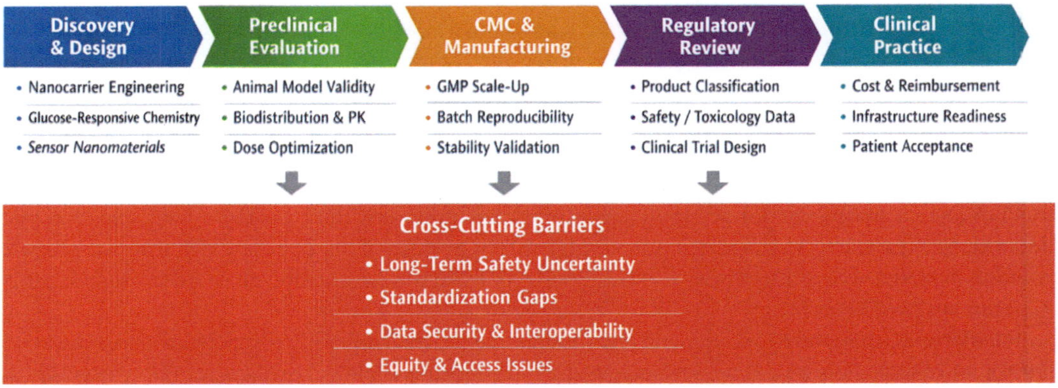

FIGURE 12.1 Translational roadmap and clinical implementation barriers for nanotechnology in diabetes.

12.4 SAFETY AND TOXICOLOGY

12.4.1 Acute and Chronic Toxicity Profiles

Acute toxicities from NP formulations typically present as infusion- or administration-related reactions (respiratory distress with inhaled systems, local irritation with transdermal/wearables, or systemic hypersensitivity with intravenous delivery). More concerning for chronic diseases such as diabetes is the evidence of sustained organ exposure: longitudinal preclinical studies report measurable NP retention in liver, spleen, and kidneys for months after administration, with associated low-grade inflammation and early fibrotic changes in some models. For example, a 2024 longitudinal study observed altered organ distribution and inflammatory markers up to 120 days after exposure, signaling that short-term rodent studies commonly used in efficacy testing may miss clinically relevant chronic effects [25].

12.4.2 Immunogenicity and Complement Activation

NPs can trigger innate immune pathways; CARPA (complement activation-related pseudo-allergy) is a well-recognized acute reaction to several nanomedicines and NP carriers. CARPA may present as transient cardiopulmonary symptoms or hypotension and is idiosyncratic, complicating preclinical prediction. Mechanistically, surface properties (charge, protein corona, PEG-density) strongly influence complement engagement. Reviews of CARPA mechanisms and animal models emphasize the need to screen candidate formulations for complement activation early in development, and to consider animal species differences (e.g., porcine models are relatively sensitive to CARPA) [26].

12.4.3 Long-Term Fate, Accumulation, Biodegradation

NP fate depends on material class: many inorganic NPs (gold, silica, metal oxides) demonstrate long residence times, whereas biodegradable polymeric carriers (PLGA, dextran derivatives) generally clear more predictably but can still leave degradation products with biological activity. Some studies of gold NPs report long-term retention without clear functional toxicity in specific contexts, but organ accumulation patterns vary with particle size, shape, and surface chemistry. Meta-analyses and biodistribution coefficient studies quantify that liver and spleen uptake dominate for many NP types, highlighting predictable sequestration by the reticuloendothelial system that may limit repeated dosing and raise cumulative exposure concerns for lifelong conditions like diabetes [27].

12.4.4 Standardized Nanotoxicology Tests Needs

Regulators and international bodies increasingly call for nanomaterial-specific toxicology frameworks. The U.S. Food and Drug Administration (FDA) now provides consolidated considerations for drug products containing nanomaterials, emphasizing characterization (size distribution, aggregation, surface chemistry), nonclinical toxicokinetics, and justification of animal models. Similarly, the Organisation for Economic Co-operation and Development (OECD) is updating guidance on toxicokinetics, sample preparation, and dosimetry to accommodate NP testing and improve interlaboratory reproducibility. These initiatives underscore two practical priorities: (1) harmonized, validated assays for complement activation, opsonization, and chronic-exposure endpoints; and (2) standardized reporting of NP physicochemical attributes and dosimetry so that safety data are comparable across studies. Adopting OECD/FDA-aligned methods will reduce regulatory uncertainty and better predict human risks for chronic indications such as diabetes [20, 28]. The multidimensional barriers impeding translation of nano-enabled diabetes technologies are summarized in Figure 12.1.

12.5 CHEMISTRY, MANUFACTURING, AND CONTROLS (CMC)

The chemistry, manufacturing, and controls (CMC) pillar is one of the critical yet under-emphasized barriers in translating nanotechnology for diabetes management into clinical products. Despite extensive academic innovation, consistent manufacturing and rigorous quality control remain major challenges that must be overcome to satisfy regulatory agencies and scale to clinical use [15, 29].

12.5.1 Batch-to-Batch Reproducibility and Scale-Up

Reproducibly manufacturing NPs with consistent physicochemical properties such as particle size distribution, drug loading, and surface chemistry is a major challenge in nanomedicine, including diabetes applications. Laboratory-scale methods (e.g., manual emulsification, batch solvent evaporation) often lack the precision needed for clinical production, causing variability between batches that can affect safety and therapeutic outcome [30].

This is particularly true for lipid NPs and polymeric carriers, where small changes in mixing speeds or temperatures can affect size and drug encapsulation efficiency. During scale-up to good manufacturing practice (GMP)-compliant processes, these discrepancies grow if process control and analytics are not rigorously implemented. Research reviews of nanomedicine manufacturing emphasize that batch variability and inconsistent critical quality attributes (CQAs) are among the principal causes of translational failure, highlighting the need for robust process design and strict controls early in development [31].

Methods such as high-throughput microfluidics and continuous manufacturing have appeared to improve scale-up reproducibility by enabling precise control over mixing and particle formation, and these strategies are increasingly explored in industrial environments to produce tens of milligrams per hour with tightly-controlled size distributions [32].

12.5.2 Characterization (Size, Surface, Release) and Analytics

Thorough characterization is essential for ensuring product quality and regulatory acceptance. NP properties such as size, surface charge, polydispersity, and drug release kinetics significantly affect the pharmacokinetics, biodistribution, and immunogenicity, yet accurate measurement of these attributes remains technically challenging. Techniques like dynamic light scattering (DLS), electron microscopy, and surface plasmon resonance are standard, but they can yield inconsistent results across instruments and laboratories if not standardized. The ability to analyze drug encapsulation efficiency and controlled release profile under physiologically relevant conditions is similarly critical. Without rigorous analytics, significant variability in performance may go undetected until later stages, risking batch failure or adverse outcomes in clinical trials [33].

Regulatory authorities are now expecting to receive detailed CMC data linking these characteristics and properties to clinical safety and efficacy, and early submissions for nanomedicines frequently fail due to a lack of this information..

12.5.3 Stability and Formulation Challenges

Nanoformulations often face stability problems in storage and handling. NPs may aggregate, change morphology, or undergo drug leakage over time, especially when temperature varies or under the influence of long shelf-life. This is accentuated in complex carriers like lipid-based NPs and multifunctional polymeric systems where multiple components can interact unpredictably. Instability can lead to reduced bioavailability or change release kinetics, undermining therapeutic goals for diabetes treatment where precise dosing and predictable performance are essential [34].

Physical and chemical stabilization approaches – lyophilization with appropriate cryoprotectants, surface PEGylation to minimize aggregation, and optimized excipients – are being examined, but they require extensive validation to ensure that they preserve product quality without introducing new safety issues [35].

12.6 REGULATORY AND APPROVAL CHALLENGES

12.6.1 Definitions and Classification Uncertainties

One of the basic regulatory barriers for nanotechnology in diabetes management is the lack of widely accepted definitions and classifications for nanomedicines. Both the U.S. Food and Drug Administration (FDA) and the European Medicines Agency (EMA) access products containing nanomaterials on a case-by-case basis rather than under a specific dedicated nanomedicine category, because no formal statutory definition of "nanomedicine" exists in either system. This ambiguity complicates early regulatory strategy and influences expectations for data generation, labeling, and oversight. In the U.S., nanotechnology regulatory thinking stems from guidance on whether FDA-regulated products involve nanotechnology, without creating a separate regulatory category, leaving developers to justify product classification and regulatory pathways [36].

Similarly, in the EU, there is no stand-alone nanomedicine regulatory route; nanotechnology-based therapeutics and diagnostics are regulated under existing medicinal products frameworks. The EMA has released reflection papers and scientific guidelines for specific nanomedicine subtypes (e.g., liposomes, iron colloids) to clarify expectations for quality, safety, and efficacy data, but product classification largely remains product-specific rather than technology-specific [37].

This lack of clear categorization creates uncertainty early in the development – developers must determine whether a product will follow drug, biologic, device, or combination pathways, each with different requirements.

12.6.2 Agency Guidance-Expectations

Regulatory agencies have responded by publishing guidance documents focused on the expectations for products containing nanomaterials rather than on nano-specific rules. For example, the FDA's 2022 guidance titles "Drug Products, Including Biological Products That Contain Nanomaterials" provides considerations for characterization, controls, testing, and risk management when nanomaterials are part of a finished dosage form. It emphasizes that the same standards for safety, efficacy, and quality apply as for conventional products, but acknowledges that nanocomponents may affect product behavior in clinical settings and require tailored evaluation [38].

Other FDA guidance documents (e.g., on liposome drug products and on whether nanotechnology is involved in a product) stress the importance of thorough physicochemical characterization, toxicology data, and robust control strategies. EMA's reflection papers similarly stress comprehensive comparability and quality of data for nanoscale products, particularly for follow-on versions, reflecting the "totality-of-evidence" approach adopted for complex medicines [39].

12.6.3 Clinical Trials Design and Endpoints for Nanomedicines

Nanomedicines and nanosensors for diabetes often have complex mechanisms of action, combining drug delivery, release modulation, and diagnostic feedback. This complexity influences clinical trial design: standard endpoints (e.g., reducing HbA1c) may not fully capture multi-functional benefits like reduced glycemic variability or improved sensor accuracy. Regulators increasingly discuss integrating surrogate endpoints (i.e., continuous glucose monitoring metrics) and further safety biomarkers relevant to nano-specifics phenomena (i.e., immunogenicity signals) into trial protocols [16, 40].

Further, given the hybrid nature of many nanotechnology products (e.g., drug-device combinations), sponsors must coordinate regulatory expectations between centers (Center for Drug Evaluation and Research [CDER], Center for Biologics Evaluation and Research [CBER], Center for Devices and Radiological Health [CDRH] in the U.S.) or seek parallel EMA scientific advice to ensure that chosen endpoints satisfy safety and efficacy standards and enable eventual approvals [41]. The multidimensional barriers hindering translation of nano-enabled diabetes technologies are outlined in Figure 12.1.

12.7 CLINICAL PRACTICE BARRIERS

Despite promising technological innovation, there are significant barriers to the translation of nanotechnology-based tools for diabetes care into practice, relating to cost and reimbursement, infrastructure, provider adoption, and patient acceptability.

12.7.1 Cost, Reimbursement, and Market Access

Nanotechnology-based therapy and devices typically entail higher manufacturing and development costs than traditional pharmaceuticals and glucose monitors. Precision NP formulations and nanomaterial-enhanced sensors require advanced materials, specialized manufacturing environments, and rigorous quality control, all of which contribute to premium pricing. In an era of constrained healthcare budgets, payers and insurers examine cost-effectiveness data before giving coverage [42].

For example, CGMs which employ increasingly advanced materials and micro/nano fabrication, have faced variable reimbursement landscapes; although many insurers now cover established CGMs, coverage criteria (e.g., documentation of frequent hypoglycemia or insulin use) differ widely, influencing adoptions. Similarly, newer nanocarrier-based insulin products or glucose-responsive systems, if approved, may struggle for formulary placement without strong evidence, showing economic value over current alternatives. Cost barriers are particularly acute in low- and middle-income countries, where even widely endorsed diabetes therapies have inconsistent access [43].

12.7.2 Healthcare Infrastructure and Provider Adoption

Effective deployment of nanotechnologies often requires compatible healthcare, infrastructure, and trained personnel. Advanced biosensors may rely on digital connectivity, cloud data integration, and sophisticated analytics platforms, which are not uniformly available across clinical settings. In many primary care environment or resource-limited regions, clinicians may lack access to real-time CGM data streams or electronic systems that integrate nanotech diagnostics with clinical decision support. Providers may also be familiar with interpreting nanotechnology-specific data outputs, such as novel biomarkers or sensor-derived metrics, slowing adoption. Without structured training and guidelines, enthusiasm among specialists may outpace comfort among general practitioners, complicating widespread diffusion [44].

12.7.3 Patient Acceptability and Adherence

Patient perspectives are central to the success of technologies intended for long-term self-management. Nanotechnology-based approaches – including implanted sensors or injectable glucose-sensitive formulations – may raise concerns about invasiveness, safety, and unfamiliar materials. Surveys of people with diabetes show that device complexity, perceived discomfort, and apprehension about new materials or algorithms can reduce willingness to adopt novel systems. Even if wearable nanomaterials-based CGMs show superior performance in studies, patients may stop using them due to calibration demands, skin irritation, or data overload. Tailored education, transparency risk communication, and user-centered design are critical to overcoming these barriers [45].

12.8 DATA, CONNECTIVITY, AND PRIVACY

The growing incorporation of nanotechnology-enhanced CGMs and wearable biosensors in diabetes care generates vast quantities of real-time physiological data. These data streams offer unprecedented information on glycemic patterns enabling closed-loop systems and personalized therapy adaptation, but also present challenges in secure data handling and systems compatibility.

12.8.1 CGM/Wearable Data Handling and Cybersecurity

Nanomaterial-based sensors transmit glucose readings to smartphones, cloud platforms, and clinical data dashboards, heightening the importance of robust cybersecurity protections. Recent analyses of medical devices security have documented vulnerabilities in connected diabetes devices, including risk of unauthorized access, data manipulation, or wireless signal interception. These risks are amplified when wearables use Bluetooth or Wi-Fi to transmit sensitive health data. Regulatory bodies such as the U.S. FDA now emphasize security by design, requiring manufacturers to implement encrypted data transmission, authenticated access controls, and routine security patching as part of the premarket submissions. Ensuring compliance with data protection regulations (e.g., health insurance portability and accountability [HIPAA] in the U.S., General Data Protection Regulation [GDPR] in the EU) is essential to maintaining patient trust and legal conformity [46].

12.8.2 Interoperability with Existing Diabetics Tech

Interoperability remains a practical barrier: nanotechnology-based systems must seamlessly communicate with the existing diabetes management tools, including insulin pumps, electronic health records (EHR), and telehealth systems. Fragmented protocols and proprietary data formats can limit integration, forcing clinicians and patients to juggle multiple apps or interfaces. To address this, industry coalitions and standards organizations are promoting common communication frameworks (e.g., IEEE 11073, FHIR) to ensure that next-generation CGMs and nanotech sensors can feed real-time data into broader care ecosystems. Achieving interoperability not only supports clinical decision-making but also enables longitudinal data analysis for outcomes research. It also enhances remote care delivery, a priority underscored by COVID-19 pandemic's expansion of telemedicine [47].

12.9 CASE STUDIES

12.9.1 Wearable Nanomaterial CGMs

Nanomaterial-enabled wearable CGMs are progressing from lab prototypes toward pilot human testing. Materials such as graphene, carbon nanotubes, and metal-NP composites enhance electrode surface area and electron transfer, enabling thinner, flexible electrochemical sensors with higher sensitivity than traditional enzyme electrodes. Recent comprehensive reviews summarize rapid advances in flexible and minimally invasive platforms while highlighting persistent problems with signal drift, biofouling, and long-term stability that limit clinical readiness. Prototype studies with graphene-platinum nanocomposites and other nanocoatings report encouraging short-term accuracy and fast response times in controlled settings, but most devices still lack the multi-week reliability required for routine outpatient use [48].

12.9.2 Oral/Transdermal Insulin Nanoparticles Efforts

Oral and transdermal NP approaches illustrate both promise and translational hurdles. A high-profile oral nanoformulation using insulin-conjugated quantum dots with a pH-responsive chitosan/glucose coating enhanced duodenal absorption in human intestinal explants and glycemic control in preclinical models, demonstrating a viable mechanism for non-injectable insulin delivery. However, such formulations still face human gastrointestinal (GI) variability, first-pass metabolism, and strict safety/CMC demands before clinical use [49].

Transdermal microneedle patches often combined with glucose-responsive chemistries (glucose oxidase, phenylboronic acid) or nanocarrier-loaded dissolving needles have shown robust, pain-minimal insulin delivery in animal models and early human feasibility work, with some designs delivering pulsatile, glucose-correlated release. Yet scale-up, sterility, regulatory classification (device vs drug), and consistent long-term dosing remain unresolved [50].

Across both domains, inhaled insulin (Technosphere/Afrezza) remains the only widely adopted non-injectable rapid-acting option and provides an important clinical benchmark for safety, dosing conversion, and patient acceptance when evaluating net-generation nanoformulations. Continued progress will require clinical endpoints, standardized durability testing, and CMC pathways that demonstrate reproducible, safe products for chronic use [51].

12.10 FUTURE PROSPECTS

Nanotechnology is poised to significantly reshape diabetes care in the coming decade by enabling personalized, highly responsive therapies and diagnostics. A key area of future growth is the integration of closed-loop systems that integrate nanoscale sensors with AI-driven decision algorithms, which could allow real-time glucose management with minimal patient input, moving closer to an "artificial pancreas." Recent findings focus on functionalized quantum dots and other optical nanomaterials for the ultra-sensitive glucose detection, potentially enabling truly non-invasive wearables in sweat or interstitial fluid [52].

On the therapeutic side, glucose-responsive and smart nanocarriers that deliver insulin or adjuvant drugs only when necessary may lessen hypoglycemia risk and lower dosing frequency, a huge improvement over regular insulin regimens. Future work will focus on clinical validation, safety profiling, and regulatory alignment aiming to translate these innovations into scalable, affordable products that can improve long-term outcomes and quality of life for the millions living with diabetes globally [53].

12.11 CONCLUSION

Nanotechnology offers transformative potential for diabetes management by enabling precise drug delivery, advanced glucose sensing, and responsive therapeutic systems that address limitations of traditional care. Across drug carriers, smart glucose-responsive materials, wearable sensors, and regenerative platforms, research indicates clear mechanistic benefits that could improve glycemic control, decreased hypoglycemia, and improved quality of life. However, realizing this potential in clinical practice requires overcoming persistent translational barriers: robust safety and toxicity profiles for chronic use, reproducible large-scale manufacturing and CMC control, clear regulatory pathways, and supportive clinical evidence.

Furthermore, cost, healthcare infrastructure, and patient acceptability must be addressed to equitable access. Ongoing advances in standardized testing methods, predictive preclinical models, and data-driven decision support systems strengthen the foundation for clinical translation. As interdisciplinary collaboration between engineers, clinicians, regulators, and patient communities grows, nanotechnology is well positioned to make enduring contributions to safe, effective, and personalized diabetes care in the coming decade.

ACKNOWLEDGMENTS

I would like to express my profound gratitude to the School of Pharmacy, ITM University, Gwalior, for providing the sophisticated infrastructure and a truly stimulating academic environment. The completion of this chapter was made possible through the unwavering support and exceptional facilities offered by the institution.

REFERENCES

1. NCD Risk Factor Collaboration (NCD-RisC). Worldwide trends in diabetes prevalence and treatment from 1990 to 2022: A pooled analysis of 1108 population-representative studies with 141 million participants. Lancet. 2024;404(10467):2077–93. https://doi.org/10.1016/S0140-6736(24)02317-1.
2. Yapislar H, Gurler EB. Management of microcomplications of diabetes mellitus: Challenges, current trends, and future perspectives in treatment. Biomedicines. 2024;12(9):1958.
3. Maurya R, Ramteke S, Guru P, Jain NK. Oral glucose-responsive nanocarrier system for management of diabetes. Journal of Endocrinology and Metabolism. 2022;12(4-5):146–60.
4. Ma J, Yang S, Yang Z, He Z, Du Z. Functional nanomaterials for advanced bioelectrode interfaces: Recent advances in disease detection and metabolic monitoring. Sensors. 2025;25(14):4412.
5. Sammut SM. Organizational Antecedents to the Implementation of Precision Medicine: Overcoming Resistance to Change. Temple University; 2020.
6. Li H, Chen X, Rao S, Zhou M, Lu J, Liang D, Zhu B, Meng L, Lin J, Ding X, Zhang Q. Recent development of micro-nano carriers for oral antineoplastic drug delivery. Materials Today Bio. 2025;30:101445.
7. Klonoff DC. Afrezza inhaled insulin: The fastest-acting FDA-approved insulin on The market has favorable properties. Journal of Diabetes Science and Technology. 2014;8(6):1071–73.
8. Marques JB *Multistage Pancreas Biomimetic Construct Based on Synergism of Nanomedicines and Stem Cell-Derived Pancreatic Cells* (Doctoral dissertation, Universidade do Porto (Portugal)). 2024.
9. Ambaye AD, Mamo MD, Zigyalew Y, Mengistu WM, Fito Nure J, Mokrani T, Ntsendwana B. The development of carbon nanostructured biosensors for glucose detection to enhance healthcare services: A review. Frontiers in Sensors. 2024;5:1456669.
10. Abbaszadeh S, Nosrati-Siahmazgi V, Musaie K, Rezaei S, Qahremani M, Xiao B, Santos HA, Shahbazi MA. Emerging strategies to bypass transplant rejection via biomaterial-assisted immunoengineering: Insights from islets and beyond. Advanced Drug Delivery Reviews. 2023;200:115050.
11. Namiot ED, Sokolov AV, Chubarev VN, Tarasov VV, Schiöth HB. Nanoparticles in clinical trials: Analysis of clinical trials, FDA approvals and use for COVID-19 vaccines. International Journal of Molecular Sciences. 2023;24(1):787.
12. Badarinadh KS, Shukla P, Chauhan SB, Singh I. A comprehensive exploration of nanomedicine's current landscape and future horizons. Lipid Based Nanocarriers for Drug Delivery. 2024;383:391–433.
13. Caturano A, Nilo R, Nilo D, Russo V, Santonastaso E, Galiero R, Rinaldi L, Monda M, Sardu C, Marfella R, Sasso FC. Advances in nanomedicine for precision insulin delivery. Pharmaceuticals. 2024;17(7):945.
14. Jamshidnejad-Tosaramandani T, Kashanian S, Omidfar K, Schiöth HB. The role of nanomaterials in the wearable electrochemical glucose biosensors for diabetes management. Biosensors. 2025;15(7):451.
15. Herdiana Y. Bridging the gap: The role of advanced formulation strategies in The clinical translation of nanoparticle-based drug delivery systems. International Journal of Nanomedicine. 2025:13039–53.
16. Liu M, Wang R, Hoi MP, Wang Y, Wang S, Li G, Vong CT, Chong CM. Nano-based drug delivery systems for managing diabetes: Recent advances and future prospects. International Journal of Nanomedicine. 2025:6221–52.
17. Karim AM. Smart antidiabetic nanomedicine: A revolutionized therapeutic approach for treatment of diabetes mellitus. Bioengineering. 2025;12(12):1309.
18. Prior H, Baldrick P, Clarke DO, Passini E, Sewell F, van Meer P. Exploring greater flexibility for chronic toxicity study designs to support human safety assessment while balancing 3Rs considerations. International Journal of Toxicology. 2024;43(5):456–63.
19. Shahapurmath S, Sharannavar BR, Koli R. Serum albumin nanoparticles: Ligand functionalization for enhanced targeted therapeutics in precision medicine. Medicine in Drug Discovery. 2025:100218.
20. Zheng N, Sun DD, Zou P, Jiang W. Scientific and regulatory considerations for generic complex drug products containing nanomaterials. The AAPS Journal. 2017;19(3):619–31.
21. Wang M, Wang C, Ren S, Pan J, Wang Y, Shen Y, Zeng Z, Cui H, Zhao X. Versatile oral insulin delivery nanosystems: From materials to nanostructures. International Journal of Molecular Sciences. 2022;23(6):3362.
22. Smoliga JM, Blanchard OL. Allometric scaling models: History, use, and misuse in translating resveratrol from basic science to human clinical applications. Functional Foods in Health and Disease-Online ISSN: 2160-3855; Print ISSN: 2378-7007. 2017;7(5):338–52.
23. Webber MJ, Anderson DG. Smart approaches to glucose-responsive drug delivery. Journal of Drug Targeting. 2015;23(7-8):651–55.
24. Retrieval EC. Late breaking abstracts. International Journal of Stroke. 2022;17(3S):289–325.
25. Cojocaru E, Petriş OR, Cojocaru C. Nanoparticle-based drug delivery systems in inhaled therapy: Improving respiratory medicine. Pharmaceuticals. 2024;17(8):1059.

26. Saxena S, Sharma S, Kumar G, Thakur S. Unravelling the complexity of CARPA: A review of emerging advancements in therapeutic strategies. Archives of Dermatological Research. 2025;317(1):439.
27. Tenchov R, Hughes KJ, Ganesan M, Iyer KA, Ralhan K, Lotti Diaz LM, Bird RE, Ivanov JM, Zhou QA. Transforming medicine: Cutting-edge applications of nanoscale materials in drug delivery. ACS Nano. 2025;19(4):4011–38.
28. Havel HA. Where are the nanodrugs? An industry perspective on development of drug products containing nanomaterials. The AAPS Journal. 2016;18(6):1351–53.
29. Ragelle H, Danhier F, Préat V, Langer R, Anderson DG. Nanoparticle-based drug delivery systems: A commercial and regulatory outlook as the field matures. Expert Opinion on Drug Delivery. 2017; 14(7):851–64.
30. Desai N. Challenges in development of nanoparticle-based therapeutics. The AAPS Journal. 2012;14(2): 282–95.
31. Osouli-Bostanabad K, Puliga S, Serrano DR, Bucchi A, Halbert G, Lalatsa A. Microfluidic manufacture of lipid-based nanomedicines. Pharmaceutics. 2022;14(9):1940.
32. Bezelya A, Küçüktürkmen B, Böncü TE, Bozkır A. Microfluidics-Based nanoparticle formulations: Preparation and evaluation of protein delivery systems. Polymers for Advanced Technologies. 2025;36(7):e70250.
33. Mehta M, Bui TA, Yang X, Aksoy Y, Goldys EM, Deng W. Lipid-based nanoparticles for drug/gene delivery: An overview of the production techniques And difficulties encountered in their industrial development. ACS Materials Au. 2023;3(6):600–19.
34. Erdoğar N, Gür B, Örgül D. Recent developments of novel nanotechnology-based drug delivery systems for dermal and transdermal applications. European Journal of Pharmaceutical Sciences. 2025: 107413.
35. King TE, Humphrey JR, Laughton CA, Thomas NR, Hirst JD. Optimizing excipient properties to prevent aggregation in biopharmaceutical formulations. Journal of Chemical Information and Modeling. 2023;64(1):265–75.
36. Lin C, Huang X, Xue Y, Jiang S, Chen C, Liu Y, Chen K. Advances in medical devices using nanomaterials and nanotechnology: Innovation and regulatory science. Bioactive Materials. 2025;48:353–69.
37. European Medicines Agency (EMA). Nanotechnology-Based Medicinal Products for Human Use: EU-IN Horizon Scanning Report. 2025.
38. Mundekkad D, Cho WC. Nanoparticles in clinical translation for cancer therapy. International Journal of Molecular Sciences. 2022;23(3):1685.
39. Tyner KM, Zou P, Yang X, Zhang H, Cruz CN, Lee SL. Product quality for nanomaterials: Current US experience and perspective. Wiley Interdisciplinary Reviews: Nanomedicine and Nanobiotechnology. 2015;7(5):640–54.
40. Wang Y, Wang C, Li K, Song X, Yan X, Yu L, He Z. Recent advances of nanomedicine-based strategies in diabetes and complications management: Diagnostics, monitoring, and therapeutics. Journal of Controlled Release. 2021;330:618–40.
41. Thor S, Vetter T, Marcal A, Kweder S. EMA-FDA parallel scientific advice: Optimizing development of medicines in the global age. Therapeutic Innovation & Regulatory Science. 2023;57(4):656–61.
42. Fortune A, Aime A, Raymond D, Kumar S. Nanotechnology in medicine: A double-edged sword for health outcomes. Health Nanotechnology. 2025;1(1):9.
43. Graham C. Continuous glucose monitoring And global reimbursement: An update. Diabetes Technology & Therapeutics. 2017;19(3_suppl)):S-60.
44. Alsabah M, Naser MA, Albahri AS, Albahri OS, Alamoodi AH, Abdulhussain SH, Alzubaidi L. A comprehensive review on key technologies toward smart healthcare systems based IoT: Technical aspects, challenges and future directions. Artificial Intelligence Review. 2025;58(11):343.
45. Shoaib A, Darraj A, Khan ME, Azmi L, Alalwan A, Alamri O, Tabish M, Khan AU. A nanotechnology-based approach to biosensor application in current diabetes management practices. Nanomaterials. 2023;13(5):867.
46. Shakeel T, Habib S, Boulila W, Koubaa A, Javed AR, Rizwan M, Gadekallu TR, Sufiyan M. A survey on COVID-19 impact in the healthcare domain: Worldwide market implementation, applications, security and privacy issues, challenges and future prospects. Complex & Intelligent Systems. 2023;9(1): 1027–58.
47. Klonoff DC, Aaron RE, Tian T, Espinoza JC. Principles of interoperability of diabetes devices. Journal of Diabetes Science and Technology. 2025;19(6):1681–86.
48. Rajamohan R, Sun S. Nanostructured materials in glucose biosensing: From fundamentals to smart healthcare applications. Biosensors. 2025;15(10):658.

49. Rial-Hermida MI, Rey-Rico A, Blanco-Fernandez B, Carballo-Pedrares N, Byrne EM, Mano JF. Recent progress on polysaccharide-based hydrogels for controlled delivery of therapeutic biomolecules. ACS Biomaterials Science & Engineering. 2021;7(9):4102–27.
50. Choi J, Jang S, Yu S, Ahn YR, Kim M, Lee H, Kim HO. Microneedle–nanoparticle hybrid platforms for metabolic syndrome: Advances in point-of-care diagnostics and transdermal therapeutics. Discover Nano. 2025;20(1):1–43.
51. KM PK, Viswanathan V, Saboo B, Sanyal D, Gangopadhyay KK, Chaudhuri T, Ayyar VS, Chawla M, Joshi A, Gupta A, Sugumaran A. Beyond the needle: Reimagining insulin delivery and the evolution of inhaled insulins. Cureus. 2026;18(2):01–11.
52. Rehan Haider ZA, Das GK, Zameer S Revolutionizing patient care: Multidimensional approaches to 21st-century diabetes management. Journal of Heart and Vasculature. 2025;4(6):01–05.
53. Zhang Y, Yu J, Kahkoska AR, Wang J, Buse JB, Gu Z. Advances in transdermal insulin delivery. Advanced Drug Delivery Reviews. 2019;139:51–70.

13 The Current Landscape of Nano-Enhanced Diabetes Care

Shweta Telang-Chaudhari
Maharashtra University of Health Sciences, Nashik, India

Jyothirmayee Devineni
KVSR Siddhartha College of Pharmaceutical Sciences, Vijayawada, India

D. Thangamani
Institute of Forest Genetics and Tree Breeding, Coimbatore, India

Nidhi Singh
Teerthanker Mahaveer College of pharmacy (TMCOP),
Teerthanker Mahaveer University, Muradabad, India

Shipra Omar
School of Pharmaceutical Sciences, Shri Guru Ram Rai University,
Dehradun, India

Shilpa Mandpe
School of Pharmacy and Technology Management, NMIMS, Shirpur, India

13.1 INTRODUCTION

Diabetes mellitus has emerged as one of the most significant global health challenges of the 21st century. According to the International Diabetes Federation (IDF) Diabetes Atlas (11th edition), approximately 589 million adults aged 20–79 years were living with diabetes worldwide in 2024, representing nearly 1 in 9 adults. This number is projected to rise dramatically to about 853 million by 2050, reflecting the continuing escalation of metabolic disorders associated with urbanization, sedentary lifestyles, and population aging [1].

Diabetes also imposes a major economic and health burden. The disease was responsible for around 3.4 million deaths globally in 2024, and global healthcare expenditure linked with diabetes was over USD 1 trillion annually [1]. Furthermore, over 80% of individuals with diabetes live in low- and middle-income countries, where access to early diagnosis and treatment remains limited. The rapid growth of diabetes prevalence has made it a major contributor of complications such as cardiovascular disease, kidney failure, neuropathy, and blindness, highlighting an urgent need for better therapeutic strategies [2].

13.1.1 Limitations of Traditional Diabetes Management

Traditional diabetes management primarily relies on insulin treatment, oral antidiabetic drugs, lifestyle change, and glucose monitoring systems. While these approaches work in terms of controlling blood glucose level, they have several limitations. Insulin therapy often requires frequent injections

DOI: 10.1201/9781003598657-13

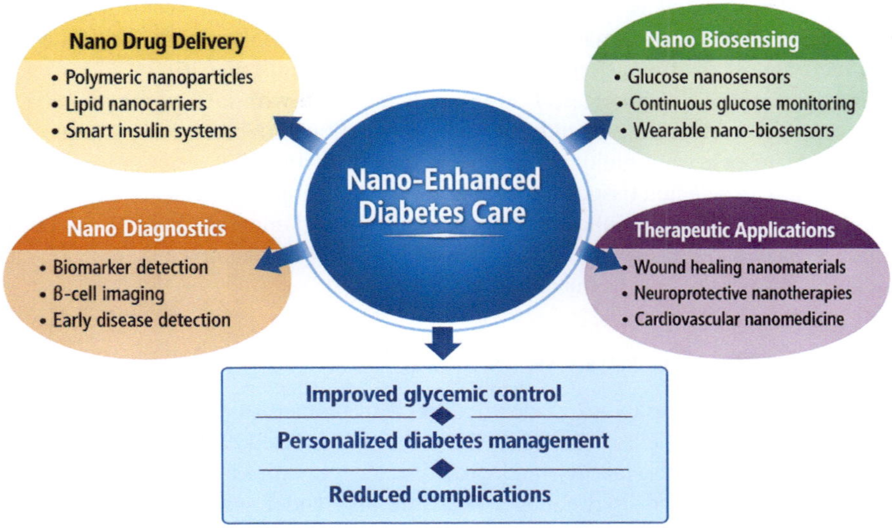

FIGURE 13.1 Nano-enabled diabetes care ecosystem.

and will have strict dosing schedules, which may result in poor patient adherence and poor glycemic control. In addition, conventional drugs are often of limited bioavailability, short-half-life, and non-specific distribution, putting one at danger of adverse effects and insufficient therapeutic response [3].

Continuous glucose monitoring technologies have improved diabetes care; however, many devices remain invasive and expensive, and their need for regular calibration limits their widespread adoption in resource-limited settings. Moreover, despite advances in pharmacotherapy, achieving precise and sustained glycemic regulation remains challenging for many patients [4].

13.1.2 Emergence of Nanotechnology in Diabetes Care

Nanotechnology has recently appeared as a revolutionary method in the field of research and treatment of diabetes. Nanomaterials including polymeric nanoparticles, liposomes, dendrimers, and metallic nanostructures can be designed to increase drug stability, targeted and controlled, or stimulus-responsive drug release. These properties make nanotechnology especially promising for overcoming the problems associated with traditional putative treatments for diabetes [5]. Nanotechnology is revolutionizing many areas of diabetes care such as drug delivery, biosensing, and diagnostics and treatment of complications (Figure 13.1).

Recent studies highlight development of glucose-responsive insulin nanocarriers, nanoparticle-based oral insulin preparations, and highly sensitive nanosensors for glucose monitoring. Such innovations aim to enable more precise glycemic control, lower dosing frequency, and better compliance. As nanomedicine continues to evolve, it is expected to play a crucial role in advancing next-generation diabetes diagnostics, therapeutics, and personalized disease management strategies.

13.2 FUNDAMENTALS OF NANOTECHNOLOGY IN MEDICINE

13.2.1 Definition and Characteristics of Nanomaterials

Nanotechnology refers to the design and application of materials with dimensions typically ranging from 1 to 100 nanometers (nm), where unique physicochemical characteristics appear due to their very small size and large surface-to-volume ratio. At this scale, materials frequently exhibit new electrical, optical, magnetic, and catalytic properties, which can be exploited for biomedical applications such as drug delivery, diagnostic, and imaging. According to the National Nanotechnology Initiative, nanomaterials are engineered materials whose functional properties arise from their nanoscale dimensions and adjustable surface properties [6].

In medical applications, nanomaterials are usually designed with surface functionalization, biocompatible coating, and targeting ligands for better interaction with biological systems. Their small size allows them to penetrate biological barriers, interact with cellular components, and deliver therapeutic agents to a selected tissue or cells. For instance, nanoparticles can be modified with antibodies, peptides, or polymers to enhance selective targeting and improve pharmacokinetics profiles. These features make nanomaterials highly attractive for addressing complex therapeutic challenges, including chronic diseases such as diabetes and cancer [7].

13.2.2 Types of Nanomaterials Used in Biomedicine

Several classes of nanomaterials are widely explored in biomedical research and medical applications. Polymeric nanoparticles are among the most widely used carriers because they provide controlled drug release, high stability, and excellent biocompatibility. Lipid-based nanocarriers, including liposomes and solid lipid nanoparticles, are also widely used as drug delivery because they can encapsulate both hydrophilic and hydrophobic drugs [8].

Another important class includes dendrimers, which are highly branched macromolecules with well-defined structures and multiple functional groups that allow precise drug loading and targeting. Inorganic nanomaterials, such as gold nanoparticles, silica nanoparticles, and iron oxide nanoparticles are often used in biomedical imaging and biosensing due to their unique optical and magnetic properties. In addition, carbon-based nanomaterials, including graphene and carbon nanotubes, are increasingly investigated for biosensing platforms and advanced treatment systems [9].

These nanomaterials have already shown some clinical relevancy. For instance, in mRNA vaccines developed by Pfizer and Moderna, lipid nanoparticle platforms were used to great success, which signifies the translational potential of nanotechnology in modern medicine [10].

13.2.3 Advantages of Nano-Based Therapeutics

Nano-based therapeutics offer several advantages over conventional drug delivery method. Their nanoscale size enables enhanced drug solubility, improved bioavailability, and prolonged circulation time in the bloodstream. Nanocarriers can also provide controlled and stimulus-responsive drug release, which allows therapeutic agents to be released only under special physiological conditions such as changes in pH or glucose concentration [11].

Another important benefit is targeted drug delivery, where nanoparticles are engineered to accumulate preferentially at specific tissues or cells, thereby minimizing systemic toxicity and enhancing therapeutic efficacy. In chronic diseases such as diabetes, nanotechnology has enabled the development of glucose-responsive insulin systems and nanosensor-based glucose monitoring devices, which may provide more precise glycemic control and reduce treatment burden for patients. Collectively, these advantages highlight the growing role of nanotechnology as a powerful platform for next-generation biomedical therapies [12].

13.3 NANO-ENABLED DRUG DELIVERY SYSTEMS

Nanotechnology has significantly transformed drug delivery through the development of nanoscale drug carriers that enhance pharmacokinetic and pharmacodynamic profiles of therapeutic agents. In diabetes management, nano-enabled delivery systems are being explored to improve drug stability, bioavailability, and targeted or controlled release of antidiabetic agents. These nanosystems can protect sensitive biomolecules such as insulin from enzymatic degradation and facilitate efficient transport across biological barriers [13].

13.3.1 Polymeric Nanoparticles

Polymeric nanoparticles are among the most commonly investigated nanocarriers for biomedical applications. They are generally prepared using biodegradable polymers as poly(lactic-co-glycolic acid) (PLGA), chitosan, and alginate. These polymers provide controlled drug release, biocompatibility, and the ability to encapsulate both hydrophilic and hydrophobic therapeutic molecules [14].

Polymeric nanoparticles have been extensively investigated for oral insulin delivery. For instance, chitosan-based nanoparticles have demonstrated enhanced intestinal absorption of insulin by increasing mucoadhesion and protecting the peptide from gastrointestinal degradation. In experimental models, PLGA-based nanoparticle systems have shown the ability to sustain insulin release for extended periods, contributing to improved glycemic control. These systems are also being investigated for delivering other antidiabetic medications including metformin and glucagon-like peptide-1 (GLP-1) analogs [15].

13.3.2 Liposomes and Nanolipid Carriers

Lipid-based nanocarriers represent another important category of nano-enabled drug delivery systems. Liposomes are spherical vesicles made of phospholipids bilayers capable of encapsulating both hydrophilic and lipophilic drugs. Their structural similarity to biological membranes enhances biocompatibility and cellular uptake. Liposomes have been widely studied for insulin delivery and targeted drug transport [16].

Solid lipid nanoparticles and nanostructured lipid carriers have also gained attention due to their improved stability and controlled release characteristics. These systems can enhance the oral bioavailability of poorly soluble drugs and protect bioactive molecules from enzymatic degradation. Lipid nanoparticle technology has also demonstrated clinical success, most notably in the lipid nanoparticle delivery systems used in mRNA vaccines developed by Pfizer and Moderna, highlighting the translational potential of lipid-based nanocarriers [16].

13.3.3 Dendrimers and Nanogels

Dendrimers are highly branched tree-like macromolecules having well-defined structures and multiple surface functional groups. These features enable the precise drug loading, surface modification, and targeted delivery. Dendrimers have been explored for delivering insulin and other peptide therapeutics because their nanoscale architecture enables high drug encapsulation efficiency and controlled release [17].

Nanogels, on the other hand, are nano-sized hydrogel networks capable of absorbing large amounts of water while maintaining structural integrity. Their soft and flexible structure enables efficient encapsulation of proteins and peptides. In diabetes research, glucose-responsive nanogels have been developed to release insulin in response to elevated glucose levels, providing a promising strategy for self-regulated insulin delivery [18].

13.3.4 Metallic and Inorganic Nanoparticles

Metallic and inorganic nanoparticles are widely used in biomedical applications due to their unique optical, magnetic, and catalytic properties. Gold nanoparticles, for example, are commonly used in biosensing and targeted drug delivery because of their high biocompatibility and surface modification ability. Iron oxide nanoparticles are regularly utilized as contrasting materials in magnetic resonance amplification and for focused treatment methods [19].

Silica-based nanoparticles have also been investigated for controlled drug release due to their porous structure and larger surface area. In diabetes research, these inorganic nanomaterials are being explored for glucose sensing platforms, targeted drug delivery systems, and imaging

TABLE 13.1
Representative Nanotechnology Platform Used in Diabetes Care and Their Applications

Nanotechnology Platform	Key Material Examples	Primary Application in Diabetes	Representative Example
Polymeric nanoparticles	PLGA, chitosan alginate	Controlled delivery and oral insulin protection	Chitosan nanoparticles improving intestinal insulin adsorption [21]
Lipid-based nanocarriers	Liposomes, solid lipid nanocarriers (SLN), nanostructured lipid carriers (NLC)	Encapsulation and sustained delivery of insulin and antidiabetic drugs	Liposomal insulin formulations for enhanced stability [22]
Dendrimers	Poly(amidoamine) (PAMAM) dendrimers	Targeted drug delivery and controlled release	Dendrimer-based carriers for peptide therapeutics [23]
Metallic nanoparticles	Gold nanoparticles, silver nanoparticles	Glucose biosensing and antimicrobial wound healing	Gold nanoparticle electrochemical glucose sensors [24]
Carbon-based nanomaterials	Graphene, carbon nanotubes	High-sensitivity glucose detection and biosensors platforms	Graphene-based wearable glucose sensors [25]
Nanofibers/Nanogels	Polymer nanofibers, hydrogel nanoparticle	Smart insulin delivery and wound healing scaffolds	Glucose-responsive nanogel insulin delivery systems [26]

techniques aimed at improving disease monitoring and therapeutic precision. Various nanomaterial platforms have been explored to improve the drug delivery, biosensing, and therapeutic performance in diabetes care. These nanosystems differ in their composition, physicochemical properties, and biomedicinal applications [20]. A comparative overview of major nanotechnology platforms currently investigated for diabetes management is presented in Table 13.1.

13.4 NANO-BASED INSULIN DELIVERY STRATEGIES

Recent researches in nanomedicine have opened new possibilities for insulin administration beyond traditional subcutaneous injections. Nano-engineered delivery platforms aim to improve insulin stability, enhance absorption across biological barriers, and enable more physiological glucose-regulated release. These strategies are designed to reduce injection frequency, boost patient adherence, and support tighter glycemic control.

13.4.1 Oral Insulin Nanocarriers

Oral insulin delivery has long been a major challenge due to enzymatic degradation in the gastrointestinal tract and poor epithelial permeability. Nanocarrier systems such as polymeric nanoparticles, lipid nanoparticles, and chitosan-based nanocomplexes have been developed to protect insulin from gastric enzymes and promote intestinal absorption. Mucoadhesive nanoparticles can temporarily open tight junctions in intestinal epithelial cells, facilitating paracellular transport of insulin. Recent preclinical studies have shown that chitosan-coated nanoparticles and PLGA-based nanocarriers enhance insulin bioavailability in animal models, indicating potential for future insulin formulations [27].

13.4.2 Transdermal and Microneedle Systems

Transdermal insulin delivery using nano-enabled microneedle arrays has emerged as a minimally invasive alternative to conventional injections. Microneedles are microscopic projections capable of penetrating the stratum corneum without reaching deeper pain receptors. When combined with insulin-containing nanoparticles or nanogels, microneedle patches can deliver controlled and sustained insulin release through the skin. Experimental microneedle systems incorporating glucose-sensitive nanomaterials have shown promising results in animal studies, enabling automated insulin release in response to rising blood glucose levels. These wearable patches may also integrate with continuous glucose monitoring systems, creating a more responsive diabetes management system [28].

13.4.3 Glucose-Responsive Smart Insulin Systems

Glucose-responsive insulin delivery systems represent one of the most innovative directions in diabetes nanotechnology. These "smart" systems use nanoscale materials that respond to change in glucose concentration. For example, nanoparticles containing glucose oxidase or phenylboronic acid derivatives can detect elevated glucose levels and trigger insulin release accordingly. In preclinical studies, glucose-responsive nanogels and polymeric vesicles have shown the ability to maintain stable glucose levels for extended periods by releasing insulin only when needed, mimicking physiological pancreatic function [29].

13.4.4 Injectable Nano-Formulations

Injectable nano-formulations remain one of the most clinically advanced approaches to nano-enabled insulin delivery. Long-acting injectable nanoparticles and nano-suspensions can prolong insulin circulation time and enable sustained release. Biodegradable polymer-based nanoformulations are being explored to provide longer glycemic control with fewer injections. These systems also offer the potential to co-deliver additional therapeutic agents, such as GLP-1 analogs, enabling combination therapy within a single nano-engineered formulation [30]. Several nano-engineered platforms have been developed to enhance insulin administration, including oral nanocarriers, microneedle patches, glucose-responsive systems, and long-acting injectable nanoparticles (Figure 13.2)

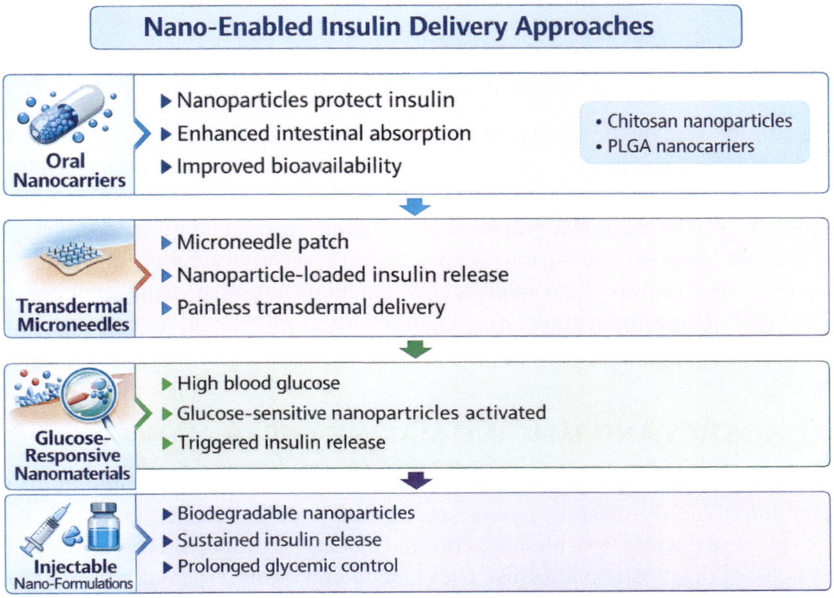

FIGURE 13.2 Nano-based insulin delivery strategies.

13.5 NANOTECHNOLOGY IN GLUCOSE MONITORING

Nanotechnology has greatly improved glucose monitoring technologies by facilitating the research of highly sensitive, miniaturized, and real-time biosensing platforms. Nanoscale materials like graphene, gold nanoparticles, and carbon nanotubes improve signal transduction and detection sensitivity, allowing rapid measurement of glucose concentrations in biological fluids. These innovations have improved the accuracy and responsiveness of modern diabetes monitoring systems.

13.5.1 Nanosensors for Glucose Detection

Nanosensors utilize nanomaterials to measure glucose by electrochemical, optical, or fluorescence-based mechanisms. Materials including gold nanoparticles, graphene, and carbon nanotubes provide large surface areas and great electrical conductivity, which improve the interaction of glucose molecules with sensing elements. These nanosensors often contain enzymes such as glucose oxidase that catalyze glucose oxidation and convert biochemical reactions into measurable electrical signals. Compared with conventional biosensors, nano-enabled sensors demonstrate higher sensitivity, faster response time, and improved detection limits, making them extremely suitable for real-time metabolic monitoring [31].

13.5.2 Continuous Glucose Monitoring (CGM) Systems

Continuous glucose monitoring (CGM) technologies represent one of the most important innovations in diabetes care. CGM devices measure glucose level in interstitial fluid using small sensors inserted beneath skin and transmit data to external receivers or mobile applications at regular intervals. These systems provide real-time glucose readings, trend analysis, and alerts for hypoglycemia or hyperglycemia, enabling improved glycemic control. Modern CGM systems, such as the Dexcom G7, can deliver glucose readings about every 5 minutes and maintain sensors for up to about 15 days with improved accuracy numbers. Such wearable monitoring technologies are increasingly integrated with insulin pumps and digital health platforms to support automatic diabetes management [32].

13.5.3 Non-Invasive Nano-Biosensors

A major research focus is the development of non-invasive glucose monitoring systems that eliminate the need to implant sensors or finger-prick blood sampling. Nanotechnology has enabled the creation of wearable biosensors capable of detecting glucose in alternative biological fluids such as sweat, saliva, or tears. For example, graphene-based nanosensors integrated into flexible wearable devices can measure glucose levels from sweat with high sensitivity. Emerging optical nanosensor using plasmonic nanostructures and fluorescence detection are also being explored for painless glucose monitoring. These innovations may significantly improve patient comfort and increasing access to continuous metabolic monitoring in the future [33].

13.6 DIAGNOSTICS AND IMAGING MAKING USE OF NANO-TECH

Nanotechnology is increasingly transforming diagnostic and imaging paradigms in diabetes by enabling detection of highly sensitive biomarkers and advanced visualization of pancreatic tissues. Nanoparticles possess tunable optical, magnetic, and electronic properties that enhance the sensitivity and specificity of diagnostic platforms. These technologies are especially useful to detect early metabolic changes, monitoring disease progression, and complications before clinical symptoms appear.

13.6.1 Nanoparticle-Based Biomarker Detection

Nanoparticle-based biosensors have become powerful tools to identify highly sensitive biomarkers related with diabetes. Nanomaterials like gold nanoparticles, graphene, quantum dots, can enhance biochemical signals and help to detect biomarkers in a biological fluid. For example, gold-nanoparticles have been used to detect biomarkers including glycated hemoglobin (HbA1c) or glycated albumin, insulin, and autoantibodies associated with diabetes with improved sensitivity compared with traditional tests [34].

Recent studies also indicate the application of nanoparticle-based portable biosensors that enable rapid, point-of-care detection of chronic diseases, including diabetes. These platforms combine miniaturized nanomaterials with electrochemical sensing systems, enabling fast and accurate detection of metabolic biomarkers even in low-resource settings.

13.6.2 Imaging of Pancreatic β-Cells

The ability to visualize pancreatic β-cells is important for understanding diabetes progression, particularly in type 1 diabetes where autoimmune destruction of β-cells occurs. Nanoparticle-based imaging agents have been created to improve the detection of the β-cell mass and function. Polymer-based nanostructures and magnetic nanoparticles can be used in fluorescence imaging and magnetic resonance imaging (MRI) to identify β-cell populations and monitor their viability [35].

Superparamagnetic iron oxide nanoparticles are especially interesting as contrast agents in MRI due to their strong magnetic properties and biocompatibility. These nanoparticles improve imaging sensitivity and allow more precise imaging of cellular structure and changes due to disease in tissues.

13.6.3 Early Detection of Diabetes and Complications

Early diagnosis of diabetes and its complications is essential for preventing irreversible organ damage. Nanotechnology-enabled diagnostic tools are being developed to detect subtle biochemical and physiological changes associated with disease onset. Nanoparticle-based imaging and biosensing systems can identify early signs of complications such as vascular damage, neuropathy, and kidney dysfunction [36].

Advanced nanodiagnostic platforms can also monitor emerging biomarkers such as microRNAs and inflammatory mediators, which are associated with metabolic dysregulation and diabetes progression. These technologies offer the potential for earlier disease detection, better risk staging, and more personalized therapeutic interventions in diabetes management.

13.7 NANOTECHNOLOGY FOR DIABETES COMPLICATIONS

Chronic hyperglycemia in diabetes causes severe complications in many organs, which include the skin, nervous system, kidney, and cardiovascular system. Conventional treatments for these complications are often poor because of poor drug targeting and side effects in the body. Nanotechnology can help in innovative therapeutic strategies through targeted drug delivery, better bioavailability, and localized treatment of damaged tissues. These nano-enabled approaches are aimed to resolve the complex pathophysiology of diabetic complications and improve therapeutic results.

13.7.1 Diabetic Wound Healing

Diabetic wound healing, specifically diabetic foot ulcers, is one of the most severe complications of diabetes and often result from impaired angiogenesis, chronic inflammation, and infection. Nanomaterials have demonstrated significant potential in accelerating wound repair by improving the local wound microenvironment. Nanoparticles such as silver, zinc oxide, and polymeric nanocarriers possess antimicrobial, antioxidant, and anti-inflammatory properties that help control infection and promote tissue regeneration. Studies indicate that nano-engineered wound dressings and nanofibers scaffolds can promote collagen deposition, stimulate angiogenesis, and support cell proliferation, thereby accelerating the healing process [37].

Recent research has also explored multifunctional hydrogels and nanozyme-based systems that release therapeutic agents directly at the wound site, while maintaining a favorable healing environment. These nano-enabled systems can simultaneously reduce bacterial load, modulate inflammation, and stimulate vascular regeneration, thereby offering promising strategy for chronic diabetic wound management [37].

13.7.2 Diabetes Neuropathy and Nephropathy

Nanomedicine is increasingly being investigated for the treatment of microvascular complications such as diabetic neuropathy and nephropathy. Nanoparticle-based drug delivery systems can improve the targeted delivery of therapeutic molecules to affected nerves and renal tissues, enhancing drug efficacy while reducing systemic toxicity. In diabetic nephropathy, nanocarriers like liposomes and polymeric nanoparticles have been investigated for delivering anti-inflammatory and antioxidant agents which help reduce renal fibrosis and oxidative stress [38].

Similarly, nano-enabled platforms are being designed for delivering neuroprotective drugs to enhance nerves regeneration and diminish neuropathic pain. These approaches aim to overcome limitations of conventional therapies by allowing sustained drug release and improved tissue targeting [39].

13.7.3 Cardiovascular Complications

Cardiovascular disease is the number one killer of diabetics. Nanotechnology has demonstrated promise in treating diabetes-associated cardiovascular complications with the help of targeted drug delivery and better diagnostic imaging. Nanocarriers can be used to deliver cardioprotective agents, antioxidants, or anti-inflammatory drugs directly to vascular tissue under hyperglycemia-induced damage [40].

Furthermore, multifunctional nanomaterials are being explored as theranostics platform, combining diagnostic and therapeutic functions to monitor inflammation and deliver treatment simultaneously. These emerging nano-based strategies may help reduce the risk of atherosclerosis, myocardial injury, and other cardiovascular complications associated with long-term diabetes [41].

13.8 EMERGING NANO-THERAPEUTIC APPROACHES

Recent advances in nanomedicine have increased therapeutic possibilities for diabetes beyond glucose control, focusing on disease-modifying strategies such as immune modulation, β-cell preservation, and regenerative therapies. These approaches aim to address underlying pathological mechanism, especially in type 1 diabetes, where autoimmune destruction of pancreatic β-cells leads to insulin deficiency.

13.8.1 Immunomodulatory Nanotherapies for Type 1 Diabetes

Type 1 diabetes is known for the destruction of insulin-producing β-cells (automatic). Nanotechnology provides novel ways of controlling immune reactions and preventing the destruction of β-cells. Nanoparticle-based delivery systems are able to deliver immunosuppressive, peptide, or antigen directly to immune cells, with less systemic toxicity and increased immune tolerance. For example, biodegradable polymeric nanoparticles have been investigated to deliver autoantigens associated with pancreatic route β-cells to dendritic cells which may cause antigen-specific immune tolerance and suppress autoimmune attack. In preclinical work, it has been demonstrated that efficacious disease progression or delay can be brought about by such targeted nanotherapies in preclinical models of autoimmune diabetes [42].

13.8.2 Nanomedicine for β-Cell Regeneration

Restoration of functional β-cell mass represents a major therapeutic goal in diabetes treatment. Nanomedicine is being explored to enhance β-cell regeneration and survival through targeted delivery of growth factors, nucleic acids, and regenerative biomolecules. Nanoparticle-based systems can deliver therapeutic genes, small interfering RNA (siRNA), or signaling molecules to stimulate β-cell proliferation and protect existing β-cells from oxidative stress and apoptosis. Additionally, nano-engineered scaffolds and hydrogels are being studied to support pancreatic tissue regeneration and improve the survival of transplanted islet cells [42].

13.8.3 Nano-Based Combination Therapies

Combination therapies that combine various therapies in one nanocarrier have also attracted interest in diabetes research. These platforms could potentially deliver insulin, anti-inflammatory compounds, and metabolic regulators simultaneously, and therefore provide synergistic therapeutic effects. For example, multifunctional nanoparticles have been developed for co-delivery of insulin and GLP-1 analogs, which can be used to improve glycemic management while promoting β-cells function [43].

Such integrated nano-therapeutic strategies characterize the growing potential of nanomedicine to acquire more than symptomatic management toward more comprehensive and disease-modifying treatments for diabetes.

13.9 SAFETY, TOXICOLOGY, AND REGULATORY CONSIDERATIONS

Despite the promising therapeutic potential of nanotechnology in diabetes care, safety and regulatory considerations remain critical for successful clinical translation. Nanomaterials may exhibit unique biological interactions due to their small size, high surface reactivity, and ability to penetrate biological barriers. These properties may affect biodistribution, cellular uptake, and accumulation in tissues, raising concerns regarding potential toxicity and immunogenicity. Therefore, thorough evaluation of nanotoxicology, pharmacokinetics, and biocompatibility is essential during the development of nano-based therapeutics [44].

Regulatory agencies like the U.S. Food and Drug Administration and European Medicines Agency have issued a guidance documents addressing the characterization, manufacturing, and safety assessment of nanomedicines. These frameworks emphasize detailed analysis of particles size, surface chemistry, and stability, and biological interactions. Establishing standardized testing protocols and long-term safety data will be crucial to ensure the safe and effective integration of nano-enabled therapies into diabetes management [45].

13.10 TRANSLATIONAL AND CLINICAL CHALLENGES

Despite significant progress in nano-enabled diabetes therapies, several translational and clinical challenges hinder their widespread adoption. One major barrier is the scale-up and reproducible manufacturing of nanomaterials with consistent physicochemical properties such as particle size, surface charge, and drug loading efficiency. Variability in these parameters can influence therapeutic performance and safety profiles. In addition, the complexity of biological interactions between nanoparticles and human tissues makes it difficult to accurately predict long-term biodistribution, metabolism, and possible toxicity [43].

Clinical translation also requires extensive preclinical validation and large-scale clinical trials, which can be costly and time-consuming. Regulatory approval pathways for nanomedicines remain evolving and often require additional characterization compared with conventional pharmaceuticals. Furthermore, cost, accessibility, and healthcare infrastructure limitations may restrict the implementation of advanced nano-therapeutic technologies, especially in low- and middle-income countries where diabetes burden is rapidly increasing [46].

13.11 FUTURE OUTLOOK

The future of nano-enhanced diabetes care is expected to be shaped by advances in precision medicine, bioresponsive materials, and digital health integration. Emerging nanotechnologies are increasingly being designed to function as multifunctional platforms, combining drug delivery. biosensors, and real-time monitoring within a single system. Such integrated approaches may enable more individualized diabetes care through continuous therapeutic intervention based on an individuals' metabolic status [47].

One promising direction is the development of closed-loop therapeutic systems, where nanosensors continuously detect glucose levels and trigger automated insulin release through glucose-responsive nanocarriers. These systems try aim to mimic physiological pancreatic function and reduce the need for frequent manual interventions. In addition, advances in nanobiomaterials and regenerative medicine may support β-cell preservation and regeneration, potentially offering disease-modifying strategies for diabetes treatment [48].

The combination of nanotechnology and wearable medical devices, AI, and mobile health platforms is likely to improve remote monitoring and predictive disease management. As interdisciplinary research continues to expand, nano-enabled technologies may play a central role in developing safer, more efficient, and patient-centered therapeutic approaches for long-term diabetes control [49].

13.12 CONCLUSION

Nanotechnology is quickly revolutionizing the face of diabetes diagnosis, monitoring, and therapy with innovative solutions that overcome many limitations of traditional treatment methods. Nano-enabled drug delivery systems, smart insulin platforms, and sophisticated biosensors have shown significant potential to improve therapeutic precision, better drug bioavailability, and real-time glucose monitoring. In addition, new nanotherapeutic strategies of β-cell protection, immune modulation, and tissue regeneration provide promising options for more complete diabetes management. Despite these developments, safety assessment issues, regulatory approval, manufacture scalability, and cost remain important considerations for clinical translation. Continued interdisciplinary research and rigorous clinical validation will be essential to ensure the safe integration of nano-based technologies into routine diabetes care, ultimately improving patient outcomes and long-term disease management.

ACKNOWLEDGMENTS

The authors express special thanks to the editors for providing necessary support and guidance.

REFERENCES

1. Duncan BB, Magliano DJ, Boyko EJ. IDF diabetes atlas 11th edition 2025: Global prevalence and projections for 2050. Nephrology Dialysis Transplantation. 2026;41(1):7–9.
2. Aschner P, Karuranga S, James S, Simmons D, Basit A, Shaw JE, Wild SH, Ogurtsova K, Saeedi P. The International Diabetes Federation's guide for diabetes epidemiological studies. Diabetes Research and Clinical Practice. 2021;172:108630.
3. Feingold KR. Oral and injectable (non-insulin) pharmacological agents for the treatment of type 2 diabetes. [Updated 2025, Dec 29]. In: Feingold KR, Adler RA, Ahmed SF, et al., editors. Endotext [Internet]. South Dartmouth (MA): MDText.com, Inc.; 2000. Available from: https://www.ncbi.nlm.nih.gov/sites/books/NBK279141/.

4. Cappon G, Vettoretti M, Sparacino G, Facchinetti A. Continuous glucose monitoring sensors for diabetes management: A review of technologies and applications. Diabetes & Metabolism Journal. 2019;43(4):383.
5. Luo X, Li N, Zhu X, Xie W, Zhang Q, Liang N, Zhang P, Zhou C. Application of nanomaterials in diabetic complication management. Colloids and Surfaces B: Biointerfaces. 2025;258:115229.
6. Shinde MU, Patwekar M, Patwekar F, Bajaber MA, Medikeri A, Mohammad FS, Mukim M, Soni S, Mallick J, Jawaid T. Nanomaterials: A potential hope for life sciences from bench to bedside. Journal of Nanomaterials. 2022;2022(1):5968131.
7. Gujjar S, Kukal S, Jayabal P, Balaji N, Sainger S, Roy S, Rallapalli S, Mahadevappa R, Minocha S, Kumar S, Mathapati S. Nanomaterials for biomedical applications: Addressing regulatory hurdles and strategic solutions. Nano Trends. 2025;11:100127.
8. Karabasz A, Bzowska M, Szczepanowicz K. Biomedical applications of multifunctional polymeric nanocarriers: A review of current literature. International Journal of Nanomedicine. 2020;6:8673–96.
9. Fateh ST, Aghaii AH, Aminzade Z, Shahriari E, Roohpour N, Koosha F, Dezfuli AS. Inorganic nanoparticle-cored dendrimers for biomedical applications: A review. Heliyon. 2024;10(9):.e29726.
10. Schoenmaker L, Witzigmann D, Kulkarni JA, Verbeke R, Kersten G, Jiskoot W, Crommelin DJ. mRNA-lipid nanoparticle COVID-19 vaccines: Structure and stability. International Journal of Pharmaceutics. 2021;601:120586.
11. John J. Advancements in nano-based drug delivery systems for therapeutics: A comprehensive review. RSC Pharmaceutics. 2025;3(1):43–59.
12. Singh J, Singh NK, Dubey S, Jaiswal G, Srivastava A, Telang SP, Srivastava SK. Novel Molecules and Materials for Drug Discovery. In Experimental and Computational Advances in Materials (pp. 439–472). Springer Nature Singapore; 2026.
13. Liu M, Wang R, Hoi MP, Wang Y, Wang S, Li G, Vong CT, Chong CM. Nano-based drug delivery systems for managing diabetes: Recent advances and future prospects. International Journal of Nanomedicine. 2025;20:6221–52.
14. Elmowafy M, Shalaby K, Elkomy MH, Alsaidan OA, Gomaa HA, Abdelgawad MA, Mostafa EM. Polymeric nanoparticles for delivery of natural bioactive agents: Recent advances and challenges. Polymers. 2023;15(5):1123.
15. Alfatama M, Choukaife H, Alkhatib H, Al Rahal O, Zin NZ. A comprehensive review of oral chitosan drug delivery systems: Applications for oral insulin delivery. Nanotechnology Reviews. 2024;13(1):20230205.
16. Mehta M, Bui TA, Yang X, Aksoy Y, Goldys EM, Deng W. Lipid-based nanoparticles for drug/gene delivery: An overview of the production techniques and difficulties encountered in their industrial development. ACS Materials Au. 2023;3(6):600–19.
17. Pérez-Ferreiro M, Abelairas AM, Criado A, Gómez IJ, Mosquera J. Dendrimers: Exploring their wide structural variety and applications. Polymers. 2023;15(22):4369.
18. Kianfar E, Kadhum WR, Mahmoud ZH. Hydrogel nanoparticles in drug delivery: A review. Intelligent Pharmacy. 2025.
19. Croitoru GA, Pirvulescu DC, Niculescu AG, Grumezescu AM, Antohi AM, Nicolae CL. Metallic nanomaterials–targeted drug delivery approaches for improved bioavailability, reduced side toxicity, and enhanced patient outcomes. Romanian Journal of Morphology and Embryology. 2024;65(2):145.
20. Janjua TI, Cao Y, Kleitz F, Linden M, Yu C, Popat A. Silica nanoparticles: A review of their safety and current strategies to overcome biological barriers. Advanced Drug Delivery Reviews. 2023;203:115115.
21. Veiseh O, Tang BC, Whitehead KA, Anderson DG, Langer R. Managing diabetes with nanomedicine: Challenges and opportunities. Nature Reviews Drug Discovery. 2015;14(1):45–57.
22. Gu Z, Dang TT, Ma M, Tang BC, Cheng H, Jiang S, Dong Y, Zhang Y, Anderson DG. Glucose-responsive microgels integrated with enzyme nanocapsules for closed-loop insulin delivery. ACS Nano. 2013;7(8):6758–66.
23. Hsu HJ, Bugno J, Lee SR, Hong S. Dendrimer-based nanocarriers: A versatile platform for drug delivery. Wiley Interdisciplinary Reviews: Nanomedicine and Nanobiotechnology. 2017;9(1):e1409.
24. Sehit E, Drzazgowska J, Buchenau D, Yesildag C, Lensen M, Altintas Z. Ultrasensitive nonenzymatic electrochemical glucose sensor based on gold nanoparticles and molecularly imprinted polymers. Biosensors and Bioelectronics. 2020;165:112432.
25. Lopes V, Abreu T, Abrantes M, Nemala SS, De Boni F, Prato M, Alpuim P, Capasso A. Graphene-based glucose sensors with an attomolar limit of detection. Journal of the American Chemical Society. 2025;147(15):13059–70.
26. Li C, Liu X, Liu Y, Huang F, Wu G, Liu Y, Zhang Z, Ding Y, Lv J, Ma R, An Y. Glucose and H_2O_2 dual-sensitive nanogels for enhanced glucose-responsive insulin delivery. Nanoscale. 2019;11(18):9163–75.

27. Han Y, Spicer J, Huang Y, Bunt C, Liu M, Wen J. Advancements in oral insulin: A century of research and the emergence of targeted nanoparticle strategies. European Journal of Lipid Science and Technology. 2024;126(7):2300271.
28. Li H, Luo Q, Zhang H, Ma X, Gu Z, Gong Q, Luo K. Nanomedicine embraces cancer radio-immunotherapy: Mechanism, design, recent advances, and clinical translation. Chemical Society Reviews. 2023; 52(1):47–96.
29. Pal S, Rakshit T, Saha S, Jinagal D. Glucose-responsive materials for smart insulin delivery: From protein-based to protein-free design. ACS Materials Au. 2025;5(2):239–52.
30. Kesharwani P, Gorain B, Low SY, Tan SA, Ling EC, Lim YK, Chin CM, Lee PY, Lee CM, Ooi CH, Choudhury H. Nanotechnology based approaches for anti-diabetic drugs delivery. Diabetes Research and Clinical Practice. 2018;136:52–77.
31. Omiyale BO, Ogbeyemi A, Zhang W, Ashraf MA, Song KY. Nanosensors as diagnostic tools: Emerging concepts, opportunities, and design barriers. Analytical Methods. 2026;18(2):238–81.
32. Mihai DA, Stefan DS, Stegaru D, Bernea GE, Vacaroiu IA, Papacocea T, Lupuşoru MO, Nica AE, Stiru O, Dragos D, Olaru OG. Continuous glucose monitoring devices: A brief presentation. Experimental and Therapeutic Medicine. 2022;23(2):174.
33. Waly Y, Hussain A, Al-Majmuei A, Alatoom M, Alaraibi AJ, Alaysereen A, Deen GR. Evolution of biosensors and current state-of-the-art applications in diabetes control. Biosensors. 2026;16(1):39.
34. Baruah A, Newar R, Das S, Kalita N, Nath M, Ghosh P, Chinnam S, Sarma H, Narayan M. Biomedical applications of graphene-based nanomaterials: Recent progress, challenges, and prospects in highly sensitive biosensors. Discover Nano. 2024;19(1):103.
35. Cristelo C, Nunes R, Pinto S, Marques JM, Gama FM, Sarmento B. Targeting β cells with cathelicidin nanomedicines improves insulin function and pancreas regeneration in type 1 diabetic rats. ACS Pharmacology & Translational Science. 2023;6(10):1544–60.
36. Huang F, Lu X, Yang Y, Yang Y, Li Y, Kuai L, Li B, Dong H, Shi J. Microenvironment-based diabetic foot ulcer nanomedicine. Advanced Science. 2023;10(2):2203308.
37. Saifullah Q, Sharma A. Current trends on innovative technologies in topical wound care for advanced healing and management. Current Drug Research Reviews Formerly: Current Drug Abuse Reviews. 2024;16(3):319–32.
38. Liu Y, Wu N. Progress of nanotechnology in diabetic retinopathy treatment. International Journal of Nanomedicine. 2021:1391–403.
39. Bhansali D, Teng SL, Lee CS, Schmidt BL, Bunnett NW, Leong KW. Nanotechnology for pain management: Current and future therapeutic interventions. Nano Today. 2021;39:101223.
40. He Y, Al-Mureish A, Wu N. Nanotechnology in the treatment of diabetic complications: A comprehensive narrative review. Journal of Diabetes Research. 2021;2021(1):6612063.
41. Wu Y, Vazquez-Prada KX, Liu Y, Whittaker AK, Zhang R, Ta HT. Recent advances in the development of theranostic nanoparticles for cardiovascular diseases. Nanotheranostics. 2021;5(4):499.
42. Addissouky TA. Beyond insulin: Advancing frontiers in cell-based and genetic therapies for type 1 diabetes management. The Egyptian Journal of Internal Medicine. 2025 ;37(1):84.
43. Karim AM. Smart antidiabetic nanomedicine: A revolutionized therapeutic approach for treatment of diabetes mellitus. Bioengineering. 2025;12(12):1309.
44. Sharma R, Borah SJ, Kumar S, Gupta A, Kumari V, Kumar R, Dubey KK, Kumar V. Emerging trends in nano-based antidiabetic therapeutics: A path to effective diabetes management. Materials Advances. 2023;4(15):3091–113.
45. Subhan MA, Subhan T. Nanomaterial's Safety Regulations in Food and Drug Industry. In Handbook of Green and Sustainable Nanotechnology: Fundamentals, Developments and Applications (pp. 641–657). Springer International Publishing; 2023.
46. Bartkowski M, Calzaferri F, Giordani S. Toward clinical translation of carbon nanomaterials in anticancer drug delivery: The need for standardisation. Beilstein Journal of Nanotechnology. 2025;16(1):2092–104.
47. Haider R, Das ZA, Zameer GK. S. Revolutionizing patient care: Multidimensional approaches to 21st-century diabetes management. Journal of Heart and Vasculature. 2025;4(6):01–05.
48. Gordijo CR, Koulajian K, Shuhendler AJ, Bonifacio LD, Huang HY, Chiang S, Ozin GA, Giacca A, Wu XY. Nanotechnology-enabled closed loop insulin delivery device: In vitro and in vivo evaluation of glucose-regulated insulin release for diabetes control. Advanced Functional Materials. 2011;21(1):73–82.
49. Adeniyi M, Ayoola VB, Samuel TE, Awosan W. Artificial intelligence-driven wearable electronics and smart nanodevices for continuous cancer monitoring and enhanced diagnostic accuracy. International Journal of Scientific Research and Modern Technology. 2024;3(11):3–18.

14 Green Frontiers
Plant-Based Nanotechnology and Molecular Insights for Next-Generation Diabetes Management

Shilpa Mandpe
School of Pharmacy and Technology Management, NMIMS, Shirpur, India

Dhananjay Pagare
University Institute of Chemical Technology, KBCNMU, Jalgaon, India

Pranita Arun Chaudhari
Shram Sadhana Bombay Trust's Institute of Pharmacy, Jalgaon, India

14.1 INTRODUCTION

Plant-mediated nanotechnology has emerged as a sustainable and biologically compatible strategy for developing next-generation therapeutics for metabolic disorders, especially diabetes mellitus. This approach integrates phytochemistry, nanoscience, and molecular pharmacology to produce nanoparticles using plant-derived biomolecules as reducing and stabilizing agents. Unlike traditional chemical synthesis, green synthesis employs plant extracts rich in flavonoids, phenolics, alkaloids, terpenoids, and tannins, which simultaneously facilitate nanoparticle formation and confer intrinsic biological activity. These phytochemicals act as natural reducing agents that convert metal ions into stable nanostructures while also providing surface functionalization that enhances biocompatibility and therapeutic efficacy [1].

Within the conceptual framework of metabolic diseases management, plant-mediated nanoparticles function through multiple interconnected mechanisms targeting glucose homeostasis, oxidative stress, and inflammatory signaling. Metallic and hybrid nanoparticles like silver (AgNPs), gold (AuNPs), zinc oxide (ZnO), selenium, and iron oxide nanoparticles have been synthesized using medicinal plant extracts and evaluated for antidiabetic activity. These nanomaterials can regulate important metabolic pathways by improving insulin sensitivity, promoting glucose uptake in peripheral tissues, and inhibiting carbohydrate-digestive enzymes such as α-amylase and α-glucosidase, which are responsible for postprandial glucose elevation [2].

Recent experimental studies illustrate the functional relevance of this framework. For example, silver nanoparticles prepared from *Allium sativum* extract have been shown to improve glucose utilization and reduce the hepatic glucose production, while inhibiting α-amylase and α-glucosidase activities, leading to significant decrease in hyperglycemia in cellular and animal models. Likewise, plant-derived nanoparticles prepared from the extracts species such as *Annona muricata*, *Leucosidea sericea*, and *Pisum sativum* show strong inhibitory activity against α-glucosidase, with inhibition values approaching 95% at low microgram concentrations, showing their interesting metabolic regulator capacity [3].

Another dimension of the conceptual framework involves the synergistic integration of phytochemicals with nanoscale delivery systems. The nanoscale size (usually 10–100 nm) increases

DOI: 10.1201/9781003598657-14

surface area and enhances cellular interactions, enabling efficient delivery of plant bioactive to metabolic tissues such as the liver, pancreas, and skeletal muscle. This enhances the pharmacokinetic profile of phytochemicals, including enhanced solubility, bioavailability, and targeted cellular uptake. In addition, the antioxidant effects of phytochemical-coated nanoparticles help mitigate oxidative stress and inflammatory signaling pathways that contribute to β-cell dysfunction and insulin resistance in diabetes [4].

Overall, the conceptual framework of plant-mediated nanotechnology positions phytogenic nanoparticles as multifunctional nanotherapeutics capable of integrating green synthesis principles with molecular-level metabolic regulation. Combining ecological sustainability with advanced nanomedicine creates a promising platform for the intervention of safer and more effective solutions for metabolic disorders, specifically for diabetes management in the future [1–4].

14.2 PHYTOCHEMICAL DRIVERS OF GREEN NANOPARTICLE FORMATION

Plant-mediated green synthesis of nanoparticles relies primarily on the diverse pool of phytochemicals present in plant extracts, which act as natural reducing, capping, and stabilizing agents. Extracts from leaves, roots, fruits, seeds, or barks contain bioactive metabolites capable of converting metal ions into nanoscale particles under mild reaction conditions. These phytochemicals transform metal ions such as Ag^{+}, Au^{3+}, or Zn^{2+} into stable nanoparticles without the need for hazardous chemical or high energy process, making the approach environmentally sustainable and biologically compatible [5].

14.2.1 Reducing and Capping Agents in Plant Extracts

In green synthesis, plant metabolites act as electron donors that reduce metal ions to their elemental nanoparticle form. At the same time, these molecules attach to the nanoparticle surface, forming a protective layer that prevents aggregation and improves stability. Such dual functionality allows plant extracts to serve as both reducing and capping agents during nanoparticle formation. Capping molecules also regulate nanoparticle growth, influencing morphology, size distribution, and surface chemistry. Stabilizing interactions between biomolecules and nanoparticle surfaces improve dispersion and enable controlled synthesis of particles typically ranging between 10 nm and 100 nm [6].

14.2.2 Role of Flavonoids, Terpenoids, Phenolics, and Alkaloids

Several classes of phytochemicals contribute directly to the biosynthesis process. Flavonoids and phenolic acids are among the most active reducing agents, capable of donating electrons to metal ions and initiating nanoparticle nucleation. Terpenoids and alkaloids also participate in stabilization and growth control due to their reactive functional groups and ability to bind metal surfaces. Experimental studies have demonstrated that phenolic compounds and flavonoids in plant extracts can reduce Ag^{+} ions in plant extracts to produce metallic silver nanoparticles, and other compounds like xanthones and phloroglucon may act as capping agents to stabilize the nanostructure [7].

14.2.3 Reaction Pathways in Biogenic Nanoparticles Synthesis

The biosynthesis of plant-mediated nanoparticles follows three distinct steps: reduction of metal ions by phytochemicals, nucleation of reduced atoms into small clusters, and stabilization of the formed nanoparticles by capping molecules. During the reduction stage, electron-rich functional groups (e.g., hydroxyl and carbonyl groups) transfer electrons to the metal ions. This is followed by nucleation and controlled growth of nanocrystals, followed by the stabilization of nanoparticles by surface-bound phytochemicals, which prevent excessive aggregation. Overall, phytochemical-based synthesis is an important mechanistic basis for greening nanotechnology that can provide controllable fabrication of biocompatible nanomaterials for biomedical applications, including advanced therapies for metabolic diseases such as diabetes [8].

14.3 GREEN NANOMATERIAL PLATFORMS DERIVED FROM MEDICINAL PLANTS

Plant-mediated nanotechnology has enabled the development of diverse nanomaterial platforms derived from medicinal plants, combining phytochemical bioactivity with nanoscale delivery systems. These green nanomaterials are increasingly explored for metabolic disease management, as they offer biocompatibility, enhanced therapeutic activity, and environmentally sustainable synthesis processes. Among the most widely studied platforms are metallic nanoparticles, polymeric phytocarriers, and carbon-based or hybrid nanostructures [9]. The development of plant-derived nanotherapeutics involves a multistep pipeline from phytochemical extraction to nanoparticle synthesis, characterization, and biological evaluation (Figure 14.1).

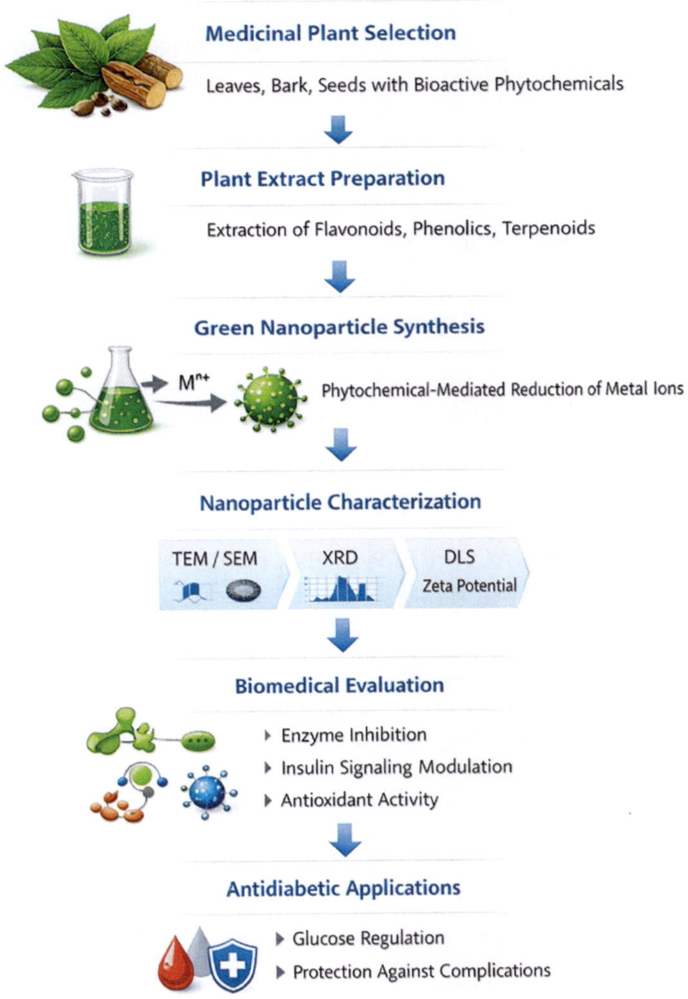

FIGURE 14.1 Green nanotechnology pipeline for plant-based antidiabetic nanomedicines.

14.3.1 Metallic Nanoparticles (Silver, Gold, Zinc Oxide)

Metallic nanoparticles synthesized using plant extracts are one of the most established categories of green nanomaterials. Silver nanoparticles (AgNPs) are particularly prominent due to strong biological activity and relatively simple biosynthesis using plant metabolites such as polyphenols and flavonoids. Several studies have demonstrated that AgNPs synthesized from medicinal plants can inhibit carbohydrate-digesting enzyme systems and improve glucose metabolism in experimental models. Gold nanoparticles AuNPs produced through plant-mediated reduction exhibit excellent stability and surface functionalization properties, enabling their use as drug carriers and biosensing platforms. Zinc oxide nanoparticles (ZnO NPs) synthesized from plant extracts have also demonstrated promising antidiabetic effects, largely due to the role of zinc in insulin synthesis and glucose metabolism [10].

14.3.2 Polymeric Phytocarriers

Polymeric phytocarriers represent another important green nanomaterial platform designed to encapsulate and deliver plant-derived bioactive compounds. Natural polymers such as chitosan, alginate, cellulose derivatives, and plant-based polysaccharides are commonly used to fabricate biodegradable nanocarriers. These systems improve the pharmacokinetic characteristic of phytochemicals by improving solubility, protecting sensitive compounds from degradation, and enabling controlled drug release. For example, nano-encapsulation of plant polyphenols has been reported to significantly improve intestinal absorption and metabolic stability, thereby enhancing their therapeutic potentials in metabolic disorders [11].

14.3.3 Carbon-Based and Hybrid Nanostructures

Carbon-based nanomaterials synthesized through green routes – including carbon dots, graphene derivatives, and biochar-derived nanostructures – have recently gained attention in biomedical applications. These nanomaterials often possess strong antioxidant properties and favorable surface chemistry that facilitate functionalization with plant bioactives. Hybrid nanostructures combining metallic nanoparticles with polymeric or carbon-based matrices further expand the functional capabilities of green nanomaterials by integrating multiple therapeutic mechanisms within a single nanosystem [12].

14.4 MOLECULAR INTERFACES BETWEEN PHYTONANOPARTICLES AND GLUCOSE METABOLISM

Plant-derived nanoparticles (phytonanoparticles) interact with multiple molecular pathways involved in glucose regulation, which makes them good candidates for advanced diabetes management. These nanosystems combine the intrinsic bioactivity of phytochemicals with enhanced cellular uptake and targeted delivery, allowing modulation of key enzymes, signaling cascades, and β-cell function associated with metabolic homeostasis [13]. Plant-derived nanomaterials interact with multiple metabolic targets including digestive enzymes, insulin signaling pathways, oxidative stress mechanisms, and tissue repair processes, highlighting their multifunctional therapeutic potential (Table 14.1).

14.4.1 Enzyme Modulation (α-Amylase, α-Glucosidase, DPP-4)

One of the main molecular mechanisms of phytonanoparticles is the inhibition of carbohydrate-digesting enzymes, such as α-amylase and α-glucosidase. These enzymes are responsible for breaking down complex carbohydrates into absorbable glucose; therefore, their inhibition slows

TABLE 14.1
Functional Roles of Plant-Derived Nanomaterials in Diabetes Management

Functional Target	Mechanistic Role of Phytonanoparticles	Therapeutic Outcome
Digestive enzymes	Inhibition of α-glucosidase	Reduced postprandial glucose levels
Insulin signaling	Activation of PI3K/Akt and AMPK pathways	Improved glucose uptake and insulin sensitivity
Oxidative stress	Scavenging reactive oxygen species (ROS)	Protection of pancreatic β-cells
Inflammatory pathways	Modulation of NF-κB signaling	Reduced metabolic inflammation
Tissue repair	Enhanced angiogenesis and collagen deposition	Improved diabetic wound healing

intestinal glucose release and reduces postprandial hyperglycemia. Experimental studies show that plant-mediated nanoparticles can achieve strong inhibitory activity against these enzymes. For instance, zinc oxide nanoparticles synthesized from *Moringa oleifera* extracts exhibited about 90% α-amylase inhibition and 96% α-glucosidase inhibition at 100 μg/mL, significantly exceeding the activity of crude plant extracts [14].

Additionally, phytochemicals present on nanoparticle surfaces can interact with dipeptidyl peptidase-4 (DPP-4), an enzyme responsible for the degradation of incretin hormones that stimulate insulin secretion. Inhibiting DPP-4 prolongs incretin activity and favors improved glycemic control [15].

14.4.2 Insulin Signaling Pathways (PI3K/Akt and AMPK)

Beyond enzyme inhibition, phytonanoparticles influence intracellular signaling pathways that regulate glucose uptake and insulin sensitivity. Phytochemicals such as polypehenols and flavonoids present in plant-based nanomaterials can activate AMP-activated protein kinase (AMPK) and PI3K/Akt signaling pathway, which promote glucose transport and metabolic regulation in skeletal muscle and adipose tissues. Activation of these pathways enhances insulin sensitivity and improves cellular glucose utilization [16].

14.4.3 Effects on Pancreatic β-Cell Preservation

Another important interface involves protection and regeneration of pancreatic β-cells. Chronic hyperglycemia produces oxidative stress and inflammatory responses that damage β-cells and impair insulin secretion. Phytonanoparticles possess strong antioxidant and anti-inflammatory properties derived from plant metabolites, enabling them to reduce oxidative damage and promote β-cells survival. Emerging studies suggest that plant-based metallic nanoparticles, including gold and silver nanoparticles, can improve insulin secretion and support β-cell regeneration in experimental diabetic models [17]. Plant-derived nanoparticles exert antidiabetic effects through multiple molecular mechanisms, including enzyme inhibition, insulin signaling modulation, antioxidant activity, and inhibition of inflammatory pathways (Figure 14.2).

14.5 ANTIOXIDANT AND ANTI-INFLAMMATORY NANOMECHANISM

Oxidative stress and low-grade chronic inflammation are the key factors in the development of diabetes and complications related to this disease. Hyperglycemia promotes the overproduction of ROS in metabolism organs like pancreas, liver, and vascular endothelium resulting in lipids, proteins, and DNA damages. Plant-derived nanoparticles (phytonanoparticles) offer a promising strategy to overcome these pathological processes since they integrate the inherent antioxidant activity of phytochemicals with enhanced interactions with the cells of nanoscale materials [18].

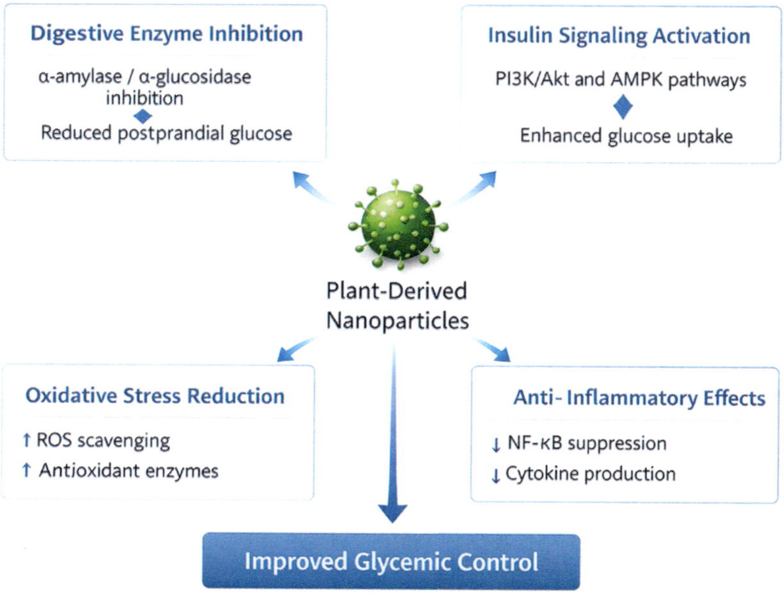

FIGURE 14.2 Mechanistic pathways of plant-derived nanoparticle in diabetes regulation.

14.5.1 Regulation of ROS and Oxidative Stress Pathways

Many phytonanoparticles exhibit strong free-radical scavenging activity due to the presence of polyphenols, flavonoids, and other antioxidant compounds on their surface. These biomolecules neutralize ROS such as superoxide radicals, hydroxyl radicals, and hydrogen peroxide, thereby reducing oxidative damage to cellular structures. Flavonoids including myricetin and related phenolic compounds can directly scavenge ROS and stimulate endogenous antioxidant enzymes such as those in the glutathione-related systems, which help maintain redox balance in metabolic tissues [19].

Recent studies also demonstrate that green-synthesized zinc oxide nanoparticles produced from medicinal plant extracts display enhanced antioxidant activity compared with crude plant extracts, highlighting the synergistic effect of nanoscale formulation.

14.5.2 NF-κB and Inflammatory Signaling Modulation

Inflammatory signaling pathways play a crucial role in insulin resistance and β-cell dysfunction. The nuclear factor-κB (NF-κB) pathway is a central regulator of inflammation gene expression, controlling cytokines such as TNF-α and IL-6 and inducible nitric oxide synthase (iNOS). Activation of NF-κB is often triggered by ROS accumulation and inflammatory cytokines in diabetic tissues [20].

Plant-derived bioactive compounds and their nanoformulations can inhibit NF-κB activation, thereby reducing inflammatory response and enhancing metabolic regulation. For example, phytochemicals such as quercetin and lignan like honokiol have been shown to reduce inflammatory mediators production through NF-κB pathways inhibition [21].

14.5.3 Protection against Diabetic Complications

By simultaneously modulating oxidative stress and inflammatory signaling, phytonanoparticles can protect against diabetes-associated complications. Experimental nanomedicine studies show that phytochemical-based nanoformulations reduce cellular apoptosis and oxidative damage in diabetic tissues, including retinal cells implicated diabetic retinopathy [22].

14.6 NANO-ENABLED ENHANCEMENT OF PLANT BIOACTIVE PHARMACOKINETICS

Many plant-derived bioactive compounds demonstrate significant antidiabetic potential; however, their clinical application is often limited by poor pharmacokinetic properties such as low aqueous solubility, limited intestinal absorption, rapid metabolism, and short systemic half-life. Nanotechnology-based delivery systems have emerged as an effective strategy to overcome these barriers by enhancing solubility, stability, and bioavailability of phytochemicals. Nano-enabled formulations, including polymeric nanoparticles, lipid-based nanocarriers, and phytochemicals-loaded nanoemulsions, provide controlled delivery platforms that enhance therapeutic efficacy in metabolic disorders such as diabetes [23].

14.6.1 Solubility Enhancement

A major challenge in phytopharmaceutical development is the poor water solubility of many plant bioactives, including flavonoids, polyphenols, and terpenoids. Nanotechnology can significantly enhance the apparent solubility of these compounds by decreasing particle size and increasing surface area. When phytochemicals are encapsulated within nanoparticles, they become dispersed in nanoscale matrices that improve dissolution in biological fluids. For example, nanoformulations of curcumin – an important plant-derived polyphenol – have been shown to increase aqueous solubility by several folds and improve systemic bioavailability compared with conventional formulations. Similar enhancements have been reported for other phytochemicals such as quercetin and resveratrol when delivering polymeric and lipid-based nanoparticles [24].

14.6.2 Targeted Delivery and Sustainable Release

Nanocarriers also facilitated delivery of plant bioactives to metabolically-relevant tissues such as the liver, pancreas, and adipose tissue. Surface functionalization of nanoparticles with natural biomolecules enables selective interaction with cellular receptors, improving therapeutic localization while reducing systemic side effects. In addition, nano-encapsulation enables sustained and controlled drug release, which maintains stable therapeutic concentrations over extended periods. For example, in experimental drug-delivery studies, chitosan-based nanoparticles loaded with plant polyphenols have shown extended release characteristics, lasting several hours to days, thereby improving glycemic control in preclinical mice [25].

14.6.3 Improved Intestinal Absorption

Another benefit of nanoscale delivery system is increased intestinal permeability. Nanoparticles can interact with epithelial cells and facilitate transcellular or paracellular transport across the gastrointestinal barrier. This improves oral bioavailability of phytochemicals that would otherwise have poor absorption. Studies have shown that nano-encapsulated polyphenols exhibit significantly higher intestinal uptake and systemic circulation levels compared with free compounds. Additionally, biodegradable nanocarriers such as chitosan nanoparticles can transiently open tight junctions in intestinal epithelium, thereby further enhancing absorption [26].

Collectively, nano-enabled delivery technologies provide a powerful platform for improving the pharmacokinetic performance of plant bioactives. By improving solubility, facilitating targeted and sustained delivery, and improving intestinal absorption, these systems drastically improve the therapeutic potential of phytochemicals for the next-generation diabetes management [27].

14.7 EXPERIMENTAL EVIDENCE OF PLANT-DERIVED NANOTHERAPEUTICS IN DIABETES

Growing experimental evidence supports the therapeutic potential of plant-derived nanotherapeutics in diabetes management. Studies conducted at both cellular and animal level demonstrate that nanoparticles synthesized using medicinal plant extracts can modulate the glucose metabolism, enhance antioxidant status, and decrease hyperglycemia more effectively than many conventional phytotherapies [28].

14.7.1 In Vitro Mechanistic Studies

In vitro investigations provide important information insights into the molecular mechanisms of phytonanoparticles. Several studies have shown that plant-mediated metallic nanoparticles can inhibit carbohydrate-digesting enzymes such as α-amylase and α -glucosidase, thereby decreasing glucose release from dietary carbohydrates. For example, biosynthesized silver nanoparticles (AgNPs) have shown high inhibition of α-amylase activity and increased glucose uptake in experimental cell-based assays, suggesting their potential role in the regulation postprandial glucose levels [29].

Another mechanistic study involving AgNPs synthesized from *Allium sativum* reported that the nanoparticles enhanced cellular glucose utilization while decreasing hepatic glucose production and inhibiting key digestive enzymes. These findings show that phytonanoparticles can directly respond with metabolic pathway responsible for glucose regulation [30].

14.7.2 In Vivo Antidiabetic Efficacy in Animal Models

Animal experiments further confirm the antidiabetic efficacy of plant-derived nanotherapeutics. Most studies employ streptozotocin (STZ)-induced diabetic rodent models, which mimic many metabolic features of human diabetes. In one investigation, silver nanoparticles synthesized using plant extracts demonstrated significant antidiabetic activity in STZ-induced diabetic rats, resulting in improved glycemic control and biochemical parameters with untreated diabetic groups [31].

Similarly, green-synthesized nanoparticles from medicinal plants such as *Azadirachta indica* and *Fagonia cretica* have been evaluated in experimental animal models. These nanoparticles reduced blood glucose levels, enhanced lipid profile, and alleviated oxidative stress markers in diabetic animals, indicating broad metabolic benefits [32].

In another experimental study, the biogenic silver nanoparticles made from plant extracts improved oxidative biomarkers and metabolic parameters in type-2 diabetic rats significantly, showing both antidiabetic and antioxidant actions [33].

14.7.3 Comparative Performance with Conventional Phytotherapy

Comparative studies indicate that nanoparticle-based formulations often outperform crude plant extracts due to enhanced increased bioavailability and cellular interaction. When phytochemicals coat nanoparticle surfaces, a synergistic effect occurs between intrinsic biological activity of plant metabolites and the nanoscale delivery system [34].

Furthermore, in laboratory experiments, certain green-synthesized nanoparticles have demonstrated stronger enzyme-inhibitory effects than conventional antidiabetic medications like acarbose, indicating their significant potential for metabolic regulation [35].

Overall, evidence from in vitro assays and in vivo animal studies demonstrates that plant-derived nanotherapeutics can effectively modulate glucose metabolism, reduce oxidative stress, and improve metabolic parameters. These findings indicate that phytonanotechnology may offer promising pathway for developing safer and more effective next-generation treatments for diabetes [34, 35].

14.8 GENE NANOTECHNOLOGY FOR DIABETIC COMPLICATION MANAGEMENT

Diabetes is frequently associated with long-term complications affecting the nervous system, kidneys, and skin, largely driven by persistent hyperglycemia, oxidative stress, and chronic inflammation. Green nanotechnology, specifically plant-derived nanoparticles, has shown promising potential in addressing these complications through antioxidant, anti-inflammatory, and tissue-regenerative mechanisms [36].

14.8.1 Diabetic Neuropathy

Diabetic neuropathy results from prolonged oxidative stress and microvascular damage that impair nerve function. Phytochemical-mediated nanoparticles have potent antioxidant functions to help lower ROS and inflammatory signaling molecules in neural tissues. Experimental studies have shown that plant-derived nanoparticles protect neuronal cells by restoring antioxidant enzyme activity and reducing inflammatory cytokines related to nerve damage [37].

14.8.2 Diabetic Nephropathy

Diabetic nephropathy is a leading cause of chronic kidney disease in diabetics and is characterized by glomerular injury, oxidative stress, and inflammatory responses. Plant-based nanoparticles containing polyphenols and flavonoids have shown nephroprotective effects in experimental models by reducing oxidative stress markers and improving renal biochemical parameters. These nanomaterials may help preserve kidney function by modulating inflammatory pathways and protecting renal cells from hyperglycemia-induced damage [38].

14.8.3 Diabetic Wound Healing

Impaired wound healing is a common complication of diabetes due to poor vascularization, infection susceptibility, and inflammation. Green-synthesized nanoparticles – especially silver nanoparticles produced using medicinal plant extracts – have demonstrated antimicrobial, anti-inflammatory, and tissue repair properties. These nanoparticles enhance collagen deposition and promote epithelial regeneration, and stimulate faster wound closure in diabetic wound models, suggesting their potential as advanced therapeutic material for diabetic wound management [39].

14.9 BIOFABRICATION CHALLENGES AND STANDARDIZATION ISSUES

Despite the growing interest in plant-mediated nanotechnology, several biofabrication challenges remain that limit the large-scale translation of green-synthesized nanoparticles into biomedical applications. These challenges are mainly associated with variability in plant extracts, reproducibility of synthesis protocols, and issues of stability and scalability, which can significantly influence nanoparticles quality and therapeutic performance.

14.9.1 Variability in Plant Extract Composition

One of the main drawbacks of plant-mediated nanoparticle synthesis is the chemical variability of plant extracts. The concentration and composition of phytochemicals – such as flavonoids, phenolics, terpenoids, and proteins – can vary depending on plant species, geographic location, seasonal changes, and extraction methods. This variability directly affects the reduction and stabilization processes during nanoparticle formation, often leading to differences in particle size, morphology, and surface chemistry. Additionally, the complexity of plant extracts makes it hard to determine what specific biomolecules are responsible for nanoparticle nucleation and stabilization, further complicating process standardization quality control [40].

14.9.2 Reproducibility of Nanoparticle Synthesis

Reproducibility is another significant challenge in green nanoparticle fabrication. Variations in synthesis parameters – such as pH, temperature, precursor concentration, reaction time, and plant extract dosage – can lead to inconsistent nanoparticle properties across experiments. Even small changes in reaction conditions may change particle size distribution, shape, and stability, thereby affecting biological performance. Furthermore, the lack of universally accepted synthesis protocols and standardized characterization methods makes it difficult to compare results across different studies or laboratories [41].

14.9.3 Stability and Scalability Concerns

Another major barrier to clinical and industrial translation is ensuring long-term stability and scalable production of plant-derived nanoparticles. Although phytochemicals can act as natural capping agents, nanoparticles may still undergo aggregation or physicochemical changes during storage, which can reduce their effectiveness. Scaling up the green synthesis process from laboratory to industrial production also presents technical challenges, including maintaining consistent nanoparticle quality, controlling reaction kinetics, and optimizing extraction procedures [42].

14.10 SAFETY, TOXICOLOGICAL PROFILING, AND ENVIRONMENTAL SUSTAINABILITY

The safety and environmental compatibility of plant-mediated nanoparticles are critical considerations for their biomedical application. Although green synthesis avoids toxic chemical reagents, nanoscale properties of these materials can still affect biological interaction and potential toxicity. Toxicological profiling therefore involves the systematic assessment of cytotoxicity, genotoxicity, biodistribution, and deposition persistence in biological systems. In vitro and in vivo studies have demonstrated that many plant-derived nanoparticles have relatively low toxicity when compared with chemically synthesized nanoparticles because of phytochemical capping layers, which increase biocompatibility and reduce oxidative stress [5].

Environmental sustainability is one of the other benefits of operating on plant-based nanotechnology. Green synthesis usually takes place under mild conditions without using dangerous solvents, which results in less environmental pollution and less energy consumption. Additionally, bio-degradable plant metabolite stabilizing agents minimize the possible ecological risks of nanoparticle production and disposal. Nevertheless, life-cycle assessment/regulatory frameworks are required to guarantee the safe large-scale application of green nanomaterials in biomedical and environmental scenarios [43].

14.11 TRANSLATIONAL CLINICAL PROSPECTS OF PLANT-BASED NANOMEDICINE

Plant-based nanomedicine represents a promising translational pathway for developing safer and more effective therapeutics for metabolic disorders such as diabetes. By integrating bioactive phytochemicals with nanoscale delivery systems, these formulations can enhance drug stability, bioavailability, and targeted tissue distribution. Such advantages may help overcome the pharmacokinetic limitations that often restrict the clinical use of many plant-derived compounds [44].

Preclinical studies have shown promising antidiabetic activity with plant-mediated nanoparticles, including improved glycemic control, enhanced antioxidant defense, and decreased inflammatory response in experimental models. These findings show great potential for translation into clinical therapeutics. In addition, the natural origin of phytochemicals and environmentally friendly synthesis methods align with the increasing demand for sustainable and biocompatible medical technologies [44].

However, successful clinical translation requires rigorous standardization of synthesis protocols, comprehensive toxicological evaluation, and compliance with regulatory frameworks to ensure consistent quality, safety, and therapeutic efficacy of plant-based nanomedicine products [44].

14.12 FUTURE DIRECTIONS IN PHYTONANOTECHNOLOGY FOR PRECISION DIABETES

Phytonanotechnology is expected to play an increasingly important role in precision medicine strategies for diabetes management. Future research is likely to focus on designing multifunctional nanoparticles that integrate plant-derived bioactives with advanced nanocarriers capable of targeted and responsive drug delivery. Such systems may enable controlled release of therapeutic agents in response to physiological triggers such as glucose levels, thereby improving treatment precision and minimizing adverse effects [31].

Another promising direction involves the integration of phytonanotechnology with emerging technologies such as artificial intelligence-assisted drug discovery and nanobiosensors. These tools can facilitate the identification of effective phytochemicals, optimize nanoparticle design, and enable personalized therapeutic strategies based on patient-specific metabolic profiles [45].

Additionally, efforts toward standardized green synthesis protocols, scalable manufacturing processes, and comprehensive safety evaluation will be essential for translating phytonanotechnology into clinical practice, ultimately supporting the development of sustainable and patient-specific nanomedicine for diabetes care [46].

14.13 CONCLUSION

Plant-based nanotechnology represents a rapidly advancing frontier in the development of innovative therapeutic strategies for diabetes management. By integrating phytochemistry with nanoscience, plant-mediated nanoparticles offer multifunctional advantages, including enhanced bioavailability of plant bioactives, enhanced antioxidant, anti-inflammatory effects, and targeted modulation of metabolic pathways involved in glucose regulation. Experimental evidences from in vitro and in vivo studies suggest that phytonanoparticles can effectively exert their effects through mechanisms such as enzyme inhibition, insulin signaling, and the protection of pancreatic β-cells.

Moreover, green synthesis approaches offer environmentally sustainable alternatives to conventional nanoparticle fabrication while enhancing biocompatibility through phytochemical surface functionalization. Despite these promising advances, challenges related to synthesis standardization, safety evaluation, and clinical translation remain. Continued interdisciplinary research will be essential to harness the full potential of phytonanotechnology for developing next-generation, precision-based therapeutics for diabetes and related metabolic disorders.

ACKNOWLEDGMENTS

The authors express special thanks to the editors for providing necessary support and guidance.

REFERENCES

1. Karnwal A, Jassim AY, Mohammed AA, Sharma V, Al-Tawaha AR, Sivanesan I. Nanotechnology for healthcare: Plant-derived nanoparticles in disease treatment and regenerative medicine. Pharmaceuticals. 2024;17(12):1711.

2. Soenen SJ, Parak WJ, Rejman J, Manshian B. Intra cellular stability of inorganic nanoparticles: Effects on cytotoxicity, particle functionality, and biomedical applications. Chemical Reviews. 2015;115(5):2109–35.
3. Jini D, Sharmila SJ. Green synthesis of silver nanoparticles from *Allium cepa* and its in vitro antidiabetic activity. Materials Today: Proceedings. 2020;22:432–38.
4. Sahoo S, Behera A, Acharya B, Patra D. Recent advances in eco-Friendly bionanocomposites for drug delivery of natural bioactive compounds: A sustainable approach. Nano Trends. 2026;13:100188.
5. Singh H, Desimone MF, Pandya S, Jasani S, George N, Adnan M, Aldarhami A, Bazaid AS, Alderhami SA. Revisiting the green synthesis of nanoparticles: Uncovering influences of plant extracts as reducing agents for enhanced synthesis efficiency and its biomedical applications. International Journal of Nanomedicine. 2023;18:4727–50.
6. Sorbiun M, Shayegan Mehr E, Ramazani A, Mashhadi Malekzadeh A. Biosynthesis of metallic nanoparticles using plant extracts and evaluation of their antibacterial properties. Nanochemistry Research. 2018;3(1):1–6.
7. Lakhani KG, Hamid R, Motamedi E, Marviya GV. A review on plant metabolite-mediated nanoparticle synthesis: Sustainable applications in horticultural crops. Frontiers in Nanotechnology. 2025;7:1545413.
8. Singaravelu S, Motsoene F, Abrahamse H, Dhilip Kumar SS. Green-synthesized metal nanoparticles: A promising approach for accelerated wound healing. Frontiers in Bioengineering and Biotechnology. 2025;13:1637589.
9. Ghosh S, Solanki R, Bhatia D, Sankaranarayanan S. Nanomaterials for delivery of medicinal plant extracts and phytochemicals: Potential applications and future perspectives. Plant Nano Biology. 2025;12:100161.
10. Morgan RN, Aboshanab KM. Green Biologically synthesized metal nanoparticles: Biological applications, optimizations and future prospects. Future Science OA. 2024;10(1):FSO935.
11. Kotenkova E, Kotov A, Nikitin M. Polysaccharide-based nanocarriers for natural antimicrobials: A review. Polymers. 2025;17(13):1750.
12. Dutta V, Verma R, Gopalkrishnan C, Yuan MH, Batoo KM, Jayavel R, Chauhan A, Lin KY, Balasubramani R, Ghotekar S. Bio-inspired synthesis of carbon-based nanomaterials and their potential environmental applications: A state-of-the-art review. Inorganics. 2022;10(10):169.
13. Chiome TJ, Srinivasan A. Phytonanotechnology: Phytonanoformulations and Their Applications in Cancer Therapy. In Medicinal Plants for Cosmetics, Health and Diseases (pp. 229–250). CRC Press; 2022.
14. Zhu J, Chen C, Zhang B, Huang Q. The inhibitory effects of flavonoids on α-amylase and α-glucosidase. Critical Reviews in Food Science and Nutrition. 2020;60(4):695–708.
15. Chhabria S, Mathur S, Vadakan S, Sahoo DK, Mishra P, Paital B. A review on phytochemical and pharmacological facets of tropical ethnomedicinal plants as reformed DPP-IV inhibitors to regulate incretin activity. Frontiers in Endocrinology. 2022;13:1027237.
16. Prakash G, Chaudhary AA, Tanu R, Ali MA, Boufahja F, Sharma PK, Lakhawat SS, Yadav T, Upadhyay NK, Kumar V. Harnessing phytochemicals and nanotechnology synergy for molecular, epigenetic, and Microbiota-driven regulation in type 2 diabetes mellitus. Pharmaceutics. 2026;18(1):113.
17. Dinić S, Arambašić Jovanović J, Uskoković A, Mihailović M, Grdović N, Tolić A, Rajić J, Đorđević M, Vidaković M. Oxidative stress-mediated beta cell death and dysfunction as a target for diabetes management. Frontiers in Endocrinology. 2022;13:1006376.
18. Cecerska-Heryć E, Engwert W, Michałów J, Marciniak J, Birger R, Serwin N, Heryć R, Polikowska A, Goszka M, Wojciuk B, Wiśniewska M. Oxidative stress markers and inflammation in type 1 and 2 diabetes are affected by BMI, treatment type, and complications. Scientific Reports. 2025;15(1):23605.
19. Zahra M, Abrahamse H, George BP. Flavonoids: Antioxidant powerhouses and their role in nanomedicine. Antioxidants. 2024;13(8):922.
20. Berbudi A, Khairani S, Tjahjadi AI. Interplay between insulin resistance and immune dysregulation in type 2 diabetes mellitus: Implications for therapeutic interventions. ImmunoTargets and Therapy. 2025;14:359–82.
21. Laurindo LF, Santos AR, Carvalho AC, Bechara MD, Guiguer EL, Goulart RD, Vargas Sinatora R, Araújo AC, Barbalho SM. Phytochemicals And regulation of NF-kB in inflammatory bowel diseases: An overview of in vitro and in vivo effects. Metabolites. 2023;13(1):96.
22. Akpoveso OO, Ubah EE, Obasanmi G. Antioxidant phytochemicals as potential therapy for diabetic complications. Antioxidants. 2023;12(1):123.
23. Yan Y, Sun Y, Li Y, Wang Z, Xue L, Wang F. Advancing cancer therapy: Nanomaterial-based encapsulation strategies for enhanced delivery and efficacy of curcumin. Materials Today Bio. 2025;33:101963.
24. Yadav H, Mahalvar A, Pradhan M, Yadav K, Sahu KK, Yadav R. Exploring the potential of phytochemicals and nanomaterial: A boon to antimicrobial treatment. Medicine in Drug Discovery. 2023;17:100151.

25. Kim M, Shin M, Zhao Y, Ghosh M, Son YO. Transformative impact of nanocarrier-mediated drug delivery: Overcoming biological barriers and expanding therapeutic horizons. Small Science. 2024;4(11):2400280.
26. Hao M, Tan X, Liu K, Xin N. Nanoencapsulation of nutraceuticals: Enhancing stability and bioavailability in functional foods. Frontiers in Nutrition. 2025;12:1746176.
27. Mehta J, Pathania K, Pawar SV. Recent overview of nanotechnology based approaches for targeted delivery of nutraceuticals. Sustainable Food Technology. 2025;3(4):947–78.
28. Sharma DK, Pattnaik G, Behera A. Recent developments in nanoparticles for the treatment of diabetes. Journal of Drug Targeting. 2023;31(9):908–19.
29. Husain S, Nandi A, Simnani FZ, Saha U, Ghosh A, Sinha A, Sahay A, Samal SK, Panda PK, Verma SK. Emerging trends in advanced translational applications of silver nanoparticles: A progressing dawn of nanotechnology. Journal of Functional Biomaterials. 2023;14(1):47.
30. Jini D, Sharmila S, Anitha A, Pandian M, Rajapaksha RM. In vitro and in silico studies of silver nanoparticles (AgNPs) from Allium sativum against diabetes. Scientific Reports. 2022;12(1):22109.
31. Sarkhel S, Shuvo SM, Ansari MA, Mondal S, Kapat P, Ghosh A, Sarkar T, Biswas R, Atanase LI, Carauleanu A. Nanotechnology-based approaches for the management of diabetes mellitus: An innovative solution to long-lasting challenges in Antidiabetic drug delivery. Pharmaceutics. 2024;16(12):1572.
32. Khan HA, Ghufran M, Shams S, Jamal A, Khan A, Abdullah, Awan ZA, Khan MI. Green synthesis of silver nanoparticles from plant *Fagonia cretica* and evaluating its anti-diabetic activity through indepth in-vitro and in-vivo analysis. Frontiers in Pharmacology. 2023;14:1194809.
33. Wahab M, Janaswamy S. A review on biogenic silver nanoparticles as efficient and effective antidiabetic agents. Functional Food Science-Online ISSN: 2767-3146. 2023;3(7):93–107.
34. Antonelli A, Palma F. Nanocarrier-based delivery systems for natural compounds across research stages. Materials. 2025;18(21):4960.
35. Rehman G, Umar M, Shah N, Hamayun M, Ali A, Khan W, Khan A, Ahmad S, Alrefaei AF, Almutairi MH, Moon YS. Green synthesis and characterization of silver nanoparticles using *Azadirachta indica* seeds extract: In vitro and in vivo evaluation of anti-diabetic activity. Pharmaceuticals. 2023;16(12):1677.
36. Xiao X, Guo Y, Msomi NZ, Islam MS, Chu M. Exosome-like nanoparticles extracted from plant cells for diabetes therapy. International Journal of Molecular Sciences. 2025;26(18):9155.
37. Ramana KV, Reddy AB, Majeti NR, Singhal SS. Therapeutic potential of natural antioxidants. Oxidative Medicine and Cellular Longevity. 2018;2018:9471051.
38. Jin Q, Liu T, Qiao Y, Liu D, Yang L, Mao H, Ma F, Wang Y, Peng L, Zhan Y. Oxidative stress and inflammation in diabetic nephropathy: Role of polyphenols. Frontiers in Immunology. 2023;14:1185317.
39. Nandhini J, Karthikeyan E, Rani EE, Karthikha VS, Sanjana DS, Jeevitha H, Rajeshkumar S, Venugopal V, Priyadharshan A. Advancing engineered approaches for sustainable wound regeneration and repair: Harnessing the potential of green synthesized silver nanoparticles. Engineered Regeneration. 2024;5(3):306–25.
40. Hanna DH, Nady DS, Wasef MW, Fakhry MH, Mohamed FS, Isaac DM, Kirolos MM, Azmy MS, Hakeem GE, Fathy CA. Plant-derived nanoparticles: Green synthesis, factors, and bioactivities. Next Materials. 2025;9:101275.
41. Kirubakaran D, Wahid JB, Karmegam N, Jeevika R, Sellapillai L, Rajkumar M, SenthilKumar KJ. A comprehensive review on the green synthesis of nanoparticles: Advancements in biomedical and environmental applications. Biomedical Materials & Devices. 2026;4(1):388–413.
42. Kumarasamy RV, Natarajan PM, Mathivanan I, Balasubramaniam M, SN S, Prabhu D, Raju K, Mironescu M, Mironescu ID. Sustainable biogenic synthesis of silver nanoparticles for oral cancer: A comprehensive review. Frontiers in Nanotechnology. 2025;7:1648900.
43. Raut SS, Sharma A, Yadav R, Kumar S, Shukla A, Singh A, Mishra A. Biological green synthesis of nanoparticles: A sustainable platform for agricultural, environmental, food, and cosmetic applications. Journal of Environmental Chemical Engineering. 2026;14(1):121102.
44. Elayaperumal S, Sivamani Y, Agarwal P, Srivastava N. Plant-based nanotherapeutics: A new frontier in disease management and prevention. Nano TransMed. 2025;4:100086.
45. Yang X, Li Q, Tang L, Huang L, Zhu C, Chen Q. Nano-reagents in acute pancreatitis: Diagnostic, therapeutic, and theranostic advances. International Journal of Nanomedicine. 2026;1(562220).
46. Lawal H, Saeed SI, Gaddafi MS, Kamaruzzaman NF. Green nanotechnology: Naturally sourced nanoparticles as antibiofilm and antivirulence agents against infectious diseases. International Journal of Microbiology. 2025;2025(1):8746754.

15 Interdisciplinary Research Approaches in Nanotechnology for Diabetes Management

K. S. Lalithaa
Vinayaka Mission's Homoeopathic Medical College & Hospital, Vinayaka Mission's Research Foundation (Deemed to be University), Salem, India

Ajay Kumar Gupta
School of Pharmaceutical Sciences (formerly University Institute of Pharmacy), C.S.J.M. University Campus (formerly Kanpur University), Kanpur, India

Pallawi P.
Patna College of Pharmacy, Patna, India

A. Rajendiran
School of Pharmaceutical Sciences, CSJM University (formerly Kanpur University), Kanpur, India

Vivek Sakthidharan
Govt. Homoeopathic Medical College, Thiruvananthapuram, India

T. Nayaki
Excel Homoeopathy Medical College, Namakkal, India

Mohammad Ali
Sri Adichunchanagiri College of Pharmacy, Adichunchanagiri University, Mandya, India

15.1 INTRODUCTION

Diabetes mellitus is a major global health challenges characterized by chronic hyperglycemia and metabolic dysregulation. According to recent global estimates, approximately 830 million adults are living with diabetes in 2024, and prevalence is projected to continue increasing in the coming decades, reaching nearly 783 million cases by 2045. This mounting burden contributes to serious complications including cardiovascular disease, kidney failure, neuropathy, and blindness, creating significant public health and economic challenges worldwide. Conventional therapeutic approaches, including insulin injection and oral hypoglycemic drugs, often face limitations such as

DOI: 10.1201/9781003598657-15

poor bioavailability, suboptimal pharmacokinetics, and challenges in maintaining tight glycemic control. Consequently, there is increasing interest in innovative technologies that can enable more precise and patient-centered diabetes management [1].

The complexity of diabetes pathophysiology requires research strategies that go beyond a single discipline. Nanotechnology has emerged as a transformative field capable of addressing several therapeutic and diagnostic challenges in diabetes through nanoscale drug carriers, biosensors, and intelligent delivery systems. These nanoscale platforms can enhance drug stability, improve targeted delivery, and provide controlled release of therapeutic agents. For example, nanoparticle-based insulin delivery systems have shown the ability to protect insulin from degradation and improve intestinal absorption in preclinical studies. Similarly, glucose-response nanoparticles capable of releasing insulin in response elevated glucose levels represent a promising strategy for mimicking physiological insulin secretion. The development of such systems requires the integration of expertise from materials science, pharmacology, biomedical engineering, and molecular biology, highlighting the importance of interdisciplinary collaboration in advancing nanomedicine for diabetic patients [2].

Recent advances in diabetes management illustrate a growing convergence between nanotechnology, medical sciences, and digital health technologies. Nanomaterials enable the fabrication of highly sensitive biosensors capable of real-time monitoring of glucose and other metabolic biomarkers. These nanosensors provide enhanced sensitivity and selectivity due to their large surface area and peculiar physicochemical features. When coupled into wearable device and data analytics platforms, such systems allow continuous glucose monitoring (CGM) and facilitate personalized therapeutic interventions. In addition, emerging closed-loop insulin delivery systems combine glucose sensing, insulin pumps, and computational algorithm to automate glycemic control. This technological convergence represents a critical step toward precision diabetes care [3].

This chapter explores the interdisciplinary research strategies driving innovations in nanotechnology for diabetes management. It emphasizes the integration of nanomaterials, biomedical engineering, and digital technologies in developing advanced therapeutic and diagnostic platforms. Particular emphasis is placed on smart nanocarriers, nano-biosensing technologies, and emerging translational strategies that aim to improve glycemic control and decrease diabetes-related complications. By synthesizing latest developments across multiple scientific domains, the chapter provides a comprehensive perspective on how interdisciplinary collaboration can lead the development of next-generation nanomedicine solutions for diabetes care.

15.2 CONVERGENCE SCIENCE IN DIABETES NANOTECHNOLOGY

The development of advanced nanotechnologies for diabetes management increasingly relies on convergence science, where multiple scientific disciplines collaborate to address complex biomedical problems. Diabetes involves multidimensional metabolic dysfunction, immune mechanisms, and long-term complications; therefore, integration of materials science, bioengineering, computational modeling, and data analytics has become fundamental for designing effective nano-enabled therapies and diagnostics platforms. Such interdisciplinary approaches trigger the development of targeted drug delivery systems, responsive therapeutic platforms, and intelligent monitoring devices that improve glycemic control and patient outcomes [4]. The mix of nanotechnology with bioengineering, computational modeling, and clinical sciences constitutes the basis of the next-generation diabetes management strategies (Figure 15.1).

15.2.1 Materials Science – Biology Interface

The interface between materials science and biology forms the foundation of modern nanomedicine for diabetes. Engineered nanomaterials such as polymeric nanoparticles, lipid nanocarriers, and inorganic nanostructures interact with biological systems at the molecular level to improve therapeutic efficiency. By manipulating nanoscale properties such as particle size, surface charge,

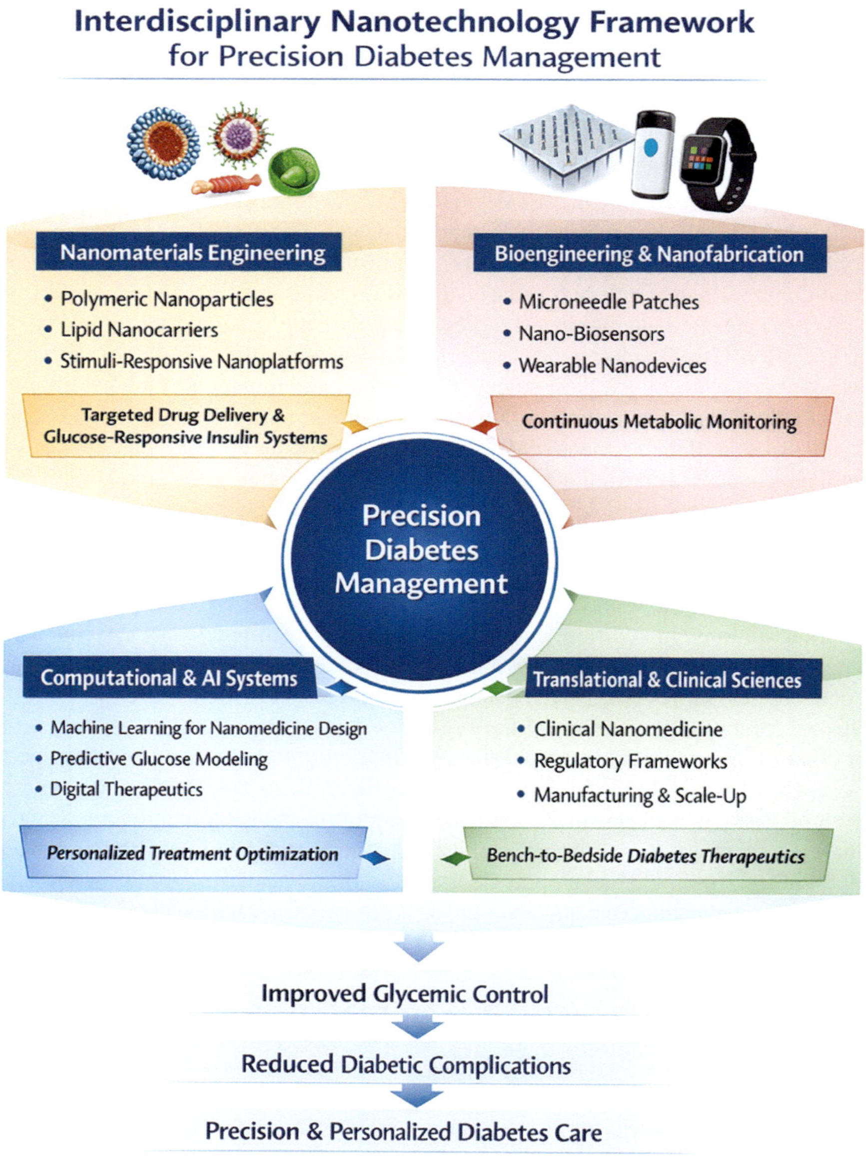

FIGURE 15.1 Interdisciplinary nanotechnology framework for precision diabetes management.

and functionalization, researchers can enhance cellular uptake, improve drug stability, and enable targeted delivery to specific tissues. For example, glucose-responsive nanoparticles with enzymes such as glucose oxidase can detect elevated glucose levels and release insulin, emulating physiological insulin secretion [5].

Recent studies have also explored smart polymeric materials and hydrogels capable of responding to physiological stimulus such as pH, temperature, or glucose concentration. These stimuli-responsive materials allow controlled release of enhanced therapeutic precision in diabetes treatments. The biological compatibility of such nanomaterials enables their application in insulin delivery, β-cell protection, and biomarker detection, demonstrating the critical role of materials science in advancing diabetes nanotechnology [6].

15.2.2 Bioengineering and Micro/Nanofabrication Strategies

Bioengineering techniques and micro/nanofabrication technologies have enabled the creation of nano-enabled devices for diabetes monitoring and therapy. Advances in microfabrication allow the production of nanoscale sensors, microneedle arrays, and wearable platforms that can continuously monitor metabolic biomarkers. For example, glucose-responsive microneedle patches integrate nanosensors with insulin reservoirs to provide automated insulin delivery in response to elevated glucose levels [7].

Nanofabrication strategies are also used to design highly sensitive biosensors capable of detecting glucose and other biomarkers with high precision. Nanostructured electrodes and enzyme-based nanosensors significantly enhance signal sensitivity due to their surface-to-volume ratio, making them suitable for CGM systems. These innovations demonstrate how bioengineering and nanofabrication contribute to the development of next-generation diagnostic and therapeutic technologies [8].

15.2.3 Computational Modeling and Systems Pharmacology

Computational modeling plays a critical role in understanding the interactions between nanomaterials and biological systems. Systems pharmacology approaches integrate pharmacokinetic and pharmacodynamic modeling to predict drug distribution, efficacy, and safety of nano-based therapeutics. Computational simulations can evaluate how different nanocarriers designs influence insulin release kinetics or tissue targeting [9].

For example, researchers have developed computational models to predict the physiological response to glucose-responsive insulin formulations, helping to optimize drug design before clinical testing. Additionally, bioinformatics and modeling tools can predict nanoparticle-cell interactions, and guide the rational design of nanocarriers for improved therapeutic outcomes [10].

15.2.4 Data Science and Artificial Intelligence Integration

The integration of data science and artificial intelligence (AI) has further accelerated advances in nanotechnology. Machine learning (ML) algorithms can analyze large biomedical datasets to identify optimal nanomaterials properties, predict drug delivery efficiency, and personalize treatment strategies. AI-driven models are increasingly used to optimize nanoparticle formulations and improve targeting accuracy in nanomedicine [11].

Furthermore, the combination of nanosensors with digital health platforms allows real-time data collection and predictive analytics for personalized diabetes management. Continuous monitoring devices integrated with AI-based decision systems can enable automated therapeutic adjustment, paving the way for precision medicine in diabetes care. Together, these interdisciplinary advances illustrate how convergence science is shaping the future of nanotechnology-enabled diabetes management [12]. The interdisciplinary combination of nanotechnology with materials science, bioengineering, digital health, and immunology has enabled the development of various therapeutic and diagnostic strategies for diabetes management (Table 15.1).

15.3 SMART NANOPLATFORMS FOR PRECISION DIABETES THERAPY

Smart nanoplatforms are the emerging tools for precision diabetes therapy offering controlled drug delivery, real-time response to physiological signals, and better therapeutic responses. Conventional insulin therapy can usually require frequent dosing and can cause blood glucose level fluctuations. Nanotechnology-based delivery systems seek to address these limitations by taking on board stimuli-responsive materials and glucose-triggered drug release mechanisms and multifunctional nanostructures, which mimic physiological regulation of insulin secretion. These advanced systems achieve greater drug stability and targeting efficacy, and allow for dynamic metabolic controlled therapeutic response [20].

TABLE 15.1
Interdisciplinary Nanotechnology Strategies for Diabetes Management

Interdisciplinary Domain	Nanotechnology Platform	Mechanism	Application in Diabetes	Representative Examples
Materials science + pharmacology	Stimuli-responsive polymeric nanoparticles	Glucose-triggered insulin release via enzyme or pH-responsive mechanisms	Precision insulin delivery	Glucose oxidase-based polymeric nanoparticles enabling glucose-responsive insulin [13]
Nanotechnology + bioengineering	Microneedle patches with nanosensors	Transdermal insulin delivery triggered by glucose sensing	Minimally invasive control glycemic	Glucose-responsive microneedle patch integrating nanosensors and insulin vesicles [13, 14]
Nanotechnology + digital health	Nano-enabled electrochemical biosensors	High-sensitivity glucose detection using nanostructured electrodes	Continous glucose monitoring	Graphene and gold nanoparticle-based glucose sensors used in wearable monitoring devices [15]
Nanotechnology + regenerative medicine	Nanofiber scaffolds and nano-hydrogels	Support β-cell survival and tissue regeneration	Pancreatic tissue engineering	Electrospun nanofibers scaffolds promoting pancreatic cell growth [16]
Nanotechnology + immunology	Nanoparticle-mediated immune modulation	Delivery of immunomodulatory agents to reduce β-cell destruction	Type 1 diabetes therapy	Antigen-loaded nanoparticles inducing immune tolerance [17]
Nanotechnology + systems pharmacology	Targeted nanocarriers	Activation of insulin signaling pathways and improved drug targeting	Treatment of insulin resistance	Nanoparticles modulating PI3K/Akt signaling and glucose uptake [18]
Nanotechnology + microbiome research	Nano-delivery systems for probiotics and bioactives	Controlled release in gastrointestinal tract	Modulation of gut microbiota regulation	Nanocarriers improving stability of probiotic delivery in metabolic disorders [19]

15.3.1 Stimuli-Responsive Nanocarriers

Stimuli-responsive nanocarriers are designed to release therapeutic agents in response to internal or external stimuli such as pH, temperature, enzymes, glucose concentration, light, or magnetic fields. These systems provide spatial and temporal control over drug delivery, which is especially beneficial for diseases like diabetes that require precise glycemic regulatory [21].

For example, polymeric hydrogels and nanoparticles, containing glucose oxidase (GOx) can respond to glucose levels by generating gluconic acid, which alters the local pH to trigger insulin release from the nanocarrier matrix. In addition, smart hydrogels composed of stimuli-responsive polymers have been developed to deliver insulin orally or transdermally while protecting the drug from enzymatic degradation in the gastrointestinal tract. Recent nanocomposite hydrogel systems have demonstrated sustained insulin release and enhanced hypoglycemic effects in experimental models [22].

15.3.2 Glucose-Triggered Drug Release Systems

Glucose-responsive drug delivery systems represent a significant development in diabetes nanomedicine because they can self-regulate insulin release in response to elevated glucose level. Several mechanisms have been explored to achieve glucose-triggered release, including enzyme-mediated reactions, glucose-binding proteins, and synthetic receptors [23].

A notable example involves nanoparticles incorporating glucose oxidase and insulin within polymeric matrices, where glucose oxidation generates gluconic acid that cleaves polymer linkages and releases insulin. Another approach utilizes lectin-based materials such as concanavalin A, which binds glucose molecules and undergoes structural changes that promote insulin release when glucose concentrations increase. Additionally, wearable glucose-responsive microneedle patches have been developed that are applied to the skin where, upon sensing high glucose levels, they automatically deliver insulin, providing a minimally invasive strategy for glycemic control [22].

15.3.3 Multifunctional and Theranostic Nanoparticles

Multifunctional nanoparticles integrate therapeutic and diagnostic capabilities within a single platform, enabling simultaneous disease monitoring and treatment. These "theranostic" systems often combine drug delivery functions with sensing or image capabilities, facilitating real-time monitoring of glucose levels and therapeutic response. Hybrid nanoparticles incorporating polymeric, lipid, or inorganic components have shown potential for oral insulin delivery and biosensing applications. Such platforms can improve treatment precision by enabling clinicians to monitor therapeutic outcomes while adjusting drug release accordingly. In diabetes care, theranostics nanoparticles may also help in detecting biomarkers related to oxidative stress or inflammation associated with diabetic complications [24].

15.3.4 Nanoformulations for Combination Therapy

Combination therapy using nanoformulations is gaining increasing attention for managing complex metabolic disorders, such as diabetes. Nanocarriers can co-deliver multiple therapeutic agents such as insulin, antioxidants, or anti-inflammatory compounds within a single formulation, enabling synergistic therapeutic effects [25].

For example, nanoparticle-based systems have been developed to deliver insulin alongside bioactive molecules that improve insulin sensitivity or reduce oxidative stress. Such multifunctional formulations can address multiple pathological pathways involved in diabetes progression. Moreover, advances in nanotechnology have enabled the design of hybrid nanoparticles capable of enhancing oral insulin bioavailability and supporting combination therapy strategies, representing an important step toward personalized diabetes treatment [26].

15.4 NANO–BIO INTERFACES FOR METABOLIC REGULATION

The interaction between nanomaterials and biological systems, commonly referred to as the nano–bio interface, plays an important role in controlling metabolism processes related to diabetes therapy. These interactions influence cellular signaling, immune responses, and tissue regrowth. In diabetes research, nano–bio interfaces enable targeted modulation of pancreatic β-cells, insulin signaling pathway, and transplanted islet cells, thereby improving therapeutic outcomes. By engineering nanoscale materials that interact precisely with cellular components, researchers can regulate glucose metabolism and restore impaired pancreatic functions [27].

15.4.1 Nano-Cell Interactions in Pancreatic β-Cells

Pancreatic β-cells are responsible for insulin secretion and maintaining glucose homeostasis. In both type 1 and 2 diabetes, β-cells dysfunction or destruction leads to inadequate insulin production. Nanotechnology tools interact directly with β-cells and enhance their functional activity [26].

For instance, mesoporous silica nanoparticles loaded with insulin-mimetic compounds have shown to stimulate insulin secretion from β-cells and enhance glucose utilization in experimental model. Additionally, nanoparticle-based drug carriers can protect β-cells from oxidative stress and inflammatory damage, which are key factors contributing to β-cells loss in diabetes. Such nano-engineered platforms facilitate controlled delivery of therapeutic agents directly to pancreatic tissues, improving treatment specificity and minimizing systemic side effects [28].

15.4.2 Targeted Nanotherapies for Insulin Signaling Pathways

Targeting intracellular insulin signaling pathways is another promising strategy for diabetes management. Insulin signaling involves receptor activation followed by downstream pathways such as IRS-1/PI3K/Akt, which regulate glucose uptake and metabolic homeostasis [29].

Nanocars functionalized with targeting ligands can deliver therapeutic molecules or genes to regulate these pathways. For example, recent studies have shown that engineered nanoparticles can regulate insulin signaling by influencing pathway associated with insulin resistance. Some nanoparticle formulations have been reported to activate the IRS/PI3K/Akt signaling pathway, thereby improving insulin sensitivity and reducing metabolic dysfunction in diabetic models. Such targeted strategies demonstrated the potential of nanomedicine to directly correct molecular defects associated with diabetes progression [30].

15.4.3 Nanotechnology in β-Cell Protection and Regeneration

Nanotechnology also plays a key role in protecting and regenerating pancreatic β-cells. Because autoimmune destruction of β-cells is the primary cause of type 1 diabetes, researchers are exploring nanoparticle-mediated delivery of immunomodulatory agents to prevent immune-mediated damage. Nanoparticles can deliver antigens, immunosuppressive drugs, or nucleic acids to immune cells, promoting immune tolerance and decreasing β-cells destruction [31].

In addition, nanomaterials have been used in regenerative medicine strategies aimed at promoting β-cell proliferation and differentiation. Nanostructured scaffolds and biomaterials can provide structural and biochemical cues that support stem cell differentiation into insulin-producing cells and improve tissue regeneration in pancreatic environments [32].

15.4.4 Nanomaterials for Islet Transplantation

Islet transplantation has emerged as a promising therapy for severe diabetes, especially type 1 diabetes, where pancreatic β-cells are destroyed. However, transplantation success is often hampered by immunological rejection, inadequate vascularization, and graft failure. Nanotechnology offers innovative solutions to address these challenges. For example, nano-thin polymer coatings and biomaterial encapsulation systems have been developed to protect transplanted islets from immune attack while allowing the diffusion of oxygen, nutrients, and insulin. Nanomaterials can also promote vascularization and improve graft survival by delivering pro-angiogenic factors or modulating the local microenvironment. Furthermore, nanoscale engineering techniques enable immune-isolation strategies to mitigate the long-term need for immunosuppressive therapy in transplant recipients [33, 34].

15.5 INTEGRATION OF NANOTECHNOLOGY WITH DIGITAL HEALTH

The convergence of nanotechnology with digital health technologies is revolutionizing diabetes management by enabling continuous physiological monitoring, automated therapeutic responses, and data-driven treatment optimization. Traditional diabetes monitoring methods often rely on intermittent blood glucose measurements, which may not fully capture dynamic metabolic fluctuations. In contrast, nano-enabled sensing technologies integrated with wearable electronics and digital platforms, allow real-time monitoring of glucose and metabolic biomarkers, supporting personalized and proactive disease management. Advances in nanosensors, wireless communication systems, and AI have enabled the progression of smart diabetes management ecosystems capable of detecting metabolic changes and adjusting therapy accordingly [34, 35].

15.5.1 Nano-Enabled Biosensing Platforms

Nanomaterials have significantly improved the sensitivity and performance of biosensors used in diabetes diagnostics. Materials such as gold nanoparticles, graphene, carbon nanotubes, and metal-oxide nanostructures offer high electrical conductivity, large surface area, and enhanced catalytic activities, enabling precise detection of glucose and other metabolic biomarkers. These nanoscale features increase enzyme immobilization and electron transfer, improving sensor responsiveness and accuracy [27].

Recent studies have demonstrated that graphene-based electrochemical nanosensors can detect glucose at very low concentrations with rapid response time, making them suitable for continuous monitoring applications. In addition to glucose sensing, nanobiosensors are also being explored for detecting biomarkers associated with diabetic complications, such as oxidative stress markers and inflammatory mediators. Such multiplexed sensing platforms offer opportunities for early detection of disease progression and improved clinical decision-making [35].

15.5.2 Wearable Nanodevices for Metabolic Monitoring

Wearable devices incorporating nanosensors are increasingly used for non-invasive or minimally invasive metabolic monitoring. These devices can detect glucose levels in interstitial fluids, sweat, or saliva, reducing the need for repeated finger-prick testing. Nanostructured electrodes and flexible materials enable the development of lightweight, skin-compatible sensors that maintain stable performance during continued use [36].

For instance, flexible graphene-based wearable sensors have been developed to monitor glucose levels in sweat while simultaneously monitoring physiological parameters such as temperature and hydration status. Such wearable nanodevices can transmit metabolic data wirelessly to smartphones or cloud-based platforms, allowing patients and healthcare providers to track glycemic patterns and adjust treatment strategies in real time [37].

15.5.3 Closed-Loop Insulin Delivery Systems

Closed-loop insulin delivery systems, often referred to as "artificial pancreas" technologies, represent major advancement in diabetes care. These systems integrate glucose sensing, insulin delivery, and control algorithms to automatically regulate blood glucose levels. CGM sensors measure glucose levels in real time, while insulin pumps deliver insulin based on algorithm-driven decisions [38].

Nanotechnology contributes to these systems by improving sensor sensitivity, stability, and miniaturization. Nanostructured sensing elements enable accurate glucose detection with reduced signal drift, which is essential for reliable automated insulin delivery. Clinical studies have shown that closed-loop systems can substantially improve the time patients spend within the target glycemic range and reduce episodes of hypoglycemia [8].

15.5.4 Artificial Intelligence-Driven Therapeutic Optimization

AI and ML are increasingly being integrated with digital diabetes management platforms to analyze large volumes of metabolic data generated by continuous monitoring systems. AI algorithms can identify patterns in glucose fluctuations, predict hyperglycemic or hypoglycemic events, and recommend personalized therapeutic adjustments [39].

In nanotechnology-enabled systems, AI can also assist in optimizing nanoparticle design, predicting drug release behavior, and enhancing targeting efficiency. By combining nanoscale sensing technologies with predictive analytics and decision-support systems, AI-driven platforms are enabling precision diabetes management, where treatment strategies are dynamically tailored to individual metabolic responses. This integration of nanotechnology, digital health, and AI represents a significant step toward more intelligent and patient-centered diabetes care [40].

15.6 NANOTECHNOLOGY FOR MODULATING METABOLIC AND INFLAMMATORY PATHWAYS

Chronic metabolic dysregulation in diabetes is especially linked with oxidative stress, low-grade inflammation, and alterations in gut microbiota composition. These interconnected processes contribute to insulin resistance and β-cell dysfunction, which accelerate the progression of diabetic complications. Nanotechnology offers innovative approaches to modulate these pathological pathways through targeted drug delivery and enhanced bioavailability of therapeutic agents. By engineered nanoparticles that selectively interact with metabolic tissues or immune cells, researchers aim to regulate oxidative damage and inflammatory signaling involved in diabetes progression [41].

15.6.1 Nanomedicine Targeting Oxidative Stress

Oxidative stress results from excessive production of reactive oxygen species (ROS), which can damage pancreatic β-cells and impair insulin signaling. Nanomedicine strategies have been developed to deliver antioxidant compounds more efficiently to affected tissues. For instance, cerium oxide nanoparticles (nanoceria) possess intrinsic redox activity and can scavenge ROS due to their reversible oxidation states. Experimental studies have shown that nanoceria can reduce oxidative damage and improve glucose metabolism diabetic models [42].

Similarly, polymeric nanoparticles have been used to encapsulate natural antioxidants such as curcumin or resveratrol, improving their stability and bioavailability. These nanoformulations enhance cellular uptake and provide sustained release, thereby reducing oxidative stress and supporting pancreatic cell function [43].

15.6.2 Nanoparticles in Inflammation Control

Chronic inflammation plays a central role in the development of insulin resistance and diabetic complications. Nanoparticle-based delivery systems can transport anti-inflammatory agents directly to target tissues, minimizing systemic side-effect. For instance, lipid nanoparticles and polymeric nanocarriers have been investigated for the delivery of anti-inflammatory drugs or small interfering RNA (siRNA) that supports pro-inflammatory cytokines such as tumor necrosis factor-α and interleukin-6. Targeted nanotherapies can also modulate immune cell activity in adipose tissues and pancreatic islets, helping restore metabolic balance and reduce tissue damage associated with prolonged inflammatory responses [44].

15.6.3 Modulation of Gut Microbiota via Nano-Delivery Systems

The gut microbiota has emerged as an important regulator metabolic health, influencing glucose metabolism, immune function, and inflammation. Alterations in microbial composition have been linked to the development of type 2 diabetes. Nanotechnology-based delivery systems are being explored to enhance the targeted delivery of probiotics, prebiotics, and bioactive compounds that support beneficial microbial populations [45].

For example, nanoparticle carriers can protect probiotic microorganisms or microbial metabolites from degradation in the gastrointestinal tract, enabling controlled release in the intestinal environment. Such strategies may help restore microbial balance and improve metabolic regulation, highlighting the potential of nano-enabled microbiome therapies in diabetes management [46].

15.7 INTERDISCIPLINARY STRATEGIES FOR DIABETIC COMPLICATION MANAGEMENT

Diabetes is frequently associated with long-term complications affecting the skin, vasculature, and nervous system. Persistent hyperglycemia promotes oxidative stress, inflammation, and impaired tissue repair, which collectively contribute to complications such as diabetic foot ulcers, microvascular dysfunction, and diabetic neuropathy. Interdisciplinary research combining nanotechnology, regenerative medicine, pharmacology, and bioengineering has led to the development of innovative therapeutic strategies aimed at preventing or treating these complications. Nanotechnology-based platforms provide targeted delivery, controlled drug release, and enhanced therapeutic stability, offering significant advantages over conventional treatment [47].

15.7.1 Nanotechnology of Diabetic Wound Regeneration

Diabetic wounds, particularly foot ulcers, represent a major clinical condition due to impaired angiogenesis, reduced collagen deposition, and chronic inflammation. Nanotechnology has enabled the development of nanofiber scaffolds, hydrogel dressing, and nanoparticle-based wound therapies that promote tissue regeneration. For example, electrospun nanofiber scaffolds composed of biocompatible polymers such as polycaprolactone or chitosan can mimic the extracellular matrix and support cell adhesion and tissue repair [48].

Silver nanoparticles incorporated into wound dressings have also demonstrated strong antimicrobial activity, decreasing bacterial infection and accelerating wound healing. In experimental and clinical studies, nanoengineered dressing capable of releasing growth factors or antimicrobial agents has shown improved wound closure rates and enhanced vascularization in diabetic wounds [49].

15.7.2 Nano-Therapeutics of Microvascular Damage

Microvascular complications are hallmark of diabetes and contribute to conditions such as diabetic nephropathy and retinopathy. These complications are largely driven by endothelial dysfunction, oxidative stress, and chronic inflammation. Nanoparticle-based drug delivery systems are being studied to target affected microvascular tissues with higher precision [50].

For example, lipid and polymeric nanoparticles have been investigated for delivering antioxidant and anti-inflammatory agents directly to endothelial cells, helping restore vascular functioning and reduce tissue damage. Targeted nanocarriers can also increase drug concentration in specific organs, such as the kidney or retina, thereby enhancing therapeutic efficacy while minimizing systemic toxicity [51].

15.7.3 Neuroprotective Nanomedicine Approaches

Diabetic neuropathy is one of the most common complications of diabetes and is characterized by progressive nerve damage caused by metabolic stress and reduced blood supply. Nanomedicine approaches aim to deliver neuroprotective agents more effectively to peripheral nerves and central nervous system tissues [52].

For example, nanoparticle formulations of neuroprotective compounds such as curcumin or antioxidants have shown improved bioavailability and enhanced therapeutic effects in experimental models of diabetic neuropathy. In addition, nanocarriers capable of crossing biological barrier may facilitate targeted delivery of therapeutic molecules that support nerve regeneration and reduce neuroinflammation. These interdisciplinary strategies highlight the potential of nanotechnology to address multiple pathways involved in diabetic complications [53].

15.8 TRANSLATIONAL AND CLINICAL INTEGRATION

The successful integration of nanotechnology in diabetes management requires successful translational and clinical integration, bridging fundamental research with real-world therapeutic applications. Because nanomedicine involves complex materials, biological systems, and advanced technologies, interdisciplinary collaboration among materials, scientists, clinicians, pharmacologist, engineers, and regulatory experts is essential for developing clinically viable solutions [54].

15.8.1 Interdisciplinary Collaboration in Nanomedicine Development

The development of nano-enabled therapies relies on the integration between various multiple disciplines. Materials scientists design functional nanomaterials, biomedical engineers develop delivery devices and biosensors, while clinicians evaluate safety and therapeutic efficacy. Such collaborative frameworks have accelerated progress in nano-based insulin delivery systems, glucose-responsive nanocarriers, and wearable biosensing technologies. Interdisciplinary research groups and international collaborations have a significant role in advancing these technologies from laboratory studies to clinical testing [55].

15.8.2 Bench-to-Beside Translation Pathways

Translating nanotechnology from the preclinical research to clinical practice includes several stages, including formulation optimization, in vitro testing, animal studies, and human clinical trials. For instance, CGM systems incorporating nanoscale sensing materials have already been integrated into clinical diabetes care. Advances in nanocarrier-based insulin delivery and glucose-responsive systems are currently undergoing extensive preclinical evaluation to assess pharmacokinetics, safety, and therapeutic performance [56].

15.8.3 Regulatory Science and Standardization Challenges

Despite promising advancements, regulatory challenges remain a significant barrier to clinical translation. Nanomedicines require detailed characterization of particle size, surface, biodistribution, and long-term safety. Regulatory agencies increasingly emphasize standardized testing protocol, quality control measures, and comprehensive toxicity evaluations to ensure the safe clinical deployment of nano-enabled therapeutics for diabetes management [57].

15.9 EMERGING FRONTIERS OF DIABETES NANOTECHNOLOGY

Rapid advances in nanoscience and digital technologies are creating new frontiers in diabetes management. Emerging concepts such as nanorobotics, biohybrid nanomaterials, and AI-assisted design are advancing the ability of nanomedicine beyond the traditional drug delivery system. These innovations are trying to develop highly precise and personalized therapeutic measures for "metabolic" diseases [58].

15.9.1 Nanorobotics and Autonomous Drug Delivery

Nanorobotics represents a futuristic approach to autonomous drug delivery, where nanoscale devices are engineered to sense physiological signals and release therapeutic agents in response to metabolic changes. Although still largely at experimental stage, researchers have proposed glucose-responsive nanorobotic systems capable of detecting increased glucose levels and delivering insulin in controlled manner. For instance, enzyme-driven nanomotors based on catalytic reactions have been explored to enhance drug transport and targeted delivery in biological environments. Such systems could potentially enable automated regulation of blood glucose without continuous patient intervention [58].

15.9.2 Biohybrid and Living Nanomaterials

Biohybrid nanomaterials combine synthetic nanostructures with biological components such as cells, proteins, or enzymes. These hybrid systems can mimic natural biological functions and improve enhance therapeutic performance. In diabetes research, biohybrid platforms incorporating pancreatic cells or glucose-responsive enzymes have been investigated for controlled insulin release and metabolic sensing. Living nanomaterials, including engineered microbial systems of cell-based nanostructures, are also being explored to modulate metabolic pathways and support regenerative therapies for pancreatic tissue repair [59].

15.9.3 AI-Guided Nanomedicine Design

AI is increasingly used to accelerate the design and optimization of nanomedicines. ML algorithms can analyze large experimental datasets to predict nanoparticle properties such as size, surface chemistry, and drug release behavior. In diabetes nanotechnology, AI-driven models are being applied to optimize nanoparticle formulations and predict therapeutic outcome. These computational tools can significantly reduce development time and enhance the precision of nano-based therapeutic systems, supporting the advancement of personalized diabetes treatment strategies [60].

15.10 CONCLUSION AND FUTURE PERSPECTIVE

Nanotechnology has emerged as a transformative approach in diabetes research by enabling innovative strategies for drug delivery, metabolic monitoring, and therapeutic intervention. The integration of nanoscale materials with biomedical engineering, digital health technologies, and computational tools has significantly expanded the possibilities for precision diabetes management. Smart nanocarriers, glucose-responsive delivery systems, and nano-enabled biosensors are demonstrating promising capabilities in improving glycemic control, enhancing drug bioavailability, and supporting real-time metabolic monitoring. Furthermore, interdisciplinary innovations such as wearable nanosensors, artificial pancreas systems, and targeted nanotherapeutics highlight the growing convergence of nanotechnology with clinical medicine and digital healthcare. Despite these advances, several challenges remain before widespread clinical implementation can be achieved. Issues related to long-term safety, large-scale manufacturing, regulatory approval, and cost-effectiveness must be carefully addressed. Continued interdisciplinary collaboration among scientists, clinicians, engineering, and regulatory authorities will be essential for translating promising laboratory discoveries into effective clinical solutions. Looking ahead, emerging technologies such as AI-guided nanomedicine design, biohybrid materials, and autonomous drug delivery platforms may further revolutionize diabetes treatment. These developments have the potential to enable highly personalized and adaptive therapeutics strategies, ultimately improving disease management and patient outcome worldwide.

REFERENCES

1. Hossain MJ, Al-Mamun M, Islam MR. Diabetes mellitus, the fastest growing global public health concern: Early detection should be focused. Health Science Reports. 2024;7(3):e2004.
2. Samuel D, Bharali D, Mousa SA. The role of nanotechnology in diabetes treatment: Current and future perspectives. International Journal of Nanotechnology. 2011;8(1–2):53–65.

3. Gulati S, Yadav R, Kumari V, Nair S, Gupta C, Aishwari M. Nanosensors in healthcare: Transforming real-time monitoring and disease management with cutting-edge nanotechnology. RSC Pharmaceutics. 2025;2(5):1003–18.
4. Haider R, Das ZA, Zameer GK. S. Revolutionizing patient care: Multidimensional approaches to 21st-century diabetes management. Journal of Heart and Vasculature. 2025;4(6):01–05.
5. Liu M, Wang R, Hoi MP, Wang Y, Wang S, Li G, Vong CT, Chong CM. Nano-based drug delivery systems for managing diabetes: Recent advances and future prospects. International Journal of Nanomedicine. 2025:6221–52.
6. Zuo H, Jiao Y, Chen J, Tong S, Li Y, Zhao W. Recent advances in smart stimulus-responsive hydrogels for precision drug delivery in tumours. Gels. 2026;12(2):98.
7. Kalantri S, Nahata AN, Godani N. A comprehensive review on the integration of microneedle technologies with biosensing platforms for advancements in fabrication, biomarker detection, and therapeutic monitoring in precision medicine. Discover Pharmaceutical Sciences. 2025;1(1):22.
8. Rajamohan R, Sun S. Nanostructured materials in glucose biosensing: From fundamentals to smart healthcare applications. Biosensors. 2025;15(10):658.
9. Alalmaie A, Alshahrani HT, Alqahtani M, Alshahrani Z, Alahmari S, Asiri A, Alqadi B, Alshahrani A, Alshahrani S, Akhter MH. Integrating computational insights in gold nanoparticle-mediated drug delivery: Enhancing efficacy and precision. Frontiers in Medical Technology. 2025;7:1528826.
10. Kaur P, Khatik G. An overview of computer-aided drug design tools and recent applications in designing of anti-diabetic agents. Current Drug Targets. 2021;22(10):1158–82.
11. Han Y, Kim DH, Pack SP. Nanomaterials in drug delivery: Leveraging artificial intelligence and big data for predictive design. International Journal of Molecular Sciences. 2025;26(22):11121.
12. Ji C, Jiang T, Liu L, Zhang J, You L. Continuous glucose monitoring combined with artificial intelligence: Redefining the pathway for prediabetes management. Frontiers in Endocrinology. 2025;16:1571362.
13. Yu J, Zhang Y, Ye Y, DiSanto R, Sun W, Ranson D, Ligler FS, Buse JB, Gu Z. Microneedle-array patches loaded with hypoxia-sensitive vesicles provide fast glucose-responsive insulin delivery. Proceedings of the National Academy of Sciences. 2015;112(27):8260–65.
14. Veiseh O, Tang BC, Whitehead KA, Anderson DG, Langer R. Managing diabetes with nanomedicine: Challenges and opportunities. Nature Reviews Drug Discovery. 2015;14(1):45–57.
15. Heller A, Feldman B. Electrochemical glucose sensors and their applications in diabetes management. Chemical Reviews. 2008;108(7):2482–505.
16. Jiang Z, Zheng Z, Yu S, Gao Y, Ma J, Huang L, Yang L. Nanofiber scaffolds as drug delivery systems promoting wound healing. Pharmaceutics. 2023;15(7):1829.
17. Getts DR, Shea LD, Miller SD, King NJ. Harnessing nanoparticles for immune modulation. Trends in Immunology. 2015;36(7):419–27.
18. Zhang L, Zhai BZ, Wu YJ, Wang Y. Recent progress in the development of nanomaterials targeting multiple cancer metabolic pathways: A review of mechanistic approaches for cancer treatment. Drug Delivery. 2023;30(1):1–8.
19. Li X, Wei H, Qi J, Ma K, Luo Y, Weng L. Interactions of nanomaterials with gut microbiota and their applications in cancer therapy. Sensors. 2023;23(9):4428.
20. Sharma DK, Pattnaik G, Behera A. Recent developments in nanoparticles for the treatment of diabetes. Journal of Drug Targeting. 2023;31(9):908–19.
21. Das SS, Bharadwaj P, Bilal M, Barani M, Rahdar A, Taboada P, Bungau S, Kyzas GZ. Stimuli-responsive polymeric nanocarriers for drug delivery, imaging, and theragnosis. Polymers. 2020;12(6):1397.
22. Pal S, Rakshit T, Saha S, Jinagal D. Glucose-responsive materials for smart insulin delivery: From protein-based to protein-free design. ACS Materials Au. 2025;5(2):239–52.
23. Volpatti LR, Matranga MA, Cortinas AB, Delcassian D, Daniel KB, Langer R, Anderson DG. Glucose-responsive nanoparticles for rapid and extended self-regulated insulin delivery. ACS Nano. 2019;14(1):488–97.
24. Parthasarathy N, Karthikeyan L, Fabiola M, Vivek R. Recent progress in multifunctional theranostic inorganic nanomaterials for cancer diagnostic imaging and therapy. Next Nanotechnology. 2025; 8:100212.
25. Kakkar S, Jha RK, Hattila D, Singh AK, Shukla PK, Yadav SP, Meena AS. Plant-derived natural product-based nanoformulations for healthcare application. Nanotheranostics. 2025;9(3):262.
26. Luo X, Li N, Zhu X, Xie W, Zhang Q, Liang N, Zhang P, Zhou C. Application of nanomaterials in diabetic complication management. Colloids and Surfaces B: Biointerfaces. 2025:115229.
27. DiSanto RM, Subramanian V, Gu Z. Recent advances in nanotechnology for diabetes treatment. Wiley Interdisciplinary Reviews: Nanomedicine and Nanobiotechnology. 2015;7(4):548–64.

28. Almatroudi A. Advances in mesoporous silica and hybrid nanoparticles for drug delivery: Synthesis, functionalization, and biomedical applications. Pharmaceutics. 2025;17(12):1602.
29. Feng Y, Ren Y, Zhang X, Yang S, Jiao Q, Li Q, Jiang W. Metabolites of traditional Chinese medicine targeting PI3K/AKT signaling pathway for hypoglycemic effect in type 2 diabetes. Frontiers in Pharmacology. 2024;15:1373711.
30. Zhang T, Tang JZ, Fei X, Li Y, Song Y, Qian Z, Peng Q. Can nanoparticles and nano–protein interactions bring a bright future for insulin delivery? Acta Pharmaceutica Sinica B. 2021;11(3):651–67.
31. Cristelo C, Nunes R, Pinto S, Marques JM, Gama FM, Sarmento B. Targeting β cells with cathelicidin nanomedicines improves insulin function and pancreas regeneration in type 1 diabetic rats. ACS Pharmacology & Translational Science. 2023;6(10):1544–60.
32. Rajendran A, Rajan RA, Balasubramaniyam S, Elumalai K. Nano delivery systems in stem cell therapy: Transforming regenerative medicine and overcoming clinical challenges. Nano TransMed. 2025;4:100069.
33. Zhang Y, Chen X, Huang Z, Qiu Y, Kou L, Yao Q. Enhancing islet transplantation outcomes in T1DM: The promise of mesenchymal stem cells and exosomes, International Journal of Pharmaceutics: X 2026:11:100498, https://doi.org/10.1016/j.ijpx.2026.100498.
34. Shoaib A, Darraj A, Khan ME, Azmi L, Alalwan A, Alamri O, Tabish M, Khan AU. A nanotechnology-based approach to biosensor application in current diabetes management practices. Nanomaterials. 2023;13(5):867.
35. Bhattacharjya T, Nalepa MA, Dědek I, Jakubec P, Panáček D, Otyepka M. Recent advances in graphene-based electrochemical biosensors for major non-communicable diseases. Current Opinion in Electrochemistry. 2025;53:101737.
36. Mansour M, Darweesh MS, Soltan A. Wearable devices for glucose monitoring: A review of state-of-the-art technologies and emerging trends. Alexandria Engineering Journal. 2024;89:224–43.
37. Qiao Y, Qiao L, Chen Z, Liu B, Gao L, Zhang L. Wearable sensor for continuous sweat biomarker monitoring. Chemosensors. 2022;10(7):273.
38. Cobelli C, Renard E, Kovatchev B. Artificial pancreas: Past, present, future. Diabetes. 2011;60(11):2672–82.
39. He Z, Li W. AI-driven management of type 2 diabetes in China: Opportunities and challenges. Diabetes, Metabolic Syndrome and Obesity. 2025;18:85–92.
40. Ingle S, Yemul M, Lavate A, Desai A. Artificial intelligence in drug delivery system. International Journal of Technology. 2024;14(2):115–24.
41. Oguntibeju OO. Type 2 diabetes mellitus, oxidative stress and inflammation: Examining the links. International Journal of Physiology, Pathophysiology and Pharmacology. 2019;11(3):45.
42. Wang J, Wang H. Oxidative stress in pancreatic beta cell regeneration. Oxidative Medicine and Cellular Longevity. 2017;2017(1):1930261.
43. Thiruvengadam R, Kondapavuluri BK, Thangavelu L, Thiruvengadam M, Hatami M, Kim JH. Nanoparticle-based strategies with bioactive compounds for targeting oxidative stress in therapeutic interventions: A comprehensive review. Industrial Crops and Products. 2025;227:120804.
44. Bakshi V, Fathima B. Solid lipid nanoparticles in metabolic disorders: A novel strategy for targeted delivery in diabetes and obesity. Journal of Bio-X Research. 2025;8:0066.
45. Scheithauer TP, Rampanelli E, Nieuwdorp M, Vallance BA, Verchere CB, Van Raalte DH, Herrema H. Gut microbiota as a trigger for metabolic inflammation in obesity and type 2 diabetes. Frontiers in Immunology. 2020 Oct 16;11:571731.
46. Kadam O, Dalai S, Chauhan B, Guru RR, Mitra S, Raytekar N, Kumar R, Kadam OR, Guru RR. Nanobiotechnology unveils the power of probiotics: A comprehensive review on the synergistic role of probiotics and advanced nanotechnology in enhancing geriatric health. Cureus. 2025 Mar 12;17(3).
47. Wang J, Yang X, Zhou T, Ma H, Yuan X, Yan S. Understanding risk factors and prognosis in diabetic foot ulcers. Open Life Sciences. 2025;20(1):20251137.
48. Wang S, Yang H, Zheng J, Tong A, Mu S, Wang D, Zhao M, Li J. Recent advances and prospects of nanoparticle-based drug delivery for diabetic ocular complications. Theranostics. 2025;15(8):3551.
49. Sedighi O, Bednarke B, Sherriff H, Doiron AL. Nanoparticle-based strategies for managing biofilm infections in wounds: A comprehensive review. ACS Omega. 2024;9(26):27853–71.
50. Yang DR, Wang MY, Zhang CL, Wang Y. Endothelial dysfunction in vascular complications of diabetes: A comprehensive review of mechanisms and implications. Frontiers in Endocrinology. 2024;15:1359255.
51. Zazuli Z, Hartati R, Rowa CR, Asyarie S, Satrialdi. The potential application of nanocarriers in delivering topical antioxidants. Pharmaceuticals. 2025;18(1):56.
52. He Z, Diao J, Hamel FG, Duan B. Innovative strategies for diabetic peripheral neuropathy: From clinical management to emerging bioengineering solutions. Bioactive Materials. 2026;61:312–38.

53. Godse S, Zhou L, Sakshi S, Singla B, Singh UP, Kumar S. Nanocarrier-mediated curcumin delivery: An adjuvant strategy for CNS disease treatment. Experimental Biology and Medicine. 2023;248(22): 2151–66.
54. Andreadi A, Lodeserto P, Todaro F, Meloni M, Romano M, Minasi A, Bellia A, Lauro D. Nanomedicine in the treatment of diabetes. International Journal of Molecular Sciences. 2024;25(13):7028.
55. Kazi RN, Hasani IW, Khafaga DS, Kabba S, Farhan M, Aatif M, Muteeb G, Fahim YA. Nanomedicine: The effective role of nanomaterials in healthcare from diagnosis to Therapy. Pharmaceutics. 2025; 17(8):987.
56. Silva DF, Melo AL, Uchôa AF, Pereira GM, Alves AE, Vasconcellos MC, Xavier-Júnior FH, Passos MF. Biomedical approach of nanotechnology and biological risks: A mini-review. International Journal of Molecular Sciences. 2023;24(23):16719.
57. Aebisher D, Dynarowicz K, Rudy I, Rogóż K, Bartusik-Aebisher D, Kawczyk-Krupka A. Applications of nanobiotechnology in medicine. Life. 2026;16(2):302.
58. Rahman MH, Liza NY, Hossain KR, Kalambhe DR, Shyeed MA, Noor DH. Additive manufacturing in nano drug delivery systems. Pharmaceutical Science Advances. 2024;2:100036.
59. Nadendla RR, Chandu UM, Rao KS. Biohybrid molecules: Integrating natural and synthetic components for advanced biochemical applications. Indian Journal of Biochemistry and Biophysics (IJBB). 2025;62(2):107–16.
60. Habeeb M, You HW, Umapathi M, Ravikumar KK, Mishra S. Strategies of artificial intelligence tools in the domain of nanomedicine. Journal of Drug Delivery Science and Technology. 2024;91:105157.

16 Symbiotic Nanomedicine
Leveraging Nano-Encapsulated Probiotics in Type 2 Diabetes Therapy

Vaishali Shirsat
Bombay College of Pharmacy (Autonomous), Mumbai, India

Neerati Prasad
University College of Pharmaceutical Sciences, Kakatiya University, Mangalore, India

Indu O. S.
Father Muller Homoeopathic Medical College, Mangalore, India

Jyothirmayee Devineni
KVSR Siddhartha College of Pharmaceutical Sciences, Vijayawada, India

Ashish Singhai
Teerthanker Mahaveer College of Pharmacy, Teerthanker Mahaveer University, Moradabad, India

Sumiti Narayan Tewari
Pranveer Singh Institute of Technology, Kanpur, India

Kamlesh Kumar Dhiwar
Century Cement College, Raipur, India

16.1 INTRODUCTION

Recent progress in metabolic research has highlighted the gut microbiome as a critical regulator of host metabolic homeostasis and a promising therapeutic target in type 2 diabetes (T2D). The human gastrointestinal tract harbors trillions of microorganisms that influence nutrient metabolism, immune signaling, and endocrine regulation. Disruptions in this microbial ecosystem, commonly referred to as gut dysbiosis, have been increasingly linked to insulin resistance, chronic inflammation, and poor glucose metabolism. Studies have shown that individuals with T2D often exhibit reduced microbial diversity, low abundance of beneficial butyrate-producing bacteria, and increased populations of opportunistic pathogens, suggesting a strong link between microbe imbalance and disease progression [1].

The metabolic influence of gut microbiota is mainly mediated through microbial metabolites such as short-chain fatty acids (SCFAs), bile acid, and amino acid metabolites. These compounds

DOI: 10.1201/9781003598657-16

modulate several metabolic pathways including insulin signaling, intestinal barrier integrity, and inflammatory responses. Dysbiosis-induced reductions in SCFA production and altered metabolite signaling have been implicated in the development of metabolic dysfunction and β-cell impairment. Consequently, targeted modulation of gut microbiota has emerged as a potential complementary approach for metabolic disease management [2].

Probiotics and synbiotic formulations have therefore gained significant attention as microbiome-directed therapeutic interventions. Beneficial bacteria strains such as *Lactobacillus* and *Bifidobacterium* have demonstrated potential to enhance glycemic control, decrease systemic inflammation, and restore microbial balance. However, conventional probiotic therapies face important limitations, including poor survival during gastrointestinal transit, instability during their storage, and inadequate colonization efficiency within the intestinal environment. These problems significantly reduce their therapeutic effectiveness in clinical applications [3].

Nanotechnology has recently emerged as a revolutionary platform capable of addressing these limitations through advanced delivery strategies. Nano-encapsulation techniques protect probiotic cells from the harsh gastric conditions, increase their stability, and ensure targeted release within the intestinal tract. Emerging nano-biomaterial systems, including polymeric nanoparticles, lipid nanocarriers, and polysaccharide-based nano-capsules, enable improved probiotic viability and controlled delivery. These innovations have given rise to the concept of symbiotic nanomedicine, where nanotechnology is combined with microbiome-based therapy to increase metabolic regulation and therapeutic effectiveness [4].

Collectively, the convergence of microbiome science and nanomedicine represents a novel paradigm in diabetes management. By combining the metabolic benefits of probiotics with advanced nano-delivery technologies, symbiotic nanomedicine offers a promising strategy to address current therapeutic restrictions to allow precision microbiome modulation for better metabolic outcomes in T2D [5].

16.2 PATHOPHYSIOLOGY OF TYPE 2 DIABETES AND GUT DYSBIOSIS

16.2.1 Insulin Resistance and Metabolic Dysregulation

T2D is primarily characterized by insulin resistance and progressive pancreatic β-cells dysfunction, leading to impaired glucose homeostasis. In insulin-resistant states, peripheral tissues such as skeletal muscle, liver, and adipose tissues exhibit reduced responsiveness to insulin signaling, resulting in decreased glucose uptake and increased hepatic gluconeogenesis. Chronic low-grade inflammation, lipotoxicity, and mitochondrial dysfunction further exacerbate metabolic dysregulation. Recent studies also indicate that metabolic biomarkers such as the triglyceride-glucose (TyG) index and metabolic score for insulin resistance (METS-IR) are increasingly used to assess the severity of insulin resistance in T2D populations. There is growing evidence that alterations in gut microbial composition contribute significantly to insulin resistance. Dysbiosis may disrupt intestinal barrier integrity and promote systemic metabolic inflammation through increased translocation of microbial products such as lipopolysaccharides, which impair insulin signaling pathways and accelerate disease progression [6].

16.2.2 Gut Microbiota Alterations in Diabetes

Individuals with T2D commonly exhibit substantial changes in gut microbial diversity and composition. Metagenomic analysis shows a reduction in beneficial butyrate-producing bacteria, such as *Faecalibacterium* and *Roseburia*, paired with a higher presence of opportunistic or pro-inflammatory bacteria. Large-scale microbiome analyses have also shown that bacterial diversity is significantly lower in individuals with T2D than in healthy controls, reflecting disrupted microbial ecosystem stability [7].

These microbial changes affect host metabolism through the production of bioactive metabolites such as SCFAs, bile acids, and amino acid derivatives. Changes in these metabolites can modify energy balance, immune signaling, and glucose metabolism, thereby contributing to metabolic dysfunction and insulin resistance [8].

16.2.3 Gut–Pancreas–Metabolic Axis

The gut microbiota communicates with metabolic organs via complex signal networks often described as the gut–pancreas–metabolic axis. Microbial metabolites, especially SCFAs including acetate, propionate, and butyrate, act as signaling molecules that regulate glucose homeostasis, insulin secretion, and inflammatory pathways. In healthy conditions, these metabolites help maintain intestinal barrier integrity and stimulate enteroendocrine hormones secretion, including glucagon-like peptide-1 (GLP-1), which enhances insulin release. However, dysbiosis-induced reductions in beneficial metabolites disrupt this regulatory network, contributing to impaired β-cell function and metabolic imbalance [9].

16.3 THERAPEUTIC POTENTIAL OF PROBIOTICS AND SYNBIOTICS FOR DIABETES

16.3.1 Probiotic Strains with Antidiabetic Activity

Probiotics are live microorganisms that confer health benefits when administrated in adequate amounts, and several strains have demonstrated potential in improving metabolic parameters associated with T2D. Among the most extensively studied probiotic genera are *Lactobacillus* and *Bifidobacterium*, which contribute to metabolic regulation through the modulation of gut microbiota composition, enhancement of intestinal barrier integrity, and production of bioactive metabolites such as SCFAs. Experimental and clinical studies suggest that these strains can improve glucose metabolism by reducing systemic inflammation, regulating bile acid metabolism, and improving insulin signaling pathways. For example, *Lactobacillus rhamnosus* LRa05 supplementation in a 12-week clinical study of individuals with T2D resulted in reduced fasting blood glucose and improved lipid profiles, highlighting the strain's metabolic benefits. Additionally, multi-strain probiotic formulations with combinations of *Lactobacillus*, *Bifidobacterium*, and *Streptococcus* species have been found to elicit greater metabolic improvements than single-strain formulations because of synergistic microbial interactions for increased microbial diversity and metabolic activity in the gut [10].

16.3.2 Synbiotic Interventions and Modulation of Microbiota

Synbiotics, defined as combinations of probiotics and prebiotics, are designed to enhance probiotic survival and functional activity in the gastrointestinal tract. Prebiotics such as inulin, fructooligosaccharides, and galactooligosaccharides selectively stimulate the growth of beneficial bacteria, thereby promoting a favorable microbial environment that supports metabolic homeostasis. In individuals with T2D, synbiotic supplementation has been associated with improved gut microbial diversity, increased production of SCFAs, and reduced intestinal inflammation. Controlled clinical studies have shown that synbiotic formulations can modulate metabolic markers including fasting blood glucose, insulin resistance indices, and lipid metabolism. In randomized trials evaluating synbiotic supplementation in adults with or at risk of diabetes, significant improvements were observed in metabolic biomarkers such as fasting glucose, HbA1c, and inflammatory markers, indicating that microbiota-targeted nutritional strategies may complement conventional pharmacological therapies [11].

16.3.3 Clinical Evidence of Glycemic Improvement

Accumulating clinical evidence from randomized controlled trials and meta-analyses supports the role of probiotic and symbiotic interventions as adjunct strategies for glycemic control in T2D. A large systematic review analyzing more than 40 randomized clinical trials involving nearly 3000 participants has reported that probiotic supplementation significantly reduced glycated hemoglobin (HbA1c), fasting plasma glucose, and circulating insulin levels, compared with placebo controls. Additional meta-analyses have confirmed that probiotic therapy can improve markers of insulin resistance, including homeostatic model assessment for insulin resistance (HOMA-IR), while also lowering fasting blood glucose and improving lipid profiles in diabetic individuals. Clinical studies further suggest that combining probiotics with standard antidiabetic medications such as metformin may improve therapeutic outcomes by improving β-cell function and metabolic regulation. Collectively, these findings demonstrate the increasing clinical relevance of microbiome-guided interventions and provide a solid scientific foundation for developing advanced delivery systems, including nano-encapsulated probiotic formulations, to improve therapeutic efficacy in diabetes management [12].

16.4 CHALLENGES IN CONVENTIONAL PROBIOTIC THERAPY

16.4.1 Gastrointestinal Degradation and Low Survival

A major limitation of traditional probiotic treatment is low survival of microorganisms during gastrointestinal transit. Following oral administration, probiotic bacteria must pass through the stomach and small intestine before reaching the colon where they have most of their metabolic and immunomodulatory effects. The stomach presents a highly acidic environment with a pH typically ranging from 1.5 to 3.0, which can damage bacterial cell membranes, denature proteins, and reduce cellular viability. In addition, digestive enzymes such as pepsin in the stomach and pancreatic enzymes in the intestine further compromise bacterial integrity. Bile salts found in the small intestine also disrupt bacterial cell membranes, leading to leakage of intracellular components and reduce metabolic activities. Experimental studies have shown that a good percentage of probiotic cells are killed during gastrointestinal passage, with survival rates often dropping below 40% of many commonly used strains. This significant loss of viable microorganisms reduces the effective dose reaching the colon and therefore limits the therapeutic benefits of conventional probiotic formulations [13].

16.4.2 Stability and Shelf-Life Limitations

Another important challenge in probiotic therapy is maintaining microbial stability and viability during storage. Probiotics are living organisms which are highly sensitive to environmental conditions such as temperature, humidity, oxygen exposure, and light. During manufacturing, transportation, and storage, these environmental factors can significantly reduce viable cell count. Many probiotic strains require refrigeration to maintain stability and exposure to higher temperatures can rapidly reduce their viability. In addition, oxygen sensitivity of certain anaerobic strains, especially *Bifidobacterium* species, complicates formulation and packaging strategies. Maintaining sufficient viable cells throughout the product's shelf life is essential because therapeutic efficacy generally requires doses ranging from 106 to 109 colony-forming units per serving. However, prolonged storage or inadequate packaging conditions can reduce viable cell counts below effective levels, resulting in reduced product efficacy [14].

16.4.3 Poor Colonization Efficiency

Even when probiotics survive gastrointestinal transit and remain viable during storage, their ability to colonize the intestinal environment is restricted. The human gut microbiome is a highly complex ecosystem with trillions of resident microorganisms competing for nutrients and ecological niches.

TABLE 16.1
Key Limitations of Conventional Probiotics and Advantages of Nano-Encapsulation Strategies

Challenge in Conventional Probiotic Therapy	Underlying Cause	Consequence for Therapy	Advantage of Nano-Encapsulation
Gastrointestinal degradation	Exposure to gastric acid, digestive enzymes, and bile salts	Significant reduction in viable probiotic cells reaching the intestine	Protective nano-coatings shield microorganisms and enable targeted intestinal release
Low survival during transit	Harsh physiological conditions in stomach and small intestine	Reduced therapeutic dose delivered to colon	Nanocarriers enhance probiotic survival and improve bioavailability
Limited storage stability	Sensitivity to temperature, moisture, oxygen, and processing conditions	Decreased viable cell counts during shelf life	Encapsulation improves stability and protects probiotics during storage and transport
Poor intestinal colonization	Competition with existing gut microbiota and limited mucosal adhesion	Transient presence of probiotic strains with reduced efficacy	Surface-modified nanocarriers enhance mucosal adhesion and retention in the gut
Inconsistent therapeutic outcomes	Variability and delivery efficiency	Reduced clinical effectiveness	Controlled and sustained release improves probiotic functionality

Newly introduced probiotic strains must compete with this established microbial community for adhesion sites on intestinal epithelial surfaces and access to metabolic substrates. Consequently, many of the probiotic strains exhibit only transient colonization, meaning they pass through the gastrointestinal tract without establishing long-term residency. Host immune responses, microbial competition, and differences in individual microbiome composition further influence colonization success. As a result, the metabolic and immunological benefits of probiotics may be short-lived unless they are administered continuously or delivered using advanced protective and targeted delivery systems [15]. The major technological barriers associated with the conventional probiotic therapy and potential benefits provided by nano-encapsulation technologies are summarized in Table 16.1.

16.5 NANO-ENCAPSULATION TECHNOLOGIES FOR PROBIOTIC DELIVERY

16.5.1 Principle of Nano-Encapsulation

Nano-encapsulation involves the entrapment of probiotic microorganisms within nanoscale protective carriers designed to enhance their survival, stability, and targeted delivery in the gastrointestinal tract. The primary principle of nano-encapsulation is to create a protective barrier around probiotic cells that shields them from harsh environmental conditions such as gastric acidity, digestive enzymes, and bile salts encouraged during oral administration. These nanostructured carriers can also enable controlled or stimuli-responsive release mechanisms, where probiotic cells remain protected in the acidic stomach but released in the more pH of the intestine. Such targeted delivery enhances the number of viable microorganisms reaching the colon, thereby improving their therapeutic potential. Nano-encapsulation additionally helps maintain microbial viability during processing and storage, addressing key limitations associated with conventional probiotic presentations [16].

16.5.2 Materials Used for Probiotic Nanocarriers

Various natural and synthetic biomaterials have been investigated for the development of probiotic nanocarriers. Biopolymers such as alginate, chitosan, pectin, and starch are generally used due to their biocompatibility, biodegradability, and ability to form protective matrices around microbial cells. Alginate-based systems are widely applied because they form gel networks capable of encapsulation probiotic cells while allowing gradual release in the intestine. Chitosan nanoparticles are especially attractive due to their mucoadhesive properties and positive surface charge, which enhance adhesion to intestinal mucosa and improve probiotic retention. In addition, lipid-based nanocarriers such as liposomes and solid lipid nanoparticles have been explored for probiotic delivery because they can protect sensitive biological materials and facilitate controlled release within the gastrointestinal tract [17].

16.5.3 Fabrication Techniques for Nano-Probiotic Systems

Several fabrication techniques have been developed to produce nano-encapsulated probiotic systems with high encapsulation efficiency and cell viability. Methods such as ionic gelation, emulsification, spray drying, and electrospinning are commonly used for encapsulation probiotics within nanoscale matrices. Ionic gelation is often employed with alginate or chitosan to form stable nanostructures under mild conditions that preserve bacterial viability. Emulsion-based techniques allow formation of nano-capsule with controlled size distribution, while spray-drying methods are commonly used in industrial probiotic formulations due to their scalability and cost-effectiveness. Advances in nanofabrication technologies are further enabling the development of multifunctional delivery systems capable of enhancing probiotic stability, gastrointestinal survival, and targeted intestinal release [18].

16.6 NANOCARRIER PLATFORMS FOR SYMBIOTIC THERAPY

16.6.1 Polymeric Nanoparticles

Polymeric nanoparticles are widely investigated for probiotic delivery due to their biocompatibility, tunable degradation, and protective capacity. Materials such as poly(lactic-co-glycolic acid) (PLGA), chitosan, and alginate are commonly used to encapsulate probiotic cells and protect them from acidic gastric environments. Recent studies demonstrate that chitosan-coated polymeric nanoparticles significantly improve survival of *Lactobacillus* species under simulated gastrointestinal conditions while enabling gradual release within the intestinal lumen [19].

16.6.2 Lipid-Based Nanocarriers

Lipid-based nanocarriers such as liposomes, solid lipid nanoparticle (SLN), and nanostructured lipid carriers (NLCs) have shown promising probiotic protection and delivery platforms. These systems have a phospholipid or lipid matrix that has the ability to encapsulate sensitive biological materials and protect them from degradation in the environment. Recent investigations show that the liposomal encapsulation can significantly increase the viability of probiotics during gastrointestinal passage while helping to control the release and increase the interaction with the intestinal mucosal surface [20].

16.6.3 Polysaccharide and Biopolymer Nanocapsules

Polysaccharide-based nanocapsules represent an important class of probiotic delivery systems because of their natural origin, biodegradability, and excellent safety profiles. Materials such as alginate, pectin, carrageenan, and starch are widely employed to form hydrogel-like nanostructures capable of entrapping probiotic cells. Alginate-based nanocapsules, often combined with chitosan coatings, have shown enhanced resistance to acidic environments and bile salts while maintaining high microbial viability during gastrointestinal transit [21].

16.6.4 Hybrid and Smart Nano-Delivery System

Hybrid nanocarriers integrate multiple biomaterials or functional components to enhance protection and target delivery. Examples include polymer-lipid hybrid nanoparticles and stimuli-responsive nanostructures that release probiotics in response to environmental triggers such as pH changes or enzymatic activity. Emerging smart nano-delivery systems are being designed to respond to intestinal microenvironment signals, enabling controlled release and improved microbial colonization, which may enhance therapeutic efficacy in metabolic disorders [22].

16.7 MECHANISTIC BASIS OF NANO-ENCAPSULATED PROBIOTICS IN DIABETES

16.7.1 Modulation of Gut Microbiota Composition

Nano-encapsulated probiotics can restore microbial balance by enhancing survival and targeted delivery of beneficial bacteria to the colon. Encapsulation technologies protect strains such as *Lactobacillus* and *Bifidobacterium* during gastrointestinal transit, allowing greater numbers of viable cells to reach the intestinal microbiota. Experimental studies demonstrate that probiotic supplementation increased microbial diversity and promotes beneficial taxa while reducing opportunistic pathogens. These microbiome shifts are associated with improved metabolic homeostasis and reduced dysbiosis commonly observed in individuals with T2D [23].

16.7.2 Short-Chain Fatty Acids Production and Metabolic Signaling

One of the major metabolic benefits of probiotics therapy is the stimulation of SCFAs production, including acetate, propionate, and butyrate, which are generated during microbial fermentation of dietary fibers. SCFAs function as signaling molecules that regulate host metabolism through activation of G-protein-coupled receptors such as GPR41 and GPR43. These pathways influence energy metabolism, intestinal barrier function, and glucose homeostasis. Enhanced SCFA production has been associated with improved insulin signaling and metabolic regulation in experimental models metabolic disease [24].

16.7.3 Anti-Inflammatory Antioxidant Effects

Chronic low-grade inflammation and oxidative stress are key contributors to insulin resistance and β-cell dysfunction in diabetes. Nano-encapsulated probiotics may reduce inflammatory responses by modulating immune signaling pathways and strengthening intestinal barrier integrity. Beneficial microbial metabolites can suppress pro-inflammatory cytokines such as tumor necrosis factor-α and interleukin 6 while promoting anti-inflammatory cytokine production. Additionally, probiotics contribute to antioxidant defense by reducing reactive oxygen species generation and increasing endogenous antioxidant enzymes, thereby supporting improved metabolic health in diabetic conditions [25].

16.7.4 Enhancement of Insulin Sensitivity and Glucose Uptake

Improved gut microbial composition and metabolite signaling ultimately influence systemic glucose metabolism. SCFAs and other microbial metabolites stimulate secretion of incretin hormones such as glucagon-like peptide-1 (GLP-1), which enhances pancreatic insulin secretion and improves glycemic regulation. Probiotic-mediated modulation of intestinal permeability also reduces metabolic endotoxemia, a factor linked to insulin resistance. Experimental and clinical studies suggest these combined mechanisms contribute to improve insulin sensitivity, enhance glucose uptake in peripheral tissues, and promote better glycemic control [26]. The proposed mechanisms through which

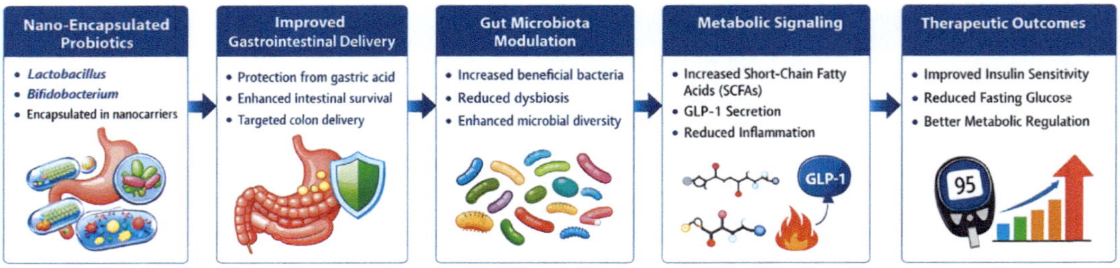

FIGURE 16.1 Mechanistic role of nano-encapsulated probiotics in T2D.

nano-encapsulated probiotics influence gut microbiota composition and the metabolic signaling pathways are shown in Figure 16.1.

16.8 PRECLINICAL EVIDENCE AND EXPERIMENTAL STUDIES

16.8.1 Animal Models of Nano-Probiotic Therapy

Preclinical animal models have been widely used to evaluate the therapeutic potential of nano-encapsulated probiotics in metabolic disorders. Studies in high-fat diet-induced diabetic mice and streptozotocin-induced diabetic rat models demonstrate that encapsulated strains such as *Lactobacillus* and *Bifidobacterium* show improved gastrointestinal survival and metabolic activity compared with free probiotics. These studies report reductions in fasting blood glucose and improved gut microbiota diversity, supporting the role of nano-delivery systems in improving probiotics' therapeutic efficacy [27].

16.8.2 Biomarkers of Metabolic Improvement

Experimental studies assessing nano-probiotic therapy often measure metabolic biomarkers to evaluate therapeutic outcomes. Improvements are often observed in indicators such as fasting blood glucose, glycated hemoglobin (HbA1c), insulin levels, and the homeostatic model assessment for insulin resistance (HOMA-IR). Additionally, increased production of SCFAs and reduced levels of inflammatory cytokines have been reported in probiotic-treated animals, suggesting that nano-encapsulation may enhance microbial metabolic activity and contribute to improved glucose regulation and metabolic homeostasis [28].

16.8.3 Safety and Biocompatibility Assessments

Safety and biocompatibility are critical aspects of the development of nano-probiotic systems. Preclinical toxicity studies typically evaluate organ histology, inflammatory responses, and systemic toxicity following administration of nanocarriers. Most biopolymer-based nanocarriers such as alginate, chitosan, and lipid nanoparticles demonstrate good biocompatibility and minimal toxicity in animal models. These findings support the feasibility of nano-encapsulation approaches for improving probiotic delivery while maintaining acceptable safety profiles [29].

16.9 CLINICAL EVIDENCE AND TRANSLATIONAL INSIGHTS

Clinical investigations increasingly support the role of microbiome-targeted interventions as complementary strategies in T2D management. Randomized controlled trials have shown that supplementation containing strains such as *Lactobacillus* and *Bifidobacterium* can modestly improve glycemic markers, including fasting plasma glucose, glycated hemoglobin (HbA1c), and insulin resistance indices such as HOMA-IR. Meta-analyses of clinical trials involving diabetic patient report consistent reductions in fasting blood glucose and improvements in lipid profiles following multi-strain probiotic supplementation. More recently, encapsulation technologies are being explored to enhance probiotic survival and therapeutic efficacy in humans, with early studies indicating improved gastrointestinal stability and metabolic outcomes compared with conventional formulations. Advances in microbiome sequencing and metabolomics are also enabling the development of personalized microbiome-based therapies, where probiotics or synbiotics interventions are tailored according to an individual's microbial composition to optimize metabolic responses and improve diabetes management [30].

16.10 INTEGRATION WITH PRECISION AND DIGITAL MEDICINE

16.10.1 Microbiome-Guided Therapeutic Design

Advances in microbiome profiling technologies have enabled microbiome-guided therapeutic strategies for metabolic diseases such as T2D. High-throughput sequencing and metagenomic analysis allow researchers to identify microbial signatures associated with insulin resistance and metabolic dysfunction. These data help guide the selection of probiotic strains capable of restoring the microbial balance. Recent studies indicate that microbiome-targeted interventions may improve metabolic regulation by increasing beneficial bacteria and reducing dysbiosis linked to diabetes progression [31].

16.10.2 AI and Omics Approaches in Symbiotic Nanomedicine

AI and multi-omic technologies are increasingly used to analyze complex host-microbiome interactions and optimize microbiome-based therapies. Integrated genomics, metabolomics, and proteomics data enable the identification of metabolic pathways influenced by gut microbes and probiotic interventions. AI-driven models can analyze large biological datasets to predict therapeutic response, helping researchers design more effective probiotic formulations and nano-delivery systems for targeted metabolic modulation in diabetes management [32].

16.11 PERSONALIZED METABOLIC INTERVENTIONS

Personalized metabolic interventions aim to tailor probiotic or synbiotic therapies to individual microbiome compositions, dietary patterns, and metabolic profiles. Emerging precision medicine approaches suggest that individualized microbiome modulation may produce better glycemic outcomes compared with generalized probiotic supplementation. Advances in digital health monitoring and microbiome analytics are supporting the development of personalized treatment approaches combining microbiome-based therapeutics with lifestyle and metabolic data for improved diabetes care [33]. The translational framework linking nanotechnology, microbiome modulation, and metabolic regulation in symbiotic nanomedicine is summarized in Figure 16.2.

16.12 REGULATORY, SAFETY, AND ETHICAL CONSIDERATIONS

16.12.1 Regulatory Landscape for Nano-Biotherapeutics

The regulatory oversight of nano-biotherapeutics, including nano-encapsulated probiotics, is evolving as nanomedicine technologies advance. Regulatory authorities such as the U.S. Food and Drug Administration (FDA) and the European Medicines Agency (EMA) require detailed characterization of nanomaterials, including particle size distribution, surface properties, stability, and biological interactions. Products combining probiotics with nanocarriers may fall under

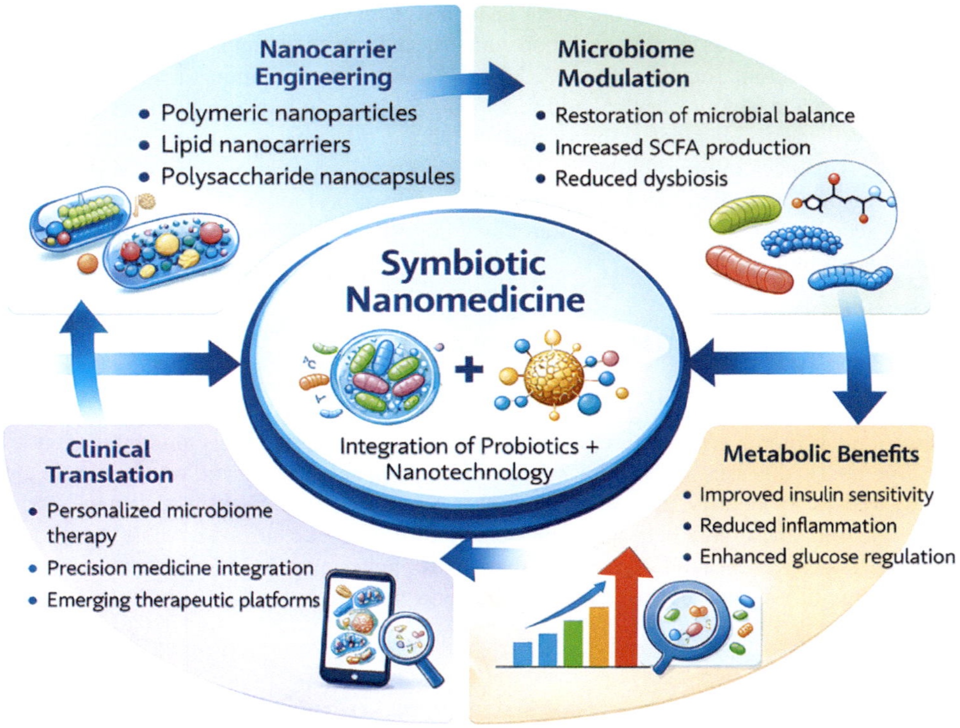

FIGURE 16.2 Translational framework of symbiotic nanomedicine for diabetes therapy.

complex regulatory categories such as biologics, drug-device combinations, or novel delivery systems, requiring rigorous quality, safety, and efficacy evaluations before clinical approval and commercialization globally [34].

16.12.2 Toxicological Evaluation of Nanocarriers

Comprehensive toxicological evaluation is essential for ensuring the safety of nanocarrier-based probiotic delivery systems. Preclinical safety assessments typically examine cytotoxicity, biodistribution, immunogenicity, and long-term tissue accumulation of nanomaterials. Biopolymer-based nanocarriers such as alginate, chitosan, and lipid nanoparticles are generally considered biocompatible and biodegradable, showing minimal toxicity in experimental models. However, variations in nanoparticle size, surface charge, and composition may alter biological interactions, necessitating standardized toxicological testing to ensure safety before clinical use [35].

16.12.3 Ethical Issues in Microbiome Engineering

Microbiome engineering and therapeutic manipulation raise several ethical considerations related to safety, data privacy, and long-term ecological impacts on the human microbiome. Personalized microbiome-based therapies often rely on genomic sequencing and microbiome profiling, which involve sensitive biological data requiring careful privacy protection. Additionally, long-term consequences of microbial ecosystems remain incompletely understood. Ethical frameworks therefore emphasize transparency, responsible innovation, informed consent, and careful clinical monitoring when implementing microbiome-targeted therapeutic technologies [36].

16.13 FUTURE OUTLOOK

Future developments in symbiotic nanomedicine are expected to focus on advanced delivery platforms and precision microbiome engineering. Smart and stimuli-responsive nano-synbiotics capable of releasing probiotics in response to environmental triggers such as pH, enzymes, or inflammatory signals may significantly improve therapeutic targeting in the gastrointestinal tract. Concurrently, engineered probiotics developed through synthetic biology are being designed to produce beneficial metabolites, regulate immune responses, or modulate glucose metabolism. Advances in scalable nanomanufacturing, microbiome analytics, and regulatory frameworks are also facilitating clinical translation. Together, these innovations may enable commercially viable microbiome-based therapeutics for personalized management of metabolic disorders, including T2D [37].

16.14 CONCLUSION

Symbiotic nanomedicine represents an emerging and promising strategy for improving microbiome-based interventions in T2D management. Conventional probiotic therapies often face limitations such as poor gastrointestinal survival, limited stability, and insufficient colonization within the intestinal environment. Nano-encapsulation technologies provide innovative solutions by protecting probiotic microorganisms from harsh physiological conditions and enabling controlled, targeted delivery in the gut. These advanced delivery systems improve microbial viability, promote beneficial microbiota modulation, and support metabolic regulation through mechanisms such as SCFA production, anti-inflammatory effects, and improved insulin sensitivity. Preclinical and early clinical evidence indicates that nano-probiotic systems may significantly enhance therapeutic outcomes compared with traditional probiotic formulations. As research advances, integration with precision medicine, microbiome analytics, and digital health technologies may further optimize probiotic-based therapies. Continued interdisciplinary research will be essential for translating these innovative approaches into safe, effective, and clinically applicable treatments for metabolic disorders.

ACKNOWLEDGMENTS

The authors express deepest gratitude to the editors for providing opportunity for writing this wonderful chapter.

REFERENCES

1. Aydin Ö, Nieuwdorp M, Gerdes V. The gut microbiome as a target for the treatment of type 2 diabetes. Current Diabetes Reports. 2018;18(8):55.
2. Liu S. Mechanisms of gut microbiota in host fat deposition: Metabolites, signaling pathways, and translational applications. Frontiers in Microbiology. 2025;16:1675155.
3. Manan MA. The role of probiotics in personalized therapeutics: Advances in gut microbe-driven interventions. The Microbe. 2025;8: [Internet]. 100497.
4. Petrovic S, Bita B, Barbinta-Patrascu ME. Nanoformulations in pharmaceutical and biomedical applications: Green perspectives. International Journal of Molecular Sciences. 2024;25(11):5842.
5. Chen A, Gong Y, Wu S, Du Y, Liu Z, Jiang Y, Li J, Miao YB. Navigating a challenging path: Precision disease treatment with tailored oral nano-armor-probiotics. Journal of Nanobiotechnology. 2025;23(1):72.
6. Dilworth L, Facey A, Omoruyi F. Diabetes mellitus and its metabolic complications: The role of adipose tissues. International Journal of Molecular Sciences. 2021;22(14):7644.
7. Harrass S, Ali S, Elshweikh M, Franco-Duarte R, Jayasinghe TN. Stage-specific gut microbiome shifts across the type 2 diabetes mellitus spectrum: A systematic review and meta-analysis. medRxiv. 2026:2026-01.
8. Gasaly N, De Vos P, Hermoso MA. Impact of bacterial metabolites on gut barrier function and host immunity: A focus on bacterial metabolism and its relevance for intestinal inflammation. Frontiers in Immunology. 2021;12:658354.

9. Zhang Y, Chen R, Zhang D, Qi S, Liu Y. Metabolite interactions between host and microbiota during health and disease: Which feeds the other? Biomedicine & Pharmacotherapy. 2023;160:114295.
10. Hosseinkhani F, Heinken A, Thiele I, Lindenburg PW, Harms AC, Hankemeier T. The contribution of gut bacterial metabolites in the human immune signaling pathway of non-communicable diseases. Gut Microbes. 2021;13(1):1882927.
11. Smolinska S, Popescu FD, Zemelka-Wiacek M. A review of the influence of prebiotics, probiotics, synbiotics, and postbiotics on the human gut microbiome and intestinal integrity. Journal of Clinical Medicine. 2025;14(11):3673.
12. Naseri K, Saadati S, Ashtary-Larky D, Asbaghi O, Ghaemi F, Pashayee-Khamene F, Yari Z, de Courten B. Probiotics and synbiotics supplementation improve glycemic control parameters in subjects with prediabetes and type 2 diabetes mellitus: A GRADE-assessed systematic review, meta-analysis, and meta-regression of randomized clinical trials. Pharmacological Research. 2022;184:106399.
13. Han S, Lu Y, Xie J, Fei Y, Zheng G, Wang Z, Liu J, Lv L, Ling Z, Berglund B, Yao M. Probiotic gastrointestinal transit and colonization after oral administration: A long journey. Frontiers in Cellular and Infection Microbiology. 2021;11:609722.
14. Mirarab A, Assadpour E, Jafari SM. Encapsulation of probiotics via electrospraying technology; Fundamentals, analysis, techniques, and applications. Future Foods. 2025;31:100897.
15. Kandari A, Odat ME, Alzaid F, Scott KP. Biotics and bacterial function: Impact on gut and host health. The ISME Journal. 2024;18(1):wrae226.
16. Silva PB, Rosales TK, Fabi JP. Nanoencapsulation of biotics: Feasibility to enhance stability and delivery for improved gut health. Pharmaceutics. 2025;17(9):1180.
17. Martău GA, Mihai M, Vodnar DC. The use of chitosan, alginate, and pectin in the biomedical and food sector—Biocompatibility, bioadhesiveness, and biodegradability. Polymers. 2019;11(11):1837.
18. Agriopoulou S, Tarapoulouzi M, Varzakas T, Jafari SM. Application of encapsulation strategies for probiotics: From individual loading to co-encapsulation. Microorganisms. 2023;11(12):2896.
19. Elmowafy M, Shalaby K, Elkomy MH, Alsaidan OA, Gomaa HA, Abdelgawad MA, Mostafa EM. Polymeric nanoparticles for delivery of natural bioactive agents: Recent advances and challenges. Polymers. 2023;15(5):1123.
20. Mall J, Naseem N, Haider MF, Rahman MA, Khan S, Siddiqui SN. Nanostructured lipid carriers as a drug delivery system: A comprehensive review with therapeutic applications. Intelligent Pharmacy. 2024;3(4):243–55.
21. Gao R, Zhao D, Zhou X, Wan Z, Wang X, Rao H, Liu X, Gao X, Hao J. Advances in polysaccharide-based biopolymers for probiotic encapsulation: From single polysaccharides to composite systems. Current Research in Food Science. 2025;11:101186.
22. Nunziata G, Pollonio D, Lacroce E, Rossi F. Smart pH-responsive polymers in biomedical applications: Nanoparticles, hydrogels, and emerging hybrid platforms. Materials Today Chemistry. 2025;49:103063.
23. Ramírez A, Bermúdez-Luque A, Román-Camacho JJ, Martín-García FJ, Moreno-García J, Güngörmüşler M, Ruiz-Castilla FJ. Exploring the future of probiotics with innovations in delivery systems and market insights. Food Bioscience. 2025;71:107029.
24. Xiong RG, Zhou DD, Wu SX, Huang SY, Saimaiti A, Yang ZJ, Shang A, Zhao CN, Gan RY, Li HB. Health benefits and side effects of short-chain fatty acids. Foods. 2022;11(18):2863.
25. Vijayaram S, Vivekanandan KE, Kandasamy S, Razafindralambo H, Ringø E, Sun YZ, Kaliyannan G. Probiotics: A multifaceted approach to health promotion-from disease prevention to food enrichment and delivery systems. AIMS Microbiology. 2025;11(3):602.
26. Kamath S, Chan NS, Joyce P. GLP-1 agonists and the gut microbiome: A bidirectional relationship. British Journal of Clinical Pharmacology. 2026;92(5):1309–125.
27. Chen X, Tan F, Yi R, Mu J, Zhao X, Yang Z. Effects of *Lactobacillus* on mice with diabetes induced by high-fat diet with streptozotocin (STZ). Applied Sciences. 2018;8(8):1249.
28. Sood R, Lee HJ. Lactiplantibacillus plantarum Ln4 attenuates streptozotocin and high-fat diet-induced type-2 diabetes. Journal of Functional Foods. 2026;138:107219.
29. Parvin N, Aslam M, Joo SW, Mandal TK. Nano-phytomedicine: Harnessing plant-derived phytochemicals in nanocarriers for targeted human health applications. Molecules. 2025;30(15):3177.
30. Ayesha IE, Monson NR, Klair N, Patel U, Saxena A, Patel D, Venugopal S, Ayesha IE. Probiotics and their role in the management of type 2 diabetes mellitus (short-term versus long-term effect): A systematic review and meta-analysis. Cureus. 2023;15(10):01–14.
31. Fang X, Zhang Y, Huang X, Miao R, Zhang Y, Tian J. Gut microbiome research: Revealing the pathological mechanisms and treatment strategies of type 2 diabetes. Diabetes, Obesity and Metabolism. 2025;27(8):4051–68.

32. Dhaarani R, Reddy MK. Progressing microbial genomics: Artificial intelligence and deep learning driven advances in genome analysis and therapeutics. Intelligence-Based Medicine. 2025;11:100251.
33. Yu J. Personalized delivery of probiotics and prebiotics via 3D food printing. Metabolites. 2025;15(11):744.
34. Stucchi F, Li M, Castellano G, Cellesi F. Regulatory framework for polymer-based nanotherapeutics in clinical translation. Frontiers in Bioengineering and Biotechnology. 2026;14:1735885.
35. Iskandar AF, Dohong AA, Widjanarko ND, Hendrawan AF, Alvianto S, Santini A, Salamah S, Iqhrammullah M, Tjandrawinata RR, Nurkolis F. Food-grade polymers as smart carriers for maternal nutrition and fetal protection. Current Research in Biotechnology. 2026;11:100369.
36. Yahya EB, Abdulsamad MA, Aburowais AS, Abogmaza AF. Insights into microbiome-based therapeutics: Engineered probiotics, bacteriophages, and microbiome-derived metabolites. Biomedical Research and Therapy. 2025;12(12):8062–71.
37. Renukadevi J, Ranjani M, Sneha P, Hussain JS, Shakthi H. Gut-targeted nutraceutical delivery: Engineering microbiome-responsive nutraceutical interfaces. Food Bioengineering. 2025;4(3):248–61.

17 Nano-Engineered Strategies for Diabetes Management

Case-Based Insights and Clinical Perspectives

Madhu B. K.
Sri Adichunchanagiri College of Pharmacy, Adichunchanagiri University, Mandya, India

Neerati Prasad
Pharmacology University College of Pharmaceutical Sciences, Kakatiya University, Warangal, India

Nidhi Singh
Teerthanker Mahaveer College of pharmacy (TMCOP), TMU, Muradabad, India

Khumanthem Deepak Singh
Asian International University, Imphal, India

Vaibhav Dagaji Aher
Maharashtra University of Health Sciences, Nashik, India

Ranjit Vinayak Gadhave
School of Health Sciences and Technology, Dr. Vishwanath Karad MIT World Peace University, Pune, India

Mohammad Ali
Sri Adichunchanagiri College of Pharmacy, Adichunchanagiri University, Mandya, India

17.1 INTRODUCTION

Diabetes mellitus remains one of the most pressing global health challenges, characterized by chronic hyperglycemia resulting from impaired insulin secretion, insulin resistance, or both. According to recent global health estimates, the prevalence of diabetes continues to rise rapidly, driven by ageing populations, sedentary lifestyles, and increasing rates of obesity. The persistent hyperglycemia contributes to a wide spectrum of long-term complications, including cardiovascular disease, nephropathy, neuropathy, and retinopathy, which considerably increase morbidity, mortality, and healthcare costs. Despite major therapeutic advances, achieving sustained glycemic control while minimizing adverse effects remains a persistent clinical challenge [1].

DOI: 10.1201/9781003598657-17

Conventional antidiabetic therapies, including oral hypoglycemic agents and insulin injections, have improved disease management but and are often associated with several limitations. These include poor drug bioavailability, short pharmacological half-life, systemic side effects, frequent dosing requirements, and poor patient adherence. Furthermore, many therapies fail to address the complex pathophysiology of diabetes at the tissue or cellular level, highlighting the need for more precise and adaptive therapeutic strategies [2].

In this context, nano-engineering approaches have emerged as promising tools to improve the delivery and therapeutic performance of antidiabetic agents. By controlling materials at the nanoscale, these systems can improve drug stability, facilitate controlled or stimuli-responsive release, and improve targeted delivery to specific tissues involved in glucose regulation. Unlikely conventional formulations, nano-engineered platform can be designed to respond dynamically to physiological cues such as glucose concentration, enabling more responsive and personalized therapeutic interventions [3].

Beyond drug delivery, nanotechnology is also contributing to broader innovations in diabetes care, including integrated therapeutic systems, biomimetic platforms, and multifunctional formulations that combine therapeutic and diagnostic capabilities. Such strategies aim not only to improve glycemic control but also to address emerging needs in precision medicine and long-term disease management [4].

This chapter covers recent nano-engineering strategies for diabetes management through a case-based and clinically oriented perspective, highlighting translational progress, practical challenges, and future opportunities for integrating nanomedicine into modern diabetes therapy.

17.2 TRANSLATIONAL GAP IN NANO-BASED DIABETES THERAPIES

Although nanotechnology has generated numerous innovative strategies for diabetes management, the successful translation of these technologies into clinical practice remains limited. Many nano-engineered formulations show promising results in laboratory and animal studies, including improved drug stability, targeted drug delivery, and controlled release of antidiabetic drugs. However, only a small proportion of these experimental systems progress to clinical testing or therapeutic approval. This discrepancy reflects a significant translational gap between preclinical innovations and real-world medical application [5].

17.2.1 Bench-to-Bedside Challenges

One of the primary challenges is the reproducibility and scalability of nanoformulations. Nanoparticles require precise control over parameters such as particle size, surface feature, and drug loading efficiency, all of which influence therapeutic performance. Achieving consistent large-scale production while maintaining these properties remains technically demanding. Additionally, the biological behavior of nanomaterials within complex physiological environments can vary considerably. Interactions with proteins, immune responses, and tissue distribution patterns may alter the efficacy and safety profile observed in preclinical models. Long-term toxicity assessment and standardized evaluation protocols are therefore essential before clinical translation [6].

17.2.2 Clinical Adoption Barriers

Beyond technical limitations, several factors hinder clinical adoption of nano-based diabetes therapies. Regulatory agencies require extensive characterization and safety data for nanomedicines, often resulting in longer approval pathways. Economic considerations, including manufacturing cost and reimbursement challenges, also influence adoption. Furthermore, clinicians need strong evidence demonstrating clear therapeutic benefits over proven therapeutic before integrating nanotechnology-based interventions into routine diabetes care [7].

17.3 PRECISION NANOMEDICINE APPROACHES IN DIABETES CARE

Precision medicine is increasingly shaping the future of diabetes management by emphasizing therapies tailored to individual patient characteristics, disease progression, and metabolic variability. In this context, nanotechnology provides special opportunities to design therapeutic systems capable of improving drug delivery accuracy and therapeutic efficiency. Nano-engineered platforms can be customized to enhance drug pharmacokinetics, enable controlled release, and improve targeting to tissues involved in glucose regulation. These capabilities support the development of more personalized treatment strategies that move beyond conventional one-size-fits-all approaches. Multiple nano-engineered methods are currently being explored to increase therapeutic precision, and improve metabolic regulation in diabetes [8]. These strategies collectively contribute to the development of integrated nanomedicine platforms aimed at improving clinical outcomes (Figure 17.1).

17.3.1 Patient-Specific Drug Delivery Strategies

Patient-specific drug delivery represents a key component of precision nanomedicine. Nanoformulations can be engineered to modulate drug release rates, protect sensitive biomolecules, and improve the stability of peptide-based therapeutics such as insulin or incretin hormones. By optimizing the particle composition, surface chemistry, and responsiveness to physiological signals, nanocarriers can be designed to respond to variations in glucose levels or metabolic conditions. Such adaptive delivery systems may reduce dosing frequency, minimize fluctuations in blood glucose, and improve overall therapeutic adherence. Furthermore, advancements in biomarker profiling and pharmacogenomics insights are expected to facilitate the development of individualized nanoformulations that align with patient-specific metabolic needs [9].

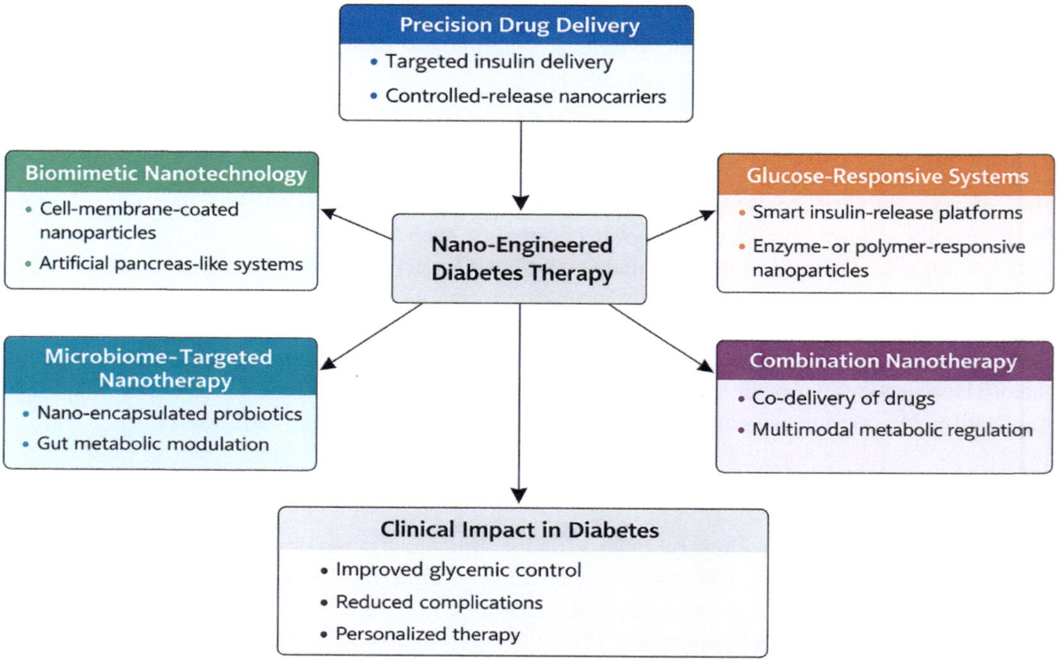

FIGURE 17.1 Translational framework of nano-engineered strategies for diabetes management.

17.3.2 Targeted Tissue Delivery

Targeted tissue delivery is another major aspect of nano-engineered diabetes therapy. Nanocarriers can be functionalized with ligands or surface modifications that promote accumulation in particular tissues involved in glucose homeostasis, such as the pancreas, the liver, or adipose tissue. This targeted approach can increase local drug concentrations while minimizing systemic exposure and potential adverse effects. By improving delivery precision, nano-engineered systems may enhance therapeutic outcomes and support more efficient metabolic regulation in patients with diabetes [10].

17.4 BIO-INSPIRED AND BIOMIMETIC NANO-SYSTEMS

Bio-inspired and biomimetic nanotechnology has been as a promising strategy for improving therapeutic performance of nanomedicine in diabetes management. Unlike conventional nanocarriers, biomimetic systems are designed to replicate biological structures or physiological processes, thereby enhancing compatibility with the human body and improving therapeutic efficiency. By integrating natural biological components such as cell membranes, enzymes, or biomolecules, these nano-systems can achieve improved circulation stability, immune system evasion, and targeted delivery. Recent studies have increasingly focused on developing biomimetic platforms that imitate pancreatic function or natural cellular interfaces involved in glucose regulation [11].

17.4.1 Cell-Membrane-Coated Nanoparticles

Cell-membrane-coated nanoparticles represent a notable advancement in biomimetic nanomedicine. In this approach, synthetic nanoparticle cores are cloaked with membranes derived from natural cells, such as red blood cells, platelets, or pancreatic β-cells. The presence of natural membrane proteins and lipids enables these nanoparticles to interact with biological environments in a more physiologically compatible manner. For example, red blood cell membrane-coated nanoparticles have shown prolonged circulation time and reduced immune clearance, which can improve the sustained delivery of therapeutic agents [12].

Recent studies have explored β-cell membrane-coated nanoparticles designed to mimic surface characteristics of pancreatic cells. These systems can enhance interactions with pancreatic tissues and may support more targeted delivery of insulin or protective agents aimed at preserving β-cell function. Additionally, macrophage membrane-coated nanoparticles have been explored for their ability to modulate inflammatory pathways associated with metabolic dysfunction, offering potential benefits in controlling diabetes-related inflammation [13].

17.4.2 Artificial Pancreas Mimetic Platforms

Artificial pancreas mimetic platforms aim to replicate the glucose-responsive behavior of natural pancreatic β-cells. These nano-engineered systems are typically designed to sense fluctuations in blood glucose levels and release insulin in a controlled and responsive manner. One widely investigated strategy involves glucose-responsive nanoparticles incorporating glucose oxidase (GOx), which catalyzes glucose conversion and triggers insulin release under hyperglycemic conditions [14].

Another emerging approach involves polymer-based vesicles or nano-networks capable of adjusting insulin release through glucose-responsive chemical interactions, such as phenylboronic acid-glucose binding mechanisms. Some experimental platforms integrate nanosensors and insulin reservoirs within injectable hydrogels or microcapsules to mimic physiological and insulin reservoirs within injectable hydrogels or microcapsules to mimic physiological insulin secretion patterns. Although most of these technologies remain in experimental stages, they represent important steps toward developing autonomous insulin delivery systems that more closely resemble the natural function of the pancreas [15].

17.5 MICROBIOME-TARGETED NANOTHERAPEUTICS IN DIABETES

Growing evidence indicates that the gut microbiome plays an important role in metabolic regulation and pathogenesis of diabetes. Alterations in intestinal microbial composition, commonly referred to as dysbiosis, have been linked to insulin resistance, chronic inflammation, and impaired glucose metabolism. Consequently, therapeutic strategies aimed at restoring microbial balance are gaining attention as complementary approaches for diabetes management. Nanotechnology has recently been explored as a tool to enhance the delivery and stability of microbiome-modulating therapeutics, enabling more precise interventions within the gastrointestinal environment [16].

17.5.1 Nanocarriers for Probiotic and Prebiotic Delivery

One emerging strategy involves the use of nanocarriers to enhance the viability and targeted delivery of probiotics or prebiotics agents. Many beneficial microbial strains are sensitive to acidic gastric conditions and digestive enzymes, which can limit their therapeutic potential. Nano-encapsulation using polymeric or polysaccharide-based carriers can protect probiotic organisms during gastrointestinal transit and promote release in intestinal tract. Recent experimental studies have reported that alginate-chitosan nano-encapsulation systems enhance the survival and colonization of probiotic strains such as *Lactobacillus* and *Bifidobacterium*, which are linked with improved glucose metabolism and reduced inflammatory signaling in metabolic disorders [17].

17.5.2 Microbiomes-Modulating Nanomedicines

Nanotechnology has also been explored for delivering bioactive compounds that influence microbial composition and metabolic activity. For instance, nanoformulations of plant-derived polyphenols, such as curcumin or resveratrol, have been investigated for their ability to modulate gut microbial diversity and improve insulin sensitivity. Encapsulation enhances the stability and intestinal bioavailability of these compounds, allowing more effective interactions with microbial communities. Such approaches may indirectly influence host metabolic pathways by promoting beneficial microbial metabolites [18].

17.5.3 Nano-Enabled Gut-Targeted Therapeutic Systems

Another promising direction involves designing nanoparticles that selectively release therapeutic agents within the intestinal microenvironment. These systems can deliver anti-inflammatory molecules, metabolic regulators, or microbial metabolites directly to the gut, where they may influence host-microbiome interactions. Emerging studies suggest that gut-targeted nanoformulations could support metabolic homeostasis, reduce intestinal inflammation, and improve glucose regulation. This highlights the growing potential of microbiome-focused nanotherapeutics in diabetes care [19].

17.6 NANOTECHNOLOGY IN METABOLIC REPROGRAMMING

Metabolic reprogramming has emerged as an important concept in diabetes research, focusing on modifying cellular metabolic pathways to restore glucose homeostasis and improve insulin sensitivity. In diabetes, key metabolic tissues including the liver, skeletal muscle, adipose tissue, and pancreatic β-cells undergo metabolic alterations in energy utilization, lipid metabolism, and inflammatory signaling. Nanotechnology offers innovative opportunities to deliver metabolic modulators with enhanced precision, stability, and tissue targeting. By enabling controlled delivery of therapeutic molecules, nano-engineered systems may help correct metabolic dysfunction and support long-term glycemic control [20].

17.6.1 Nanocarriers for Modulating Insulin Signaling Pathways

Several nanoformulations have been developed to enhance the delivery of agents that influence insulin signaling pathways. For example, nanoparticles encapsulating metformin or AMP-activated protein kinase (AMPK) have been investigated for improving cellular glucose uptake and regulating hepatic glucose production. Polymeric nanoparticles composed of biodegradable materials such as poly(lactic-co-glycolic) acid (PLGA) have been shown in experimental studies to increase the bioavailability of antidiabetic drugs and sustain their metabolic effects. Such targeted delivery strategies may improve therapeutic efficiency while minimizing systemic side effects associated with conventional dosing [21].

17.6.2 Nanoparticles Targeting Adipose Tissue Metabolism

Adipose tissue plays a crucial role in metabolic regulation and insulin sensitivity. Recent nanotechnology-based approaches aim to deliver bioactive molecules that modulate adipocytes functions and inflammatory signaling within adipose tissue. For example, lipid-based nanoparticles have been explored for delivering small interfering RNA (siRNA) to suppress genes associated with insulin resistance or lipid accumulation. Experimental studies have also reported the use of nano-encapsulated polyphenols, such as resveratrol-loaded nanoparticles, to influence adipocyte metabolism and improve insulin responsiveness [22].

17.6.3 Nano-Enabled Delivery of Metabolic Regulatory Molecules

Nanotechnology also facilitates the delivery of metabolic regulators such as peptides, nucleic acids, or mitochondrial-targeted antioxidants. These molecules can influence pathways involved in oxidative stress, mitochondria function, and cellular energy balance. For example, cerium oxide nanoparticles and other nano-antioxidants have been studied for reducing oxidative stress in metabolic tissues. By increasing the stability and targeted delivery of metabolic modulators, nanotechnology may support emerging therapeutic approaches aimed at reprogramming dysfunctional metabolic networks in diabetes [23].

17.7 NANO-ENGINEERED COMBINATION THERAPIES

Combination therapy is commonly used in diabetes management to address the multifactorial nature of the disease, which involves impaired insulin signaling, inflammation, oxidative stress, and metabolic dysregulation. Traditional combination treatments often require multiple medications administered separately. Nano-engineered combination therapies provide an innovative solution by enabling co-delivery of multiple therapeutic agents within a single nanoscale platform. Such systems can improve pharmacokinetic compatibility, enhance therapeutic synergy, and enable controlled release of drugs with different mechanisms of action. Several innovative nano-engineered strategies are currently being explored to improve therapeutic outcomes in diabetes management [24]. These methods range from glucose-responsive insulin delivery systems to biomimetic nanoparticles and combination nanotherapies that address multiple metabolic pathways simultaneously (Table 17.1).

17.7.1 Co-Delivery of Antidiabetic Drugs

Nanocarriers can be designed to encapsulate concurrently two or more antidiabetics that enhance therapeutic efficiency by complimentary action. For example, polymeric nanoparticles have been studied for contemporaneous improvement of insulin sensitivity and hepatic glucose production by combined delivery of metformin and pioglitazone. Lipid-based nanocarriers and nanostructured lipid carriers have also been explored for the delivery of combinations of insulin with oral

TABLE 17.1
Emerging Nano-Engineered Strategies for Diabetes Management and Their Clinical Relevance

Nano-Engineered Strategy	Key Functional Concept	Representative Example	Potential Clinical Benefit
Glucose-responsive nanocarriers	Insulin release triggered by glucose-sensitive components (e.g., glucose oxidase or phenylboronic acid)	GOx-integrated polymeric nanoparticles [25]	Automated insulin delivery and reduced hypoglycemia risk
Biomimetic nanoparticles	Nanoparticles coated with natural cell membranes to improve biological compatibility	Red blood cell membrane-coated insulin nanocarriers [26]	Prolonged circulation and reduced immune clearance
Microbiome-targeted nanoformulations	Nano-encapsulation of probiotics or bioactive compounds to modulate gut microbiota	Alginate-chitosan nano-encapsulated *Lactobacillus* [27]	Improved metabolic regulated and reduced inflammation
Combination nanotherapy	Co-delivery of multiple therapeutic agents within a single nanocarrier	Metformin-curcumin co-loaded polymeric nanoparticles [28]	Synergistic metabolic and anti-inflammatory effects
Nano-enabled wound therapy	Nanomaterial-based dressings delivering antimicrobial or regenerative agents	Silver nanoparticle hydrogel dressings [29]	Accelerated healing of diabetic foot ulcers

anti-diabetic agents. These integrated systems could increase the glycemic control while decreasing the drug dose needed for reducing systemic side effects [30].

17.7.2 Integration of Therapeutic and Anti-Inflammatory Agents

Chronic low-grade inflammation is a recognized contributor to insulin resistance and diabetes progression. Nano-engineered platforms have therefore been designed to deliver antidiabetic drugs alongside anti-inflammatory or antioxidant compounds. For example, curcumin-loaded nanoparticles combined with traditional antidiabetic drugs have shown improved metabolic outcomes in experimental studies due to curcumin's ability to regulate inflammatory pathways and oxidative stress. Similarly, resveratrol-loaded nanocarriers have explored for their combined metabolic and anti-inflammatory effects [10].

17.7.3 Hybrid Nanoplatforms for Multimodal Therapy

Recent advances in nanomedicine have enabled the development of hybrid nanoplatforms that integrate therapeutic agents with biological molecules such as peptides, nucleic acids, or metabolic regulators. For example, lipid nanoparticles delivering siRNA that target metabolic genes have been used in combination with traditional antidiabetic drugs to improve therapeutic outcomes. Such multimodal strategies aim to address multiple disease pathways simultaneously, representing a promising direction for more comprehensive personalized diabetes treatment [31].

17.8 CLINICAL-BASED CLINICAL INSIGHTS

Recent advances in nanotechnology have generated several experimental and early translational approaches aimed at improving diabetes management. Case-based analyses of these emerging technologies provide valuable insights into how nano-engineered systems may address limitations of conventional therapies. Although many of these innovations remain under investigation, they demonstrate the potential of nanomedicine to increase therapeutic precision, improve drug delivery, and address complications associated with diabetes [3].

17.8.1 Glucose-Responsive Insulin Systems

Glucose-responsive insulin delivery platforms represent one of the most actively explored nanotechnological strategies for diabetes treatment. These systems are designed to release insulin in response to fluctuations in blood glucose levels, thereby mimicking the physiological function of pancreatic β-cells. A notable example involves polymeric nanoparticles incorporating glucose oxidase (GOx), an enzyme that converts glucose into gluconic acid and hydrogen peroxide. This biochemical reaction triggers structural changes within the nanoparticle matrix, enabling controlled insulin release during hyperglycemic conditions. Experimental studies in diabetic animal models have shown that such glucose-responsive nano-systems can maintain more stable glycemic levels and reduce the risk of hypoglycemia compared with conventional insulin administration [32].

17.8.2 Oral Insulin Nanotechnology

Oral insulin delivery has long been a major challenge due to enzymatic degradation and poor intestinal absorption of peptide drugs. Nanotechnology has offered promising solutions through protective nano-encapsulation and mucoadhesive delivery strategies. For example, chitosan-based nanoparticles have been investigated for their ability to protect insulin from gastrointestinal degradation while improving permeability. Some studies have also explored lipid-based nanocarriers that facilitate insulin transport across intestinal epithelial barriers. Preclinical research suggests these nanoformulations can improve insulin bioavailability and achieve measurable reductions in blood glucose levels following oral administration [33].

17.8.3 Nano-Enabled Wound Repair

Chronic wounds, particularly diabetic foot ulcers, represent a serious complication of diabetes. Nanotechnology-based wound therapies have been developed to accelerate healing by delivering antimicrobial, anti-inflammatory, or regenerative agents. For example, silver nanoparticle-embedded hydrogels and nanofiber dressing have demonstrated antimicrobial activity and enhanced tissue regeneration in diabetic wound models. Such nano-enabled wound care platforms may improve outcomes while reducing infection risk in patients with diabetes [34].

17.9 MANUFACTURING AND SCALABILITY OF NANO-THERAPEUTICS

The successful clinical maneuvering of nano-therapeutics in diabetes management is not only dependent on biological efficacy but also on reliable biological manufacture and large-scale productions. While many of these nano-engineered formulations have shown promising findings in laboratory and pre-clinical studies, getting such systems into a commercial form requires robust production processes to ensure consistency, stability, and regulatory compliance. Scalable manufacturing must ensure that critical physicochemical properties such as particle size distribution, surface charge, drug loading efficiency, and release kinetics are not changed since these properties have a direct impact on therapeutic performance and safety [3].

17.9.1 Scalability Production Technologies

Several advanced manufacturing technologies have been developed to support the large-scale production of nanomedicines. Techniques such as high-pressure homogenization, microfluidic synthesis, and nanoprecipitation have gained attention for their ability to produce nanoparticles with uniform characteristics. For example, microfluidic platforms have been increasingly used to generate lipid nanoparticles and polymeric nanocarriers with improved reproducibility and controlled particle sizes. Continuous manufacturing approaches are also emerging as efficient alternatives to traditional batch production, enabling better process control and reduced variability. These technologies are especially pertinent for scaling nano-formulations designed for insulin delivery or peptide-based therapeutics [35].

17.9.2 Quality Control and Regulatory Compliance

Consistency of quality during nano-therapeutic production is a major requirement for regulatory approval. Regulatory agencies put a strong emphasis on detailed characterization of nanomedicines on the basis of particle morphology, surface chemistry, stability, and drug release behavior. Analytical methods like dynamic light scattering, electron microscopy, and chromatography analysis are common for quality evaluation. Additionally, good manufacturing practice (GMP) guidelines need to be strictly adhered to for reproducibility as well as for product safety. Establishing standard measures of characterization and well-established production procedures are still crucial for facilitating the mass clinical adoption of nano-engineered diabetes treatments [36].

17.10 REGULATORY AND ETHICAL CONSIDERATIONS

The development of nano-engineered therapies for diabetes introduces important regulatory and ethical considerations that must be addressed before widespread clinical implementation. Because nanomedicines possess unique physicochemical properties compared with conventional pharmaceuticals, regulatory agencies require additional characterization and safety evaluation. Agencies such as the U.S. Food and Drug Administration (FDA) and the European Medicines Agency (EMA) have issued guidance documents emphasizing detailed assessment of nanoparticle composition, surface properties, biodistribution, and long-term toxicity. These requirements seek to assure that nano-therapeutics have consistent quality, safety, and therapeutic efficacies before entering clinical practice [37].

A major regulatory challenge involves the lack of universally standardized assessment frameworks for nanomedicine. Variability in nanoparticle design, manufacturing processes, and biological interactions can complicate regulatory assessment. For example, lipid nanoparticle platforms used for drug delivery require careful evaluation of stability, immune responses, and pharmacokinetics. Recent regulatory experiences with lipid nanoparticle-based therapeutics have helped inform safety evaluation strategies that may also guide the approval of future nano-enabled diabetes treatments [36, 37].

Ethical considerations are important in the development of nanotechnology-based healthcare solutions. Issues related to long-term safety, patient consent, and equitable access to advanced therapies will need to be carefully addressed. Since nano-engineered treatments may have higher costs of production, fairness of accessibility in different healthcare systems is also a key issue. Transparent communication regarding benefits, risks, and uncertainties will be essential to build patient trust and support the responsible integration of nanomedicine into diabetes care.

17.11 FUTURE CLINICAL LANDSCAPE OF NANO-ENGINEERED DIABETES THERAPY

The future clinical universe of nano-engineered diabetes therapy is expected to be shaped by advances in precision medicine, smart drug delivery systems, and integrated therapeutic technologies. Nanotechnology offers the potential to move diabetes management beyond conventional drug administration toward more adaptive and patient-centered treatment strategies. Emerging nanoformulations are being designed to respond dynamically to physiological signals such as glucose fluctuations, enabling more precise and automated regulation of insulin delivery [38].

One promising direction involves the integration of nanomedicine with digital health technologies. Nano-enabled biosensors and drug delivery platforms may eventually be combined with continuous glucose monitoring systems and algorithm-based control mechanisms to support closed-loop diabetes management. Such integrated systems could enhance real-time therapeutic adjustments and improve long-term glycemic control [39].

Another important area of development is the use of multifunctional nanoplatforms capable of addressing multiple aspects of diabetes simultaneously. For example, next-generation nanotherapeutics are being investigated for their ability to deliver metabolic regulators, anti-inflammatory agents, or gene-modulating molecules in a targeted manner. These strategies may help address underlying metabolic dysfunction rather than only controlling blood glucose levels [10].

Although several technological and regulatory challenges remain, continued interdisciplinary research and improved manufacturing strategies are expected to accelerate the clinical translation of nano-engineered therapies, potentially transforming future approaches to diabetes care.

17.12 CONCLUSION

Nano-engineered approaches are emerging as potential tools for improving diabetes management by addressing several limitations associated with conventional treatments. Through advances in targeted drug delivery, glucose-responsive systems, and multifunctional nanoplatforms, nanotechnology has the potential to enhance therapeutic precision, improve drug stability, and mitigate systemic side effects. Recent developments in biomimetic systems, microbiome-targeted approaches, and combination nanotherapies further highlight the expanding scope of nanomedicine in metabolic disease management. Despite encouraging progress in preclinical studies, important challenges remain in terms of large-scale manufacturing, regulatory approval, long-term safety, evaluation, and cost-effectiveness. Bridging the translational gap between experimental research and clinical implementation will require coordinated efforts from scientists, clinicians, regulatory agencies, and industrial partners. With continued technological and rigorous clinical validation, nano-engineered therapies may play increasingly important role in shaping the future of precision diabetes care.

REFERENCES

1. Goyal R, Singhal M, Jialal I. Type 2 Diabetes. StatPearls [Internet]; 2023.
2. Feingold KR. Oral and injectable (non-insulin) pharmacological agents for the treatment of type 2 diabetes. [Updated 2025, Dec 29]. In: Feingold KR, Adler RA, Ahmed SF, et al., editors. Endotext [Internet]. South Dartmouth (MA): MDText.com, Inc.; 2000. Available from: https://www.ncbi.nlm.nih.gov/sites/books/NBK279141/.
3. Sarkhel S, Shuvo SM, Ansari MA, Mondal S, Kapat P, Ghosh A, Sarkar T, Biswas R, Atanase LI, Carauleanu A. Nanotechnology-based approaches for the management of diabetes mellitus: An innovative solution to long-lasting challenges in antidiabetic drug delivery. Pharmaceutics. 2024;16(12):1572.
4. Haider R, Das ZA, Zameer GK. S. Revolutionizing patient care: Multidimensional approaches to 21st-century diabetes management. Journal of Heart and Vasculature. 2025;4(6):01–05.
5. Karim AM. Smart antidiabetic nanomedicine: A revolutionized therapeutic approach for treatment of diabetes mellitus. Bioengineering. 2025;12(12):1309.
6. Petrovic S, Bita B, Barbinta-Patrascu ME. Nanoformulations in pharmaceutical and biomedical applications: Green perspectives. International Journal of Molecular Sciences. 2024;25(11):5842.
7. Eze UV, Eze CE, Alaneme GU, Mirembe NF, Paul-Chima UO, Ogenyi FC, Ugwu CN, Okon MB, Ugwu JN. Systematic review of nanoelectronic drug delivery systems advancing technological innovation, clinical integration, and personalized therapy. Frontiers in Nanotechnology.2026;7:1686599.
8. Raghav A, Ashraf H, Ahmad J. Nanogenomic synergy in diabetes care: Precision therapeutics for patients with multiple long-term conditions. Frontiers in Endocrinology. 2026;17:1767858.

9. Xiao W, Jiang W, Chen Z, Huang Y, Mao J, Zheng W, Hu Y, Shi J. Advance in peptide-based drug development: Delivery platforms, therapeutics and vaccines. Signal Transduction and Targeted Therapy. 2025;10(1):74.
10. Luo X, Li N, Zhu X, Xie W, Zhang Q, Liang N, Zhang P, Zhou C. Application of nanomaterials in diabetic complication management. Colloids and Surfaces B: Biointerfaces. 2025;258:115229.
11. Issaka E, Tornyeava B, Agyekum EA, Enyan M, Okai Amu-Darko JN, Chimuza HT. Nature-inspired solutions: A comprehensive review of biomimetic nanoparticles in nanomedicine. Journal of Thermoplastic Composite Materials. 2025;38(4):1637–72.
12. Shen H, Ouyang Y, Zhang L, Li J, Wang S. Blood cell membrane-coated nanomaterials as a versatile biomimetic nanoplatform for antitumor applications. Nanomaterials. 2024;14(21):1757.
13. Saleem H, Zaidi SJ. Developments in the application of nanomaterials for water treatment and their impact on the environment. Nanomaterials. 2020;10(9):1764.
14. Daly LA. The 'designer' artificial pancreas: How does current technology mimic pancreatic physiology? Cureus. 2025;17(6):01–09.
15. Loushambam B, Krishnaswami V, Kumar M, Vijayaraghavalu S. Advances in nanomedicine-enabled transdermal patches for insulin delivery: From design to clinical translation. Journal of Pharmaceutical and BioTech Industry. 2026;3(1):5.
16. Sadagopan A, Mahmoud A, Begg M, Tarhuni M, Fotso M, Gonzalez NA, Sanivarapu RR, Osman U, Kumar AL, Mohammed L, Fotso MN. Understanding the role of the gut microbiome in diabetes and therapeutics targeting leaky gut: A systematic review. Cureus. 2023:15(7):01–12.
17. Arratia-Quijada J, Nuño K, Ruíz-Santoyo V, Andrade-Espinoza BA. Nano-encapsulation of probiotics: Need and critical considerations to design new non-dairy probiotic products. Journal of Functional Foods. 2024;116:106192.
18. Adefegha SA, Ogundare PO, Oboh G, Esatbeyoglu T, Papenbrock J. An overview on the mechanisms of encapsulation of polyphenols used to help fight diabetes mellitus. Discover Food. 2025;5(1):185.
19. Renukadevi J, Ranjani M, Sneha P, Hussain JS, Shakthi H. Gut-targeted nutraceutical delivery: Engineering microbiome-responsive nutraceutical interfaces. Food Bioengineering. 2025;4(3):248–61.
20. Khoshnejat M, Banaei-Moghaddam AM, Moosavi-Movahedi AA, Kavousi K. A holistic view of muscle metabolic reprogramming through personalized metabolic modeling in newly diagnosed diabetic patients. Plos One. 2023;18(6):e0287325.
21. Liu M, Wang R, Hoi MP, Wang Y, Wang S, Li G, Vong CT, Chong CM. Nano-based drug delivery systems for managing diabetes: Recent advances and future prospects. International Journal of Nanomedicine. 2025:6221–52.
22. Chang W, Meng Z, Zhao Y, Qi Y, Li Z, Lian H. Emerging nanotechnology strategies for obesity therapy. Advanced Science. 2025;12(32):e01813.
23. Padmanaban S, Pully D, Samrot AV, Gosu V, Sadasivam N, Park IK, Radhakrishnan K, Kim DK. Rising influence of nanotechnology in addressing oxidative stress-related liver disorders. Antioxidants. 2023;12(7):1405.
24. "9. Pharmacologic approaches to glycemic treatment: Standards of care in diabetes—2025. Diabetes Care. 2025;48(Supplement_1):S181–S206.
25. Wong CY, Al-Salami H, Dass CR. Recent advancements in oral administration of insulin-loaded liposomal drug delivery systems for diabetes mellitus. International Journal of Pharmaceutics. 2018; 549(1-2):201–17.
26. Zhang Q, Dehaini D, Zhang Y, Zhou J, Chen X, Zhang L, Fang RH, Gao W, Zhang L. Neutrophil membrane-coated nanoparticles inhibit synovial inflammation and alleviate joint damage in inflammatory arthritis. Nature Nanotechnology. 2018;13(12):1182–90.
27. Yao M, Xie J, Du H, McClements DJ, Xiao H, Li L. Progress in microencapsulation of probiotics: A review. Comprehensive Reviews in Food Science and Food Safety. 2020;19(2):857–74.
28. Zhang Y, Chan HF, Leong KW. Advanced materials and processing for drug delivery: The past and The future. Advanced Drug Delivery Reviews. 2013;65(1):104–20.
29. Mihai MM, Dima MB, Dima B, Holban AM. Nanomaterials for wound healing and infection control. Materials. 2019;12(13):2176.
30. Yadav NK, Mazumder RU, Rani AN, Kumar AR. Current perspectives on using nanoparticles for diabetes management. International Journal of Applied Pharmaceutics. 2024;16(5):38–45.
31. Sun X, Setrerrahmane S, Li C, Hu J, Xu H. Nucleic acid drugs: Recent progress and future perspectives. Signal Transduction and Targeted Therapy. 2024;9(1):316.
32. Xiao Y, Tang Z, Huang X, Joseph J, Chen W, Liu C, Zhou J, Kong N, Joshi N, Du J, Tao W. Glucose-responsive oral insulin delivery platform for one treatment a day in diabetes. Matter. 2021;4(10):3269–85.

33. Al Tahan MA, Al-Khattawi A, Russell C. Oral Peptide delivery systems: Synergistic approaches using polymers, lipids, nanotechnology, and needle-based carriers. Journal of Drug Delivery Science and Technology. 2025;112:107205.
34. Elshazly EM, Arafa MG, Nour SA. Exploration of recent advancements of nanoparticle-based therapeutics emphasis on diabetic-related chronic wound management: A comprehensive review. Archives of Pharmacal Research. 2025:1–33.
35. Gimondi S, Ferreira H, Reis RL, Neves NM. Microfluidic devices: A tool for nanoparticle synthesis and performance evaluation. ACS Nano. 2023;17(15):14205–28.
36. Mazahir F, Bhogale D, Palai AK, Yadav AK Nanomedicine: Principles, Properties, and Regulatory Issues. In Smart Polymeric Nano-Constructs in Drug Delivery (pp. 523–565). Academic Press; 2023.
37. Fortune A, Aime A, Raymond D, Kumar S. Nanotechnology in medicine: A double-edged sword for health outcomes. Health Nanotechnology. 2025;1(1):9.
38. Al Saidi AK, Al-Shannaq R, Ul-Islam M, Shehzad A, Ahmad MW, Farid M, Kamal T, Alshammari FH. Future aspects of nanotechnology in therapeutics: A comprehensive review of materials, applications, and future directions. Materials Research Express. 2025;12(12):122001.
39. Barbosa AI, Rebelo R, Reis RL, Bhattacharya M, Correlo VM. Current nanotechnology advances in diagnostic biosensors. Medical Devices & Sensors. 2021;4(1):e10156.

18 The Nano-Intervention
Severing the Molecular Links between Obesity and Diabetes

M. Jayakumar
Excel Homoeopathy Medical College, Namakkal, India

Khumanthem Deepak Singh
Asian International University, Imphal, India

D. Thangamani
Institute of Forest Genetics and Tree Breeding, R. S. Puram, Coimbatore, India

Jyothirmayee Devineni
KVSR Siddhartha College of Pharmaceutical Sciences, Vijayawada, India

Ashish Singhai
Teerthanker Mahaveer College of Pharmacy, Teerthanker Mahaveer University, Moradabad, India

Aparna Sanjay Deshmukh
Thakur College of Science and Commerce, Mumbai, India

Neerati Prasad
Pharmacology University College of Pharmaceutical Sciences, Kakatiya University, Warangal, India

18.1 INTRODUCTION

Obesity and type 2 diabetes mellitus (T2DM) are increasingly recognized as interconnected metabolic disorders that share a complex molecular and physiological continuum. Rather than existing as separate diseases, obesity often acts as a primary metabolic trigger that progressively disrupts glucose homeostasis and culminates in diabetes. This continuum is driven by a network of molecular events involving adipose tissue dysfunction, chronic inflammation, hormonal imbalance, and impaired insulin signaling pathways [1].

A defining feature of obesity-associated metabolic dysfunction is the transformation of adipose tissue from a passive energy storage organ into an active endocrine and immunological organ. As adipocytes enlarge and adipose depots expand, they begin to release bioactive molecules known as adipokines. These include pro-inflammatory mediators such as tumor necrosis TNF-α, IL-6, and adipokines like resistin and chemerin, which collectively disrupt insulin signaling and promote systemic insulin resistance. Conversely, protective adipokines such as adiponectin, which normally enhance

DOI: 10.1201/9781003598657-18

insulin sensitivity and regulate lipid metabolism, are often reduced in obesity, further aggravating metabolic imbalance [2].

Another central mechanism linking obesity and diabetes is chronic low-grade inflammation within adipose tissue. Excess nutrient availability and adipocyte hypertrophy stimulate infiltration of immune cells, especially macrophages, which secret inflammatory cytokines that interfere with insulin receptor signaling in the liver, muscle, and adipose tissue. This inflammatory environment creates a positive feedback loop of metabolic stress and insulin resistance, a hallmark precursor to T2DM [3].

Recent research further highlights the involvement of additional molecular drivers, including mitochondrial dysfunction, lipotoxicity, and ectopic lipid deposition in organs such as the liver and the pancreas. These processes impair cellular energy metabolism and β-cell function, accelerating the transition from insulin resistance to overt diabetes [4].

Understanding this obesity-diabetes molecular continuum has become essential for developing next-generation therapeutic approaches. Conventional pharmacological approaches often target single metabolic pathway, which may limit long-term efficacy. Emerging technologies, especially nanomedicine and precision metabolic interventions, aim to disrupt various pathogenic nodes simultaneously by delivering targeted therapeutics to adipose tissue, inflammatory cells, or metabolic organs. Such approaches hold promise for serving the molecular links that connect obesity to diabetes and may redefine future strategies for metabolic disease management [5].

18.2 MOLECULAR NODES FROM OBESITY TO DIABETES

The progression from obesity to T2DM is governed by interconnected molecular disturbances that disrupt metabolic homeostasis. These molecular nodes represent critical biological interfaces where excess nutrient availability, hormonal imbalance, and cellular stress converge to impair glucose regulation. Understanding these mechanisms provide important insight into how obesity predisposes individuals to insulin resistance and metabolic disease [6]. The progression from obesity to diabetes is driven by several interconnected molecular disturbances affecting adipose tissue function, inflammatory signaling, mitochondrial metabolism, and gut microbial balance (Figure 18.1).

18.2.1 Adipose Tissue Dysfunction

Adipose tissue plays a central role in metabolic regulation, functioning not only as an energy reservoir but also as a dynamic endocrine organ. In obesity, adipocyte hypertrophy and hyperplasia lead

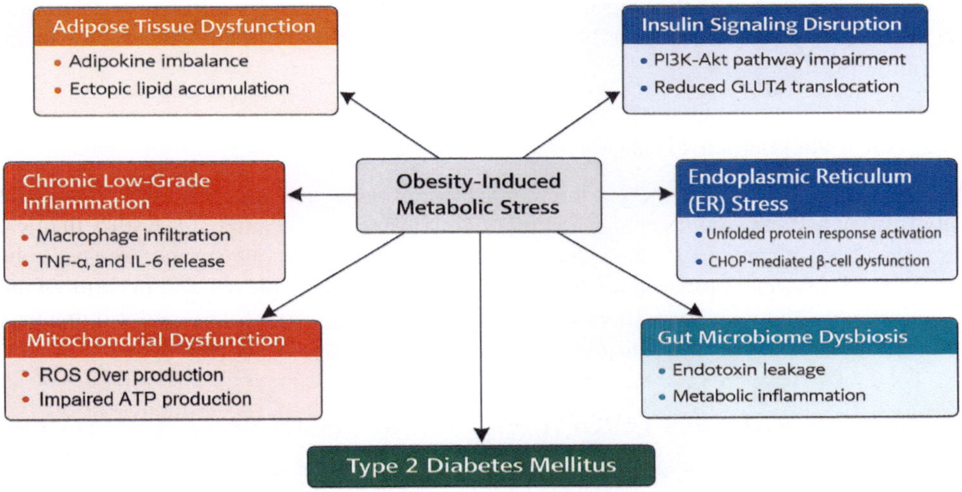

FIGURE 18.1 Molecular pathways linking obesity to the development of T2DM.

to structural and functional alterations within adipose tissue. Enlarged adipocytes exhibit impaired lipid storage capacity and release excessive free fatty acids into circulation. At the same time, the secretion profile of adipokines shifts toward a pro-diabetic pattern characterized by increased levels of resistin, leptin, and inflammatory mediators, alongside reduced adiponectin. This dysregulated adipokine signaling promotes systemic insulin resistance and contributes to ectopic lipid accumulation in metabolic organs such as the liver and skeletal muscles [7].

18.2.2 Chronic Low-Grade Inflammation

A hallmark feature of obesity-associated metabolic disease is persistent low-grade inflammation within adipose tissue. As adipocytes enlarge, they attract immune cells infiltration, especially macrophages and T lymphocytes. These immune cells release cytokines such as tumor necrosis factor-α (TNF-α), interleukin-6 (IL-6), and monocyte chemo attractant protein-1 (MCP-1), which interfere with insulin receptor signaling pathways. The resulting inflammatory environment amplifies metabolic stress and further aggravates adipose dysfunction. Recent studies have also identified activation of the NLRP3 inflammation as an important molecular driver of obesity-induced metabolic inflammation [8].

18.2.3 Insulin Signaling Disruption

Insulin resistance represents a pivotal molecular link between obesity and diabetes. Under normal physiological conditions, insulin binding to its receptor then activates downstream signaling cascades, such as the PI3K/Akt pathway, enabling glucose uptake in peripheral tissues. In obesity, inflammatory cytokines, lipid intermediates, and oxidative stress impair these signaling pathways by inducing serine phosphorylation of insulin receptor substrates. This disruption reduces glucose transporter (GLUT4) translocation and limits cellular glucose uptake, ultimately leading to chronic hyperglycemia [9, 10].

18.2.4 Mitochondrial Dysfunction and Lipotoxicity

Excess nutrient intake in obesity places significant metabolic pressure on mitochondria. Overloaded mitochondrial oxidative pathways lead to increased generation of reactive oxygen species (ROS) and reduced oxidative efficiency. Concurrently, excess fatty acids are deposited as toxic lipid intermediary such as ceramides and diacylglycerols. These molecules interfere with insulin signaling and damage pancreatic β-cells, impairing insulin secretion and accelerating metabolic deterioration [9, 10].

18.2.5 Gut Microbiome Dysbiosis

Emerging evidence highlights the gut microbiome as an important regulator of metabolic health. Obesity is often associated with changes in microbial diversity and composition, specifically shifts in the ratio of *Firmicutes* to *Bacteroidetes* species. Dysbiotic microbiota can increase intestinal permeability and systemic inflammation through increased endotoxins release. In addition, altered microbial metabolites, including short-chain fatty acids and bile acid derivatives, influence host glucose metabolism and insulin sensitivity and contribute to diabetogenesis [11].

18.3 NANO-STRATEGIES TARGETING ADIPOSE TISSUE PATHOPHYSIOLOGY

Nanotechnology has emerged as a promising approach for selectively modulating adipose tissue dysfunction, a central driver of obesity-related metabolic disorders. Conventional pharmacological agents often lack tissue specificity, resulting in systemic side-effects and limited therapeutic

TABLE 18.1
Nanotechnology Strategies Targeting Molecular Links between Obesity and Diabetes

Molecular Target	Pathological Role in Obesity-Diabetes Axis	Nano-Intervention Strategy	Representative Examples	Therapeutic Outcome
Adipose tissue dysfunction	Adipocyte hypertrophy and altered adipokine secretion leading to insulin resistance	Adipocyte-targeted polymeric nanoparticles	Prohibitin-targeted nanoparticles delivering metabolic modulators	Improved adipose tissue metabolism and insulin sensitivity [13]
Chronic inflammation	Macrophage infiltration and cytokine release (TNF-α, IL-6) impair insulin signaling	Macrophage-targeted nanocarriers	Mannose-functionalized nanoparticles delivering anti-inflammatory siRNA	Reduced adipose inflammation and improved glucose tolerance [14]
Insulin signaling disruption	Impaired PI3K/Akt signaling and GLUT4 translocation	Glucose-responsive nanocarriers	Phenylboronic acid-based insulin nanocarriers	Controlled insulin release and glycemic regulation [15]
Lipotoxicity and mitochondrial dysfunction	Accumulation of toxic lipid intermediate and oxidative stress	Mitochondria-targeted nanoparticles	Triphenylphosponium-modified nanoparticles delivering antioxidants	Reduced ROS and improved mitochondrial function [16]
Gut microbiome dysbiosis	Altered microbial composition and endotoxin-mediated inflammation	Microbiome-modulating nanocarriers	Chitosan nanoparticles delivering probiotic or prebiotic compounds	Restoration microbial balance and metabolic improvement [17]
Gene dysregulation	Abnormal expression of metabolic and inflammation genes	RNA-based delivery systems	Lipid nanoparticles delivering siRNA or miRNA modulators	Targeted gene silencing and improved metabolic regulation [18]

efficiency. In contrast, nano-based delivery systems enable targeted transport of bioactive molecules to adipose depots, allowing precise intervention in adipocyte metabolism, inflammatory signaling, and energy regulation [12]. The important molecular targets and related nano-intervention approaches described throughout this chapter are summarized in Table 18.1.

18.3.1 Adipocytes-Targeted Nanocarriers

Adipocyte-specific nanocarriers are engineered to enhance drug accumulation within adipose tissue while minimizing off-target effects. These systems typically employ surface ligands that recognize adipocyte-associated receptors or transport proteins. For instance, peptide-modified polymeric nanoparticles targeting prohibiting receptors expressed on adipose vasculature have been explored to deliver metabolic modulators directly to adipocytes. Similarly, liposomal and poly(lactic-co-glycolic acid) (PLGA)-based nanocarriers have been investigated for the targeted delivery of anti-inflammatory drugs, improving therapeutic localization within visceral fat depots [19].

18.3.2 Nanoparticles for Adipose Tissue Remodeling

Another emerging strategy involves the use of nanoparticles to remodel dysfunctional adipose tissue and restore metabolic balance. Nanocarriers can deliver small molecules, peptides, or nucleic acids that regulate adipogenesis, lipid metabolism, or inflammatory pathway. For example, recent studies have shown that polymeric nanoparticles deliver macrophage infiltration and cytokine production within adipose tissue. Such nano-interventions help restore adipose tissue functionality and enhance systemic insulin sensitivity [20].

18.3.3 Nanotechnology-Mediated Browning of White Adipose Tissue

Promoting the conversion of energy-storing white adipose tissue into metabolically active brown-like adipocytes represents an innovative therapeutic concept. Nanotechnology platforms have been explored to deliver browning-inducing agents such as β3-adrenergic agonists, mitochondrial activators, or gene-regulating molecules. For instance, lipid-based nanoparticles carrying browning regulators have been shown to stimulate thermogenetic gene expression, including uncoupling protein-1 (UCP1), thereby enhancing energy expenditure and improving metabolic control. These strategies emphasize the promise of nanomedicine to reprogram adipose tissues physiology and interrupt the pathological link between obesity and diabetes [21].

18.4 NANOMEDICINE FOR INFLAMMATION MODULATION

Chronic low-grade inflammation is a critical mediator linking obesity to insulin resistance and the subsequent development of T2DM. In obese adipose tissue, infiltrating immune cells (especially macrophages) secrete inflammatory cytokines and ROS that inhibit insulin signaling. Nanomedicine provides innovative strategies to selectively modulate these inflammatory pathways by enabling targeted delivery of anti-inflammatory agents and antioxidants to metabolically active tissues [3, 22].

18.4.1 Macrophage-Targeted Nanotherapeutics

Macrophages play a central role in obesity-induced inflammation by shifting from an anti-inflammatory M2 phenotype to a pro-inflammatory M1 phenotype within adipose tissue. Nanoparticle-based delivery systems have been designed to specifically target these immune cells and reprogram their inflammatory profile. For example, mannose-functionalized nanoparticles have been explored to selectively bind macrophage surface receptors and deliver anti-inflammatory medicines or small interfering RNA (siRNA). Recent experimental studies have demonstrated that polymeric nanoparticles delivering siRNA against inflammatory mediators such as NF-κB can suppress macrophage activation and reduce adipose tissue inflammation in metabolic disease models [23].

18.4.2 Nanoparticle-Based Cytokine Regulation

Another promising strategy involves the use of nanocarriers to regulate the production or activity of pro-inflammatory cytokines. Liposomal and polymeric nanoparticles have been designed to deliver cytokine inhibitors or anti-inflammatory peptides directly to inflamed metabolic tissues. For example, nanoparticle-mediated delivery of anti-TNF-α agents has shown potential in reducing inflammatory signaling pathways that impair insulin receptor activity. Similarly, nanocarriers transporting IL-10 mimetics or gene modulators have demonstrated the ability to restore anti-inflammatory signaling and improve metabolic outcomes in preclinical models [24].

18.4.3 ROS-Scavenging Nano-Antioxidants

Oxidative stress generated by excessive ROS further amplifies inflammatory responses and contributes to insulin resistance. Nano-engineered antioxidants including cerium oxide nanoparticles and polymer-based ROS-responsive nanocarriers have been studied for their ability to neutralize oxidative stress in metabolic tissues. These nano-antioxidants can mimic endogenous antioxidant enzymes and reduce ROS-mediated damage, thereby protecting insulin signaling pathways and mitigating inflammation associated with obesity-related dysfunction [25].

18.5 RESTORING INSULIN SIGNALING THROUGH NANO-INTERVENTION

Disruption of Insulin signaling is a central molecular event connecting obesity with the onset of T2DM. Excess lipid accumulation, inflammatory mediators, and oxidative stress impair key signaling pathways responsible for glucose uptake and metabolism regulation. Nanotechnology-based therapeutic systems have emerged as innovative tools to restore insulin sensitivity by enabling targeted delivery metabolic regulators and controlled drug release at specific physiological site [26].

18.5.1 Nano-Enabled Insulin Sensitizers

Nanoformulations have been widely explored to enhance the bioavailability and tissue targeting of insulin-sensitizing agents. Encapsulation of drugs such as metformin, rosiglitazone, or natural polyphenols within polymeric or lipid-based nanoparticles enhances their stability and controlled release. For example, PLGA nanoparticles loaded with metformin have shown improved cellular uptake and enhanced glucose-lowering efficacy in experimental models of insulin resistance. Similarly, curcumin- and resveratrol-loaded nanocarriers have shown potential to improve insulin sensitivity by reducing oxidative stress and inflammatory signaling with metabolic tissues [27].

18.5.2 Glucose-Responsive Nanocarriers

Glucose-responsive nanocarriers represent an advanced strategy for self-regulated therapeutic delivery. These systems are designed to sense elevated glucose concentrations and release insulin or insulin-mimetic drugs accordingly. Materials incorporating glucose oxidase, phenylboronic acid, or glucose-binding polymer have been developed to create "smart" nanocarriers capable of adjusting drug release in response to blood glucose levels. Recent research has shown that glucose-responsive polymeric nanoparticles can provide controlled insulin release, reducing the risk of hypoglycemia while maintaining stable glycemic control [28].

18.5.3 Nanoparticle-Mediated AMPK and PI3K/Akt Activation

Key metabolic signaling pathways, particularly AMP-activated protein kinase (AMPK) and PI3K/Akt, play critical roles in glucose uptake and energy homeostasis. Nanoparticle-based delivery systems have been studied to promote the activity of these pathways. For example, nanocarriers delivering AMPK-activating compounds such as berberine, or mitochondrial modulators have been shown to enhance glucose utilization in skeletal muscles and liver tissues. Similarly, targeted nanoparticles delivering signaling modulators can restore PI3K/Akt pathway activity, thereby enhancing GLUT4 translocation and promoting cellular glucose uptake. These nano-interventions highlight the potential of nanomedicine to precisely reprogram impaired insulin signaling networks [29].

18.6 NANOTECHNOLOGY TARGETING LIPOTOXICITY AND MITOCHONDRIAL DYSFUNCTION

Lipotoxicity and mitochondrial impairment are increasingly recognized as key metabolic drivers connecting obesity with insulin resistance and T2DM. Excess nutrient intake leads to the accumulation of free fatty acids and toxic lipid intermediates in metabolic organs such as the liver, the pancreas, and skeletal muscles. These lipid species disrupt mitochondrial oxidative phosphorylation, increase ROS production, and impair insulin signaling. Nanotechnology offers innovative strategies to deliver metabolic regulators directly to the affected tissues, thereby mitigating lipid-induced cellular stress and restoring mitochondrial function [30].

18.6.1 Mitochondria-Targeted Nanoparticles

Targeting mitochondria has become an important therapeutic strategy for correcting the metabolic dysfunction. Nanoparticles functionalized with mitochondria-targeting molecules, like triphenylphosphonium (TPP) or mitochondrial-penetrating peptides can selectively accumulate within mitochondrial membranes. These systems enable the delivery of antioxidants, metabolic modulators, or gene-regulating molecules directly to the mitochondrial compartment. For example, TPP-modified polymeric nanoparticles carrying mitochondrial antioxidants such as coenzyme Q10 or mitoquinone have shown ability to reduce oxidative stress and improve mitochondrial respiration in experimental models of metabolic disease. Such targeted approaches help restore mitochondrial bioenergetics and protect pancreatic β-cells from oxidative damage [31].

18.6.2 Lipid-Modulating Nanoformulations

Nanocarriers have also been explored to regulate lipid metabolism and reduce lipotoxicity. Lipid-modulating nanoformulations can deliver small molecules, peptides, or nucleic acids that influence fatty acid oxidation, lipid storage, or lipid transport pathways. For example, nanoparticle-mediated delivery of siRNA targeting genes involved in lipid synthesis, such as sterol regulatory element-binding protein-1c (SREBP-1c), has shown the potential to alleviate hepatic lipid accumulation. Similarly, nanoformulated natural compounds such as berberine or curcumin have been investigated for their ability to improve lipid metabolism and reduce inflammatory lipid signaling [32].

18.6.3 Nano-Regulation of Cellular Energy Metabolism

Beyond lipid regulation, nanotechnology can modulate broader cellular energy pathways that control metabolic balance. Nano-delivery systems carrying AMPK activators, mitochondrial cofactors, or metabolic enzymes, have been investigated to enhance fatty acid oxidation and improve glucose utilization. Recent studies have shown that nanocarriers delivering mitochondrial cofactors such as nicotinamide adenine dinucleotide (NAD+) precursors can enhance mitochondrial efficiency and metabolic flexibility. Through these approaches, nanotechnology provides a platform for reprogramming cellular energy metabolism and interrupting the pathological cascade linking obesity, lipotoxicity, and diabetes [33].

18.7 GUT-METABOLIC AXIS: NANO-MODULATION OF THE MICROBIOME

The gut-metabolic axis has emerged as a critical regulator of host metabolism, linking intestinal microbial composition with obesity and T2DM. Dysbiosis in obese individuals is often associated with altered microbial diversity, increased intestinal permeability, and elevated endotoxin levels that promote systemic inflammation and insulin resistance. Nanotechnology offers innovative tools to selectively modulate the gut microbiome and restore metabolic balance through targeted delivery of therapeutic agents and microbial modulators [34].

18.7.1 Nanocarriers for Microbiome Restoration

Nanocarriers can protect bioactive compounds from degradation in the gastrointestinal environment and enable targeted delivery to specific regions of the intestine. Polymeric and lipid-based nanoparticles have been explored to deliver prebiotics, antimicrobial peptides, or microbiota-modulating molecules that enhance beneficial microbial populations. For example, chitosan-based nanoparticles have been investigated for their ability to improve intestinal stability of microbiome-modulating compounds and improve metabolic parameters in experimental models of obesity [35].

18.7.2 Probiotic-Nanoparticles Hybrid Systems

Hybrid systems combining probiotics with nanomaterials represent a novel strategy to improve microbial survival and colonization in the gut. Encapsulation of probiotic strains such as *Lactobacillus* or *Bifidobacterium* within protective nano-shells has been shown to improve their resistance to gastric acidity and bile salts, thereby improving therapeutic effects. Such nano-enabled probiotics may help restore microbial balance and reduce inflammation associated with metabolic disorders [36].

18.7.3 Nano-Enhanced Delivery of Microbial Metabolites

Microbial metabolites, particularly short-chain fatty acids such as butyrate and propionate, play important roles in regulating glucose metabolism and intestinal barrier integrity. Nanocarrier systems have been developed to deliver these metabolites or their precursors in a controlled manner, enhancing their bioavailability and metabolic impact. These approaches highlight the potential of nano-modulation to harness the therapeutic benefits of the gut microbiome in metabolic disease management [37].

18.8 GENE AND RNA-BASED NANO-THERAPEUTICS

Gene and RNA-based therapeutics are emerging as powerful tools addressing the molecular drivers of obesity-associated diabetes. Unlike conventional drugs that target downstream metabolic effects, nucleic acid therapies can directly regulate gene expression involved in insulin signaling, inflammation, lipid metabolism, and β-cell survival. However, RNA molecules and gene-editing components are unstable and susceptible to enzymatic degradation in biological environments. Nanotechnology has therefore become essential for protecting nucleic acids, delivering them to specific targets, and enhancing therapeutic efficacy in metabolic tissues such as the liver, adipose tissue, and the pancreas [38].

18.8.1 siRNA and miRNA Nanodelivery

Small interfering RNA (siRNA) and microRNA (miRNA) therapies aim to silence or regulate genes implicated in metabolic dysfunctions. Nanocarriers such as lipid nanoparticles, polymeric nanoparticles, and lipid-polymer hybrid systems are widely studied for enhanced intracellular delivery of these molecules. For instance, lipid nanoparticle-mediated delivery systems of siRNA targeting pro-inflammatory genes such as TNF-α or NF- κB have demonstrated the ability to reduce inflammatory signaling in the adipose tissue, thereby improving insulin sensitivity in experimental models of obesity. Similarly, miRNA-based therapies have gained attention due to their ability to regulate multiple metabolic pathways simultaneously. Nanocarriers delivering miR-33 inhibitors, for example, have shown promise in improving lipid metabolism and reducing hepatic steatosis, a key factor contributing to insulin resistance. Polymeric nanoplates with miR-223 or miR-146a have also been explored for their ability to inhibit macrophage-mediated inflammation in metabolic tissues [39].

18.8.2 CRISPR-Enabled Nano-Platforms

Clustered regularly interspaced short palindromic repeats (CRISPR) technology has revolutionized gene editing by enabling precise modification of disease-related genes. Nanoparticle-based delivery systems provide a non-viral alternative for transporting CRISPR components such as Cas9 proteins and guide RNAs into target cells. Lipid nanoparticles and gold nanoparticles have been investigated as carriers for CRISPR systems targeting genes involved in lipid metabolism or insulin resistance. Experimental studies have demonstrated that nanoparticle-mediated CRISPR editing of metabolic regulators such as PCSK9 or genes involved in lipid synthesis can improve lipid profile and metabolic function. These approaches highlight the potential of nano-enabled gene editing for long-term correction of metabolic abnormalities [40].

18.8.3 Epigenetics Modulation via Nanotechnology

Epigenetic mechanisms, including DNA methylation, histone modification, and chromatin remodeling, play a significant role in regulating metabolic gene expression in obesity and diabetes. Nanotechnology offers innovative platforms for delivering epigenetic modulators that can reprogram metabolic pathways. For example, nanoparticles delivering histone deacetylase (HDAC) inhibitors or DNA methylation regulators have been studied to restore normal gene expression patterns associated with insulin sensitivity and mitochondrial function. Additionally, nano-enabled delivery of epigenetic-modulation RNAs has shown promise in regulating genes involved in adipogenesis and energy metabolism. By influencing epigenetic regulations, nanomedicine offers the possibility of durable metabolic reprogramming and represents a promising frontier in precision therapy for obesity-induced diabetes [41].

18.9 PRECISION NANO-THERAPEUTICS FOR METABOLIC REPROGRAMMING

The complexity of metabolic diseases like obesity-associated diabetes calls for treatment strategies that can simultaneously act on a number of pathological pathways. Precision nanomedicine has become an interesting strategy to reprogram faulty metabolic networks by allowing targeted delivery, controlled drug delivery, and patient-specific therapeutic design. By combining the advances in nanotechnology, molecular biology, and systems metabolism, nano-therapeutics can enter into key molecular nodes that cause insulin resistance, inflammation, and lipid dysregulation [42].

18.9.1 Multi-Target Nanoplatforms

Metabolic diseases involve interconnected pathways including inflammation, oxidative stress, lipid accumulation, and abnormal insulin signaling. Multi-target nanoplatforms are designed to deliver combinations of therapeutic agents that act on several pathways simultaneously. For example, polymer-lipid hybrid nanoparticles have been studied to target anti-inflammatory drugs and insulin sensitizers, improving metabolic outcomes in experimental obesity models. Similarly, nanocarriers encapsulating both antioxidants and mitochondrial modulators have shown the ability to reduce oxidative stress and increase energy metabolism in cells. Such integrated approaches allow the coordinated modulation of metabolism pathway rather than addressing individual targets in isolation [43].

18.9.2 Stimuli-Responsive Nanocarriers

Stimuli-responsive nanocarriers are engineered to release therapeutic payloads in response to specific biological signals associated with metabolic dysfunction. These triggers can be increased glucose levels, increased oxidative stress, inflammatory enzymes, or pH changes in diseased tissues. For instance, glucose-responsive polymeric nanoparticles containing derivatives of phenylboronic acid have been developed to release insulin in response to increasing glucose concentration to accomplish more physiologic glycemic control. Similarly, nanoparticles that respond to redox-responsive (RP) have been designed to release antioxidant molecules specifically in inflamed metabolic tissues, which helps in oxidative damage reduction as well as insulin signaling restoration [44].

18.9.3 Personalized Nano-Intervention Strategies

The heterogeneity of metabolic diseases among people has stimulated the development of personalized nano-therapeutic strategies. Advances in genomic profiling, metabolomics, and digital health technologies allow identification of patient-specific metabolic signatures that can guide targeted

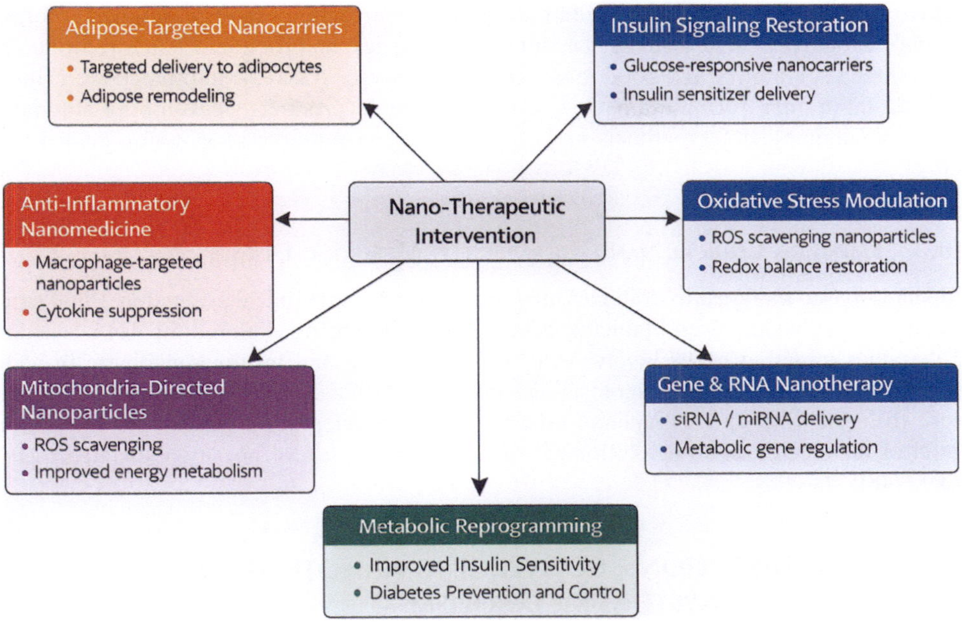

FIGURE 18.2 Nano-intervention strategies to disrupt the obesity diabetes axis.

nanomedicine intervention. For instance, RNA-based nanocarriers can be designed to silence genes associated with individual metabolic risk profiles, while nano-diagnostic systems may monitor metabolic biomarkers in real time. Such personalized approaches may allow more precise and effective treatment of obesity-related diabetes for the path toward truly individualized metabolic medicine [45]. Precision nanomedicine allows multi-target approaches that may simultaneously modulate multiple metabolic pathways in the obesity–diabetes continuum (Figure 18.2).

18.10 TRANSLATIONAL AND CLINICAL PERSPECTIVES

Despite promising preclinical advances, translating nanotechnology-based therapies into clinical applications for metabolic diseases remains a complex process. Several scientific, regulatory, and manufacturing challenges must be addressed to safely and effectively implement nano-based treatments for obesity and diabetes.

18.10.1 Safety and Nanotoxicology Considerations

Safety evaluation is a critical component of nanomedicine development. Nanoparticles may interact with biological systems in specific ways depending on their size, surface chemistry, and composition. Potential concerns include immune system activation, oxidative stress, and long-term accumulation in organs such as the liver or spleen. Recent studies emphasize the importance of comprehensive nanotoxicological assessments, including biodistribution analysis, metabolic clearance studies, and long-term safety monitoring. Advances in biodegradable nanomaterials, such as polymeric nanoparticles composed of PLGA or lipid based nanocarriers, have enhanced their safety profile and lowered the risk of chronic toxicity [46].

18.10.2 Regulatory and Manufacturing Challenges

Regulatory approval of nano-therapeutics presents additional challenges due to the complexity of nanomaterial characterization and quality control. Agencies such as the U.S. Food and Drug

Administration and the European Medicines Agency increasingly require detailed information regarding nanoparticle size distribution, surface properties, stability, and batch reproducibility. Manufacturing scalability and good manufacturing practice (GMP) compliance are critical for translating laboratory formulations into clinically viable products. Developing standardized protocols for nanoparticle synthesis and characterization remains an ongoing priority in the field [47].

18.10.3 Emerging Clinical Nano-Therapies for Metabolic Disease

Several nano-based therapeutic strategies are progressing toward clinical evaluation. Lipid nanoparticle technologies, widely used in nucleic acids delivery, are being explored for RNA-based metabolic therapies targeting genes involved in lipid metabolism and insulin sensitivity. In addition, nanoformulated GLP-1 receptor agonists and insulin delivery systems are under investigation to increase drug stability and therapeutic efficacy. These developments underscore the increasing potential of nanomedicine to revolutionize treatment approaches of obesity-associated metabolic disorders [48].

18.11 FUTURE DIRECTIONS: CONVERGING NANOTECHNOLOGY WITH AI AND SYSTEMS METABOLISM

The future of treatment of metabolic diseases will probably come out of the convergence of nanotechnology, AI, and systems metabolism. AI-based modeling can be used to analyze complex metabolic data such as genomics, metabolomics, and microbiome profiles to determine personalized targets for therapies related to obesity and diabetes. When combined with nanotechnology, such insights allow precision nanocarriers to be designed for the delivery of drugs, RNA molecules, or metabolic modulators to adherent tissue, liver or pancreatic β-cells [49].

Recent research has demonstrated the use of machine learning algorithms to optimize nanoparticle size, surface chemistry, and drug-loading efficiency for targeted metabolic therapy. AI-supported screening platforms are also accelerating the discovery of nanomaterials capable of modulating insulin signaling or reducing metabolic inflammation. In parallel, systems metabolism approaches integrate multi-omics data to better understand the interconnected pathways driving metabolic dysfunction. Together, these technologies may enable adaptive, patient-specific nano-therapeutic strategies for more effective management of obesity-associated diabetes [50].

18.12 CONCLUSION

Obesity and diabetes are closely interconnected metabolic disorders driven by complex molecular interactions involving adipose tissue dysfunction, chronic inflammation, insulin resistance, mitochondrial impairment, and microbiome imbalance. Traditional therapeutic strategies often address symptoms rather than the underlying molecular mechanisms that sustain this metabolic continuum. Nanotechnology offers a transformative approach by enabling delivery of therapeutic agents to specific tissues and molecular targets involved in metabolic dysregulation. Emerging nano-enabled strategies including gene RNA delivery systems, mitochondria-targeted nanoparticles, microbiome-modulating nanocarriers, and stimuli-responsive metabolic nanomedicine demonstrate the potential to disrupt multiple pathogenic pathways simultaneously. Although challenges related to safety, regulatory approval, and large-scale manufacturing remain, continued advances in nanomaterials, precision medicine, and computational tools are expected to accelerate clinical translation. Ultimately, nano-intervention strategies may provide innovative solutions for serving the molecular links between obesity and diabetes and improving long-term metabolic health.

REFERENCES

1. Ruze R, Liu T, Zou X, Song J, Chen Y, Xu R, Yin X, Xu Q. Obesity and type 2 diabetes mellitus: Connections in epidemiology, pathogenesis, and treatments. Frontiers in Endocrinology. 2023;14:1161521.
2. Clemente-Suárez VJ, Redondo-Flórez L, Beltrán-Velasco AI, Martín-Rodríguez A, Martínez-Guardado I, Navarro-Jiménez E, Laborde-Cárdenas CC, Tornero-Aguilera JF. The role of adipokines in health and disease. Biomedicines. 2023;11(5):1290.
3. Zatterale F, Longo M, Naderi J, Raciti GA, Desiderio A, Miele C, Beguinot F. Chronic adipose tissue inflammation linking obesity to insulin resistance and type 2 diabetes. Frontiers in Physiology. 2020;10:1607.
4. Wang G, Sun B, Liu H, Hu M, Xu H, Li H, Wang X, Tong M. Interactions between lipid droplets and mitochondria in metabolic diseases. Lipids in Health and Disease. 2025;24(1):357.
5. Kannan S, Chellappan DK, Kow CS, Ramachandram DS, Pandey M, Mayuren J, Dua K, Candasamy M. Transform diabetes care with precision medicine. Health Science Reports. 2023;6(11):e1642.
6. Galicia-Garcia U, Benito-Vicente A, Jebari S, Larrea-Sebal A, Siddiqi H, Uribe KB, Ostolaza H, Martín C. Pathophysiology of type 2 diabetes mellitus. International Journal of Molecular Sciences. 2020;21(17):6275.
7. Choe SS, Huh JY, Hwang IJ, Kim JI, Kim JB. Adipose tissue remodeling: Its role in energy metabolism and metabolic disorders. Frontiers in Endocrinology. 2016;7:30.
8. Saltiel AR, Olefsky JM. Inflammatory mechanisms linking obesity and metabolic disease. The Journal of Clinical Investigation. 2017;127(1):1–4.
9. Huang X, Liu G, Guo J, Su Z. The PI3K/AKT pathway in obesity and type 2 diabetes. International Journal of Biological Sciences. 2018;14(11):1483.
10. Taheri R, Mokhtari Y, Yousefi AM, Bashash D. The PI3K/Akt signaling axis and type 2 diabetes mellitus (T2DM): From mechanistic insights into possible therapeutic targets. Cell Biology International. 2024; 48(8):1049–68.
11. Aznou A, Drenth JP, Nieuwdorp M, Meijnikman AS. Exploring the role of the gut microbiome across the lifespan: Implications for aging and metabolic disorders. Journal of the Endocrine Society. 2025; 9(10):bvaf130.
12. Xu K, Wang L, Lv T, Jin C, Wu Q, Zhou Y, Xu G, Duan Z, Luo K, Yang J. Nanomedicines against mitochondrial dysfunction-induced metabolic diseases. Advanced Science. 2025;12(48):e14522.
13. Wang J, Li L, Zhang Z, Zhang X, Zhu Y, Zhang C, Bi Y. Extracellular vesicles mediate the communication of adipose tissue with brain and promote cognitive impairment associated with insulin resistance. Cell Metabolism. 2022;34(9):1264–79.
14. Zhao X, Zhang W, Jiang F, Chen X, Chen C, Wang M, Chen B, Cannon RD, Saffery R, Han TL, Zhang H. Excessive palmitic acid disturbs macrophage α-ketoglutarate/succinate metabolism and causes adipose tissue insulin resistance associated with gestational diabetes mellitus. Free Radical Biology and Medicine. 2024;222:424–36.
15. Yang C, Sheng T, Hou W, Zhang J, Cheng L, Wang H, Liu W, Wang S, Yu X, Zhang Y, Yu J. Glucose-responsive microneedle patch for closed-loop dual-hormone delivery in mice and pigs. Science Advances. 2022;8(48):eadd3197.
16. Wang T, Xu P, Yuan J, Chen H, Guo X, Gao J, Wang Y, Yao D, Li X, Liu B, Liu Y. Mitochondrial dysfunction in oocytes: Implications for fertility and ageing. Journal of Ovarian Research. 2025;18(1):186.
17. Lu ZX, Wang P, Ou HB, Wei SX, Wu LC, Jiang Y, Wang RJ, Liu XS, Wang ZH, Chen LJ, Liu ZM. Effects of different vegetation restoration on soil nutrients, enzyme activities, and microbial communities in degraded karst landscapes in southwest China. Forest Ecology and Management. 2022;508:120002.
18. Kulkarni V, Jayakumar S, Mohan M, Kulkarni S. Aid or antagonize: Nuclear long noncoding RNAs regulate host responses and outcomes of viral infections. Cells. 2023;12(7):987.
19. Luo T, Chen L, Tu K, Jiang L, Liang S, Wang S, Huang Y, Yang X. Adipose tissue-targeted drug delivery for treating obesity: Current opportunities and challenges. Drug Delivery. 2025;32(1):2547751.
20. Uti DE, Omang WA, Alum EU, Ugwu OP, Wokoma MA, Oplekwu RI, Atangwho IJ, Egbung GE. Targeting CD44-hyaluronic acid signalling in obesity treatment: Insights from small molecules and nanobioconjugates. Nutrition and Metabolic Insights. 2026;19:11786388251408961.
21. Lin C, Chen J, Hu M, Zheng W, Song Z, Qin H. Sesamol promotes browning of white adipocytes to ameliorate obesity by inducing mitochondrial biogenesis and inhibition mitophagy via β3-AR/PKA signaling pathway. Food & Nutrition Research. 2021;65:10–29219.
22. Kohlgruber A, Lynch L. Adipose tissue inflammation in the pathogenesis of type 2 diabetes. Current Diabetes Reports. 2015;15(11):92.

23. Hu G, Guo M, Xu J, Wu F, Fan J, Huang Q, Yang G, Lv Z, Wang X, Jin Y. Nanoparticles targeting macrophages as potential clinical therapeutic agents against cancer and inflammation. Frontiers in Immunology. 2019;10:1998.
24. Ismail EA, Nyandoro VO, Omolo CA, Govender T. Nanocarrier-based targeting of pattern recognition receptors as an innovative strategy for enhancing sepsis therapy. Advanced Healthcare Materials. 2025;14(23):2501146.
25. Padmanaban S, Pully D, Samrot AV, Gosu V, Sadasivam N, Park IK, Radhakrishnan K, Kim DK. Rising influence of nanotechnology in addressing oxidative stress-related liver disorders. Antioxidants. 2023;12(7):1405.
26. Choo YN, Ravi RN, Subramaniyan V. Insulin resistance induced by obesity: Mechanisms, metabolic implications and therapeutic approaches. Molecular Biology Reports. 2026;53(1):357.
27. Nie X, Chen Z, Pang L, Wang L, Jiang H, Chen Y, Zhang Z, Fu C, Ren B, Zhang J. Oral Nano drug delivery systems for the treatment of type 2 diabetes mellitus: An available administration strategy for Antidiabetic phytocompounds. International Journal of Nanomedicine. 2020;15:10215–40.
28. Volpatti LR, Matranga MA, Cortinas AB, Delcassian D, Daniel KB, Langer R, Anderson DG. Glucose-responsive nanoparticles for rapid and extended self-regulated insulin delivery. ACS Nano. 2019;14(1):488–97.
29. Schultze SM, Hemmings BA, Niessen M, Tschopp O. PI3K/AKT, MAPK and AMPK signalling: Protein kinases in glucose homeostasis. Expert Reviews in Molecular Medicine. 2012;14:e1.
30. Sergi D, Naumovski N, Heilbronn LK, Abeywardena M, O'Callaghan N, Lionetti L, Luscombe-Marsh N. Mitochondrial (dys) function and insulin resistance: From pathophysiological molecular mechanisms to the impact of diet. Frontiers in Physiology. 2019;10:449821.
31. Ali MS, Gowda BJ, Shukla R, Kesharwani P. Triphenylphosphine-based mitochondrial targeting nanocarriers: Advancing cancer therapy. Clinical Pharmacology: Advances and Applications. 2025; 31:119–41.
32. Sun Y, Yan K, Zhang Y, Han YQ, Hao LH, Gao Y, Wang HL, Chu HQ, Ye J, Liu YL, Yang YF. Advanced multifunctional nano-delivery platform focusing on treating diseases related to lipid metabolism via targeted intervention in various lipid metabolic processes. Military Medical Research. 2025;12(1):87.
33. Balasubramani SP, Armstead SA, Buggs AT, Bell MS. Mito-Nutraceutical potential of plant secondary metabolites fortune. Journal of Health Sciences. 2025;8:217–44.
34. O'Riordan KJ, Moloney GM, Keane L, Clarke G, Cryan JF. The gut microbiota-immune-brain axis: Therapeutic implications. Cell Reports Medicine. 2025;6(3):101982.
35. Zhang Z, Chang R, Yue Q, Liu B, Li Z, Yuan Y, Liang S, Li Y. Nanoparticle delivery systems of functional substances for precision nutrition. Advances in Food and Nutrition Research. 2024;112:51–88.
36. Arratia-Quijada J, Nuño K, Ruíz-Santoyo V, Andrade-Espinoza BA. Nano-encapsulation of probiotics: Need and critical considerations to design new non-dairy probiotic products. Journal of Functional Foods. 2024;116:106192.
37. Nogal A, Valdes AM, Menni C. The role of short-chain fatty acids in the interplay between gut microbiota and diet in cardio-metabolic health. Gut Microbes. 2021;13(1):1897212.
38. Thi YV, Ho TT, Caglayan S, Ramasamy TS, Chu DT. RNA therapeutics for treatment of diabetes. Progress in Molecular Biology and Translational Science. 2024;203:287–300.
39. Zhang J, Chen B, Gan C, Sun H, Zhang J, Feng L. A comprehensive review of small interfering RNAs (siRNAs): Mechanism, therapeutic targets, and delivery strategies for cancer therapy. International Journal of Nanomedicine. 2023;31:7605–35.
40. Wang S, Zeng X, Jiang Y, Wang W, Bai L, Lu Y, Zhang L, Tan GY. Unleashing the potential: Type I CRISPR-Cas systems in actinomycetes for genome editing. Natural Product Reports. 2024;41(9):1441–55.
41. Chen P, Wang Y, Chen F, Zhou B. Epigenetics in obesity: Mechanisms and advances in therapies based on natural products. Pharmacology Research & Perspectives. 2024 ;12(1):e1171.
42. Karim AM. Smart antidiabetic nanomedicine: A revolutionized therapeutic approach for treatment of diabetes mellitus. Bioengineering. 2025;12(12):1309.
43. Manful CF, Fordjour E, Ikumoinein E, Abbey L, Thomas R. Therapeutic strategies targeting oxidative stress and inflammation: A narrative review. BioChem. 2025;5(4):35.
44. Das SS, Bharadwaj P, Bilal M, Barani M, Rahdar A, Taboada P, Bungau S, Kyzas GZ. Stimuli-responsive polymeric nanocarriers for drug delivery, imaging, and theragnosis. Polymers. 2020;12(6):1397.
45. O'Sullivan S, Qi L, Zalloua P. From omics to AI—Mapping the pathogenic pathways in type 2 diabetes. FEBS Letters. 2025;599(22):3244–80.
46. Fortune A, Aime A, Raymond D, Kumar S. Nanotechnology in medicine: A double-edged sword for health outcomes. Health Nanotechnology. 2025;1(1):9.

47. Allan J, Belz S, Hoeveler A, Hugas M, Okuda H, Patri A, Rauscher H, Silva P, Slikker W, Sokull-Kluettgen B, Tong W. Regulatory landscape of nanotechnology and nanoplastics from a global perspective. Regulatory Toxicology and Pharmacology. 2021;122:104885.
48. Mukai H, Ogawa K, Kato N, Kawakami S. Recent advances in lipid nanoparticles for delivery of nucleic acid, mRNA, and gene editing-based therapeutics. Drug Metabolism and Pharmacokinetics. 2022;44:100450.
49. Singh S, Sarma DK, Verma V, Nagpal R, Kumar M. Unveiling the future of metabolic medicine: Omics technologies driving personalized solutions for precision treatment of metabolic disorders. Biochemical and Biophysical Research Communications. 2023;682:1–20.
50. Tantray J, Khadam VK, Patel A, Nagdev S, Prajapati B. From detection to intervention: Nanotechnology-driven precision strategies in obesity management. Bulletin of the National Research Centre. 2026; 50(1):15.

Index

Note: Page numbers followed by f and t indicate figures and tables, respectively.